INTRODUCTION TO

Research and Medical Literature

for Health Professionals

Edited by

J. Glenn Forister, MS, PA-C

Adjunct Associate Professor
Department of Physician Assistant Studies
School of Health Professions
UT Health Science Center San Antonio
San Antonio, Texas

J. Dennis Blessing, PhD, PA

Distinguished Teaching Professor (Retired)
Department of Physician Assistant Studies
Associate Dean (Retired)
School of Health Professions
UT Health Science Center San Antonio
San Antonio, Texas

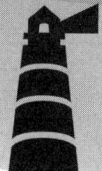

JONES & BARTLETT
LEARNING

World Headquarters
Jones & Bartlett Learning
5 Wall Street
Burlington, MA 01803
978-443-5000
info@jblearning.com
www.jblearning.com

Jones & Bartlett Learning books and products are available through most bookstores and online booksellers. To contact Jones & Bartlett Learning directly, call 800-832-0034, fax 978-443-8000, or visit our website, www.jblearning.com.

Substantial discounts on bulk quantities of Jones & Bartlett Learning publications are available to corporations, professional associations, and other qualified organizations. For details and specific discount information, contact the special sales department at Jones & Bartlett Learning via the above contact information or send an email to specialsales@jblearning.com.

Copyright © 2016 by Jones & Bartlett Learning, LLC, an Ascend Learning Company

All rights reserved. No part of the material protected by this copyright may be reproduced or utilized in any form, electronic or mechanical, including photocopying, recording, or by any information storage and retrieval system, without written permission from the copyright owner.

The content, statements, views, and opinions herein are the sole expression of the respective authors and not that of Jones & Bartlett Learning, LLC. Reference herein to any specific commercial product, process, or service by trade name, trademark, manufacturer, or otherwise does not constitute or imply its endorsement or recommendation by Jones & Bartlett Learning, LLC and such reference shall not be used for advertising or product endorsement purposes. All trademarks displayed are the trademarks of the parties noted herein. *Introduction to Research and Medical Literature for Health Professionals, Fourth Edition* is an independent publication and has not been authorized, sponsored, or otherwise approved by the owners of the trademarks or service marks referenced in this product.

There may be images in this book that feature models; these models do not necessarily endorse, represent, or participate in the activities represented in the images. Any screenshots in this product are for educational and instructive purposes only. Any individuals and scenarios featured in the case studies throughout this product may be real or fictitious, but are used for instructional purposes only.

07243-3

Production Credits
VP, Executive Publisher: David Cella
Executive Editor: Nancy Duffy
Associate Editor: Sean Fabery
Senior Production Editor: Nancy Hitchcock
Marketing Manager: Grace Richards
Art Development Editor: Joanna Lundeen
Art Development Assistant: Shannon Sheehan
VP, Manufacturing and Inventory Control: Therese Connell
Composition: Cenveo Publisher Services
Cover Design: Kristin E. Parker
Photo Research, Rights & Permissions: Amy Rathburn
Cover Image: (horizontal wave) © oconner/Shutterstock; (background) © LeonART/Shutterstock
Printing and Binding: Edwards Brothers Malloy
Cover Printing: Edwards Brothers Malloy

Library of Congress Cataloging-in-Publication Data
Introduction to research and medical literature for health professionals / [edited by] J. Glenn Forister and J. Dennis Blessing. — 4th edition.
   p. ; cm.
Includes bibliographical references and index.
ISBN 978-1-284-03464-6
I. Forister, J. Glenn, editor. II. Blessing, J. Dennis, editor.
[DNLM: 1. Biomedical Research. 2. Health Personnel—education. 3. Research Design. W 20.5]
R727
610.73'7069—dc23
                                        2014038444

6048
Printed in the United States of America
19 18 17 16 15   10 9 8 7 6 5 4 3 2

Contents

DEDICATION v
PREFACE vii
FOREWORD ix
CONTRIBUTORS xi
REVIEWERS xv

SECTION I Getting Started 1

    Chapter 1 Introduction 3
                J. Glenn Forister, MS, PA-C
                J. Dennis Blessing, PhD, PA

    Chapter 2 Regulatory Protection of Human Subjects in Research 11
                Rhonda Oilepo, MS, CIP
                Kimberly K. Summers, PharmD
                Joseph O. Schmelz, PhD, RN, CIP, FAAN

    Chapter 3 The Research Problem 23
                Salah Ayachi, PhD, PA-C
                J. Dennis Blessing, PhD, PA

    Chapter 4 Review of the Literature 33
                Linda Levy, MSW, MLS, AHIP
                J. Dennis Blessing, PhD, PA
                Richard Dehn, MPA, PA-C

    Chapter 5 The Systematic Review 45
                Margaret J. Foster, MS, MPH

SECTION II The Research Process: Design 59

    Chapter 6 Methodology 61
                Christopher E. Bork, PhD
                Robert W. Jarski, PhD, PA-C
                J. Glenn Forister, MS, PA-C

    Chapter 7 Survey Research 79
                J. Dennis Blessing, PhD, PA

Chapter 8 Qualitative Research 97
Elsa M. González, PhD
J. Glenn Forister, MS, PA-C

Chapter 9 Community-Based Participatory Research 111
Scott D. Rhodes, PhD, MPH
Christina J. Sun, PhD, MS

Chapter 10 Clinical Investigations 133
J. Glenn Forister, MS, PA-C

SECTION III The Research Process: Analysis 141

Chapter 11 Data Analysis 143
Meredith A. Davison, PhD, MPH
Bruce R. Niebuhr, PhD
J. Glenn Forister, MS, PA-C

Chapter 12 Exploring Statistics Comparing Differences in Health Care 155
J. Glenn Forister, MS, PA-C

Chapter 13 The Results Section 169
Anthony A. Miller, MEd, PA-C
J. Dennis Blessing, PhD

Chapter 14 The Discussion Section 177
Richard R. Rahr, EdD, PA-C
J. Dennis Blessing, PhD, PA

SECTION IV The Research Process: Writing and Interpretation 183

Chapter 15 References 185
Christine S. Gaspard, MSLS
Katherine A. Prentice, MSIS
Eric Willman, MSIS
Albert Simon, DHSc, MEd, PA-C

Chapter 16 Writing and Publishing in the Health Professions 193
James F. Cawley, MPH, PA-C, DHL (hon)

Chapter 17 Interpreting the Literature 215
J. Glenn Forister, MS, PA-C
J. Dennis Blessing, PhD, PA

Appendix Funding Research: Grants 227
J. Dennis Blessing, PhD
William D. Hendricson, MA, MS

Glossary 229

Index 241

Dedication

This book is dedicated to all the people who made it happen. The contributors to this book have put forth their effort to improve the research capabilities of all healthcare professionals, present and future. It is rare for authors from so many professions to collaborate on such an effort.

We further dedicate this book to our friends and colleagues at Jones & Bartlett Learning. They work behind the scenes to make us look good.

Ultimately, the contributors and publishers want this to be a successful book that helps every reader in their understanding of research and what it means to the people who benefit from our healthcare efforts.

JGF

JDB

Preface

The editors of and contributors to this book are dedicated teachers, researchers, administrators, and practitioners in healthcare professions. They have worked tirelessly to make this book readable, understandable, and useful for students and practitioners in healthcare professions. Our intent is to provide a tool that can be the first step in understanding research and, perhaps, the first step in a research career. We hope this book places that first step on a sound footing without intimidation.

Research articles, news flashes, and advertisements bombard us daily. To make sense of it all, we must be able to interpret and apply the information in our patients' best interests. This skill is a critical requirement of clinical practice in today's world, and it requires an understanding of the research process.

CONCEPTUAL APPROACH

We have tried to present our material in stepwise order, beginning with the protection of human subjects and the formation of a research question. Next, we consider different types of literature review and research methodologies. The analysis, results, and discussion sections follow. We also consider the writing and publication process. Finally, a chapter on the interpretation of the literature covers the skills a health professional must develop to be a consumer of the literature.

Ultimately, understanding the research process and interpretation of the research literature are inextricable—this book addresses both at the basic level. Our contributors represent a wide range of healthcare and education professionals with expertise in different aspects of research; however, each contributor has written with the novice researcher or clinician in mind. Prior knowledge of research is not assumed.

ORGANIZATION AND FEATURES

Each chapter begins with a Chapter Overview designed to relate the essential information covered in the chapter. Basic Learning Objectives for the chapter are also provided. The important key terms for each chapter are highlighted in bold font, with definitions provided in the glossary. In most chapters, tables and figures are used to help summarize key information. The overall scheme allows the reader to move naturally through the research process, ending with concepts needed to interpret the research of others.

NEW TO THIS EDITION

The changes in this edition are based on the feedback from readers of the previous edition. A newly revised chapter on the regulatory protection of human subjects provides readers with a comprehensive look at the workings of the institutional review board. We have added new chapters covering systematic reviews, qualitative research, and statistics. Along with these new chapters, the editing and reorganization of the chapters from the previous edition provides the reader enhanced content without expanding the scope of the book beyond the beginner stage.

INSTRUCTOR RESOURCES

Qualified instructors can receive the full suite of Instructor Resources, including the following:

- Slides in PowerPoint format, featuring more than 350 slides
- Test Bank, containing more than 250 questions
- Instructor's Manual, including suggestions for classroom discussions and activities
- Sample Syllabus, providing guidance for structuring a course around this text

To gain access to these valuable teaching materials, contact your Health Professions Account Specialist at http://go.jblearning.com/findarep.

J. Glenn Forister

J. Dennis Blessing

Foreword

Douglas L. Murphy, PhD
Dean, College of Health Related Professions
University of Arkansas for Medical Sciences
Little Rock, Arkansas

Over the past two decades, I have devoted thousands of hours, as a teacher, advisor, and thesis or dissertation committee member, to working with scores of students dealing with a research project of some type. These students in the allied health professions, nursing, dentistry, and biomedical sciences requested assistance with refining research questions, tying theories together, laying out research designs, planning for data collection and analyses, and relating their research findings to their research goals and specific aims. Other students required assistance in interpreting published research and applying the results to their anticipated practice. In the process, I often scoured my personal library of references on research methods and statistics to find just the right chapter or article that would enable the student to gain the insight they required to become more independent as a "consumer" of research literature or fledgling researcher. I often came up short because the book wasn't exactly what the student needed. The examples were from a different discipline, making the information difficult to apply; the content was too basic and theoretical, making the information difficult to understand; or the information was outdated, not taking into account technological advances that make the conduct of research easier.

I wish now that I had had a book such as *Introduction to Research and Medical Literature for Health Professionals, Fourth Edition,* to lend. It would have made my task simpler and would have enlightened the student far better than what I was able to provide at the time. This book, edited by my colleagues J. Glenn Forister and J. Dennis Blessing, is the first research methods textbook written specifically for students in the allied health professions. Both gentlemen are respected physician assistant educators, researchers, and scholars. Dr. Blessing has received numerous national awards for his contributions to education and research, and Mr. Forister is recognized as an outstanding teacher and researcher.

Why a book on allied health research methods? On the one hand, one may argue that research methods are research methods and data analysis techniques are data analysis techniques, regardless of the discipline, and that is true to some extent. On the other hand, there are many good reasons for a book specifically for allied health professions students.

First, the allied health professions are maturing at a rapid rate and are evolving into distinctive professions in their own right, with their own professional concerns, clinical techniques, roles within healthcare systems, and practice traditions. These factors often lead to research questions that can and should be answered and, in turn, research findings must be understood and applied by students and practitioners.

Second, as the allied health professions evolve, greater demands are placed on practitioners for responsibility and accountability in health care. Increasingly, practitioners are expected to participate as full members of healthcare teams who contribute expertise on par with physicians, nurses, dentists, and other team members. Therefore, allied health professionals must stay current on the research in their disciplines and must understand how research finding A or technique X applies to the care of their patients or clients, because it is unlikely that other members of the team will be able to contribute that same expertise.

Third, allied health professionals must demonstrate the efficacy of their contributions to health and wellness. Evidence-based care, economic imperatives, and professional ethics require us to show concretely that research finding A or technique X actually does result in better outcomes or reduce costs. The days of justifying a procedure or clinical practice by invoking tradition are quickly fading away.

Finally, allied health research tends to be grounded in the real-life experiences of allied health clinicians, many of whom have extended therapeutic care relationships with patients, clients, and their families. Other allied health personnel such as laboratory scientists and health information professionals may have no or limited direct contact with patients or clients. Their vital contributions lead to other research opportunities that range from basic scientific mechanisms to investigations into human factors (person–program or person–machine interfaces) that result in more accurate laboratory tests or more efficient, productive, and useful information systems. The nature of these relationships and their role in treatment, healing, and wellness can and should shape the kinds of research questions that are posed, methods used for answering the questions, and even the theory that shapes practice.

Fulfilling as a research career may be, it is unlikely that a large proportion of students reading *Introduction to Research and Medical Literature for Health Professionals, Fourth Edition*, will pursue a career in allied health research. Some will practice in clinical settings as clinician-researchers, research partners, or research participants. The majority, however, will be informed consumers of research as they apply new knowledge, new procedures, and new techniques to day-to-day clinical care. All will require competencies in reading and comprehending research reports, interpreting and applying results, judging the adequacy of research practices, and drawing justifiable conclusions.

The editors and authors of this book are expert educators, researchers, and academics who have "been there and done that." They speak from experience in guiding students and conducting research. This book is a valuable introduction to the major considerations in planning and carrying out research projects, guidelines for judging the quality of investigations, cautions for interpreting and applying findings, and essential resources. The topics range from the process for identifying a "researchable" problem and focusing research questions to finding the appropriate journal for your manuscript. Research techniques are explained from positivist and postpositivist paradigms to qualitative methods. Ethical considerations of human research are described, and guidelines for writing a research report are provided. Community-based participatory research, an emerging expectation in biomedical research, is explained and guidelines are provided for planning and conducting such research. Chapters and sections that describe the full array of study types that fall under the term *research* are particularly valuable because they can stimulate creative thinking about options for answering research questions and, even, what kinds of questions are "legitimate."

Regardless of the ultimate career aspirations of the allied health professions student reading this book, this is one that you will keep on your shelf and refer to often. I know that I will keep a copy (or two or three) handy for that student who knocks on my door asking for some advice about a perplexing research project.

Contributors

Salah Ayachi, PhD, PA-C
Associate Professor (retired)
Department of Physician Assistant Studies
School of Health Professions
University of Texas Medical Branch
Galveston, Texas

Christopher E. Bork, PhD
Professor (retired)
Department of Public Health and Preventive Medicine
College of Medicine
The University of Toledo
Toledo, Ohio

James F. Cawley, MPH, PA-C, DHL (hon)
Professor
Department of Prevention and Community Health
School of Public Health and Health Services
Professor
Department of Physician Assistant Studies
School of Medicine and Health Sciences
The George Washington University
Washington, D.C.

Meredith A. Davison, PhD, MPH
Associate Dean of Academic Services
School of Community Medicine
Associate Program Director
Physician Assistant Program
College of Medicine
The University of Oklahoma–Tulsa
Tulsa, Oklahoma

Richard Dehn, MPA, PA-C
Professor and Founding Chair
Department of Physician Assistant Studies
College of Health and Human Services
Northern Arizona University
Flagstaff, Arizona

Margaret J. Foster, MS, MPH
Assistant Professor
Systematic Reviews and Research Coordinator
Medical Sciences Library
Texas A&M University
College Station, Texas

Christine S. Gaspard, MSLS
Head of Access Services and Interlibrary Loan
Instructional Librarian, Briscoe Library
UT Health Science Center San Antonio
San Antonio, Texas

Elsa M. González, PhD
Assistant Professor
Department of Educational Leadership, Higher Education Administration
College of Education and Human Development
Texas A&M University–Corpus Christi
Corpus Christi, Texas

Robert W. Jarski, PhD, PA-C
Professor (retired)
School of Health Sciences
The OU William Beaumont School of Medicine
Director
Complementary Medicine and Wellness Program
Oakland University
Rochester, Michigan

Linda Levy, MSW, MLS, AHIP
Assistant Library Director (retired)
Briscoe Library
UT Health Science Center San Antonio
San Antonio, Texas

Anthony A. Miller, MEd, PA-C
Chief Policy Officer, Head of Research
Physician Assistant Education Association
Alexandria, Virginia

Bruce R. Niebuhr, PhD
Susan Brown Logan Distinguished Professor in Teaching Excellence
Distinguished Teaching Professor (retired)
Department of Physician Assistant Studies
School of Health Professions
University of Texas Medical Branch
Galveston, Texas

Rhonda Oilepo, MS, CIP
Associate Director
Office of the Institutional Review Board
UT Health Science Center San Antonio
San Antonio, Texas

Katherine A. Prentice, MSIS
Associate Director for User Experience and Assessment
Schusterman Library
The University of Oklahoma–Tulsa
Tulsa, Oklahoma

Richard R. Rahr, EdD, PA-C
Professor Emeritus
Department of Physician Assistant Studies
School of Health Professions
University of Texas Medical Branch
Galveston, Texas

Scott D. Rhodes, PhD, MPH
Professor
Division of Public Health Sciences
School of Medicine
Wake Forest University
Winston-Salem, North Carolina

Joseph O. Schmelz, PhD, RN, CIP, FAAN
Assistant Vice President for Research Operations
UT Health Science Center San Antonio
San Antonio, Texas

Albert Simon, DHSc, MEd, PA-C
Chair
Department of Physician Assistant Studies
Arizona School of Health Sciences
Mesa, Arizona

Kimberly K. Summers, PharmD
Director, Research Regulatory Programs
UT Health Science Center San Antonio
San Antonio, Texas

Christina J. Sun, PhD, MS
Research Fellow
Division of Public Health Sciences
School of Medicine
Wake Forest University
Winston-Salem, North Carolina

Eric Willman, MSIS
Library Technology Coordinator
Briscoe Library
UT Health Science Center San Antonio
San Antonio, Texas

Reviewers

Allison Bernknopf, PharmD, BCPS
Associate Professor
College of Pharmacy
Ferris State University
Big Rapids, Michigan

Vera C. Brancato, EdD, MSN, BSN, RN
Professor of Nursing
Alvernia University
Reading, Pennsylvania

Pamela J. Bretschneider, PhD
Faculty
Massachusetts College of Pharmacy and Health Sciences University
Boston, Massachusetts

Kim Cavanagh, DHSc, MPAS, PA-C
Associate Professor
Physician Assistant Program
Morosky College of Health Professions and Sciences
Gannon University
Erie, Pennsylvania

Sara M. Denning, MPA, PA-C
Academic Instructor, Clinical Science Instructor
Physician Assistant Program
The College of Health Professions
The University of Findlay
Findlay, Ohio

Michael L. Rowland, PhD
Assistant Professor
Department of Leadership, Foundations, and Human Resource Education
School of Medicine
University of Louisville
Louisville, Kentucky

Michele L. Shade-McCay, MPH, DrPH
Visiting Assistant Professor
College of Science and Health
DePaul University
Chicago, Illinois

Daniel T. Vetrosky, PA-C, PhD, DFAAPA
Associate Professor and Director of Didactic Education
Department of Physician Assistant Studies
College of Allied Health Professions
University of South Alabama
Mobile, Alabama

SECTION I

Getting Started

CHAPTER 1

CHAPTER OVERVIEW

This chapter is designed to introduce health professionals and students to research. The chapter introduces readers to the basic definitions and sources of research. An outline is offered to aid in the development of a project or research agenda. Each small piece of research that can add to the body of medical knowledge results in improvement in the healthcare professions and in the physical, mental, and social health of those for whom care is provided.

Introduction

J. Glenn Forister, MS, PA-C
J. Dennis Blessing, PhD, PA

Learning Objectives

- Define *research*.
- Describe types of research.
- Describe and discuss the importance of research in the healthcare professions.
- Begin to develop a scientific approach to study and practice.

INTRODUCTION

The bottom line is that research determines almost everything that is practiced now and in the future. The word *research* often evokes a panic reaction. Students may see research as a mysterious process that is difficult to understand and difficult to conduct. Often students cannot make the connection between a required research assignment and their future healthcare careers. Similarly, many clinicians may not connect research to their work. Research, however, provides an opportunity to explore, understand, and explain practice. By mastering research, healthcare professionals can enhance their clinical careers and improve patient outcomes.

Many clinical practices are becoming involved with clinical trials and studies. This involvement makes understanding the scientific process and research a practice requirement. Beyond the possibility of being directly involved in research, every healthcare professional must understand research processes in order to interpret healthcare literature. The decision to incorporate a new treatment modality depends on the ability to assess and understand the research that led to that modality. Additionally, healthcare professionals must be able to evaluate the literature in terms of how it relates to patients and to evaluate the best treatment options.

RESEARCH AND STUDENTS IN HEALTHCARE PROFESSIONS

The word *research* conjures up many images:

- Socially inept individuals hidden away in a lab doing something that seems to have little relationship to everyday life
- Dr. Frankenstein
- Boring work forced on students
- The pursuit of information that has little application in the real world
- Not something a health professional does in clinical practice

For many people, the research process is difficult to understand. Research requires manipulations of impossible-to-learn formulations that end up in a language that only other researchers comprehend. Research sometimes produces contradictory results that often leave healthcare professionals wondering what to do. Research frightens clinicians and keeps educators from taking tenure-track positions. Research conjures up an image of boring, regimented work that may have little to do with the "real world."

In reality, the very opposite is true. Research provides the basis for practice of the healthcare profession. Research is the key to the present and future, regardless of one's profession, position, or function in health care. The practice of medicine, nursing, and health care is based in scientific research that is applied to every patient. The only way health care can advance is by research, that is, developing evidence of what works and applying the results. Practitioners who are not actively involved in research must possess a basic understanding of the processes and what research results mean to practice. This understanding allows practitioners to interpret results, to differentiate between conflicting results, and to discern what is useful *and* best for patients. As evidence-based medicine becomes the basis for health care, understanding and conducting research also has become more important. More and more practicing healthcare professionals are finding that research or some aspect of research has become part of their day-to-day job.

RESEARCH EQUALS CURIOSITY

Whether they realize it or not, everyone has done research in some manner. Seeking an answer to a question is a form of research. Even looking up a word in a dictionary can be considered a form of research. Curiosity and the need for information create the drive to find answers in health care and daily life. Finding those answers is research. Certainly, much "research" is informal and without the systematic constraints required in formal research, but it occurs every day. A parent's admonition to "Look it up!" sends children off on a research effort whether they realize it or not. Practitioners do research every day as they investigate the literature for solutions to patients' problems. Students do research as part of their education and preparation to enter their profession. The very act of study is an investigation in some ways, regardless of what it is called. Exam preparation is a form of research.

Research occurs in the laboratory, classroom, office, practice, and society at large. It may be directly applicable to a problem or only a small piece of larger solutions. Research can help practitioners prepare for what will happen and understand what has happened. Individual needs and desires direct how research is used and the part it plays in careers and lives. Research is a tool to be used. Learning to use this tool helps relieve anxieties and increases the ability to appreciate and enjoy the process. Application is likely to improve the lives of patients.

Research that involves interests or needs for discovery is most important. In some ways research may be more important to the practitioner than to the student, but research skills are introduced during education. Similarly, what interests a healthcare practitioner or student may be mundane but necessary to the profession or livelihood. For example, an occupational therapist may have little interest in the differences in practice census flows by disability type, but that information may have a great impact on patient scheduling and clinical assignments. Research may provide answers that allow for the most efficient use of time and expertise in practice. Many questions about one's practice can be answered by research. It may or may not require statistical analysis, but it requires the systematic gathering, analysis, and interpretation of information (data).

Another example of research application in practice is patient outcomes. What is the difference in practice outcomes if a disease is treated with regimen A versus regimen B? There may be a wealth of information in texts and the literature, but what about a particular practice? Personal research is needed to determine the answer, whether a formal or informal process is used. The values of informal versus formal research may be equal, but a formal investigation might lead to benefits beyond a single setting if the investigation yields significant information.

RESEARCH AND THE STUDENTS OF HEALTHCARE PROFESSIONS

For a student, research is part of the task of discovery and learning. Research provides the information needed to build a fund of knowledge that guides what a student will do as a healthcare provider. Every student must become an informed consumer and learn to interpret the medical research and healthcare literature. At a minimum, learning how to interpret research findings is a necessary skill for a professional career. Effective interpretation skills allow healthcare practitioners to deliver an acceptable level of care. In many ways, the research process is comparable to clinical reasoning and critical thinking skills. Much of the discipline needed to develop and conduct research is the same as the discipline needed to assess and manage disease processes.

Education in the healthcare professions should be consistent with adult learning theory. All healthcare practitioners should be lifelong learners; the healthcare professional that stops building his or her knowledge base and abilities will soon be hopelessly behind. Experience is part of that knowledge base, but continuing to understand and interpret the literature is the foundation for maintaining, redefining, and increasing that base. Research can help meet future healthcare challenges. Research is one tool that helps practitioners to "learn how to learn."

RESEARCH AND HEALTHCARE PROFESSIONALS

The unknowns and seemingly complex methods of systematic research and its processes frighten many people. Analysis, statistics, and interpretation can be daunting, as well. Research as a discipline even has its own language. Research may be held in high regard by many and in low regard (almost thought of as a dirty word?) by others. Many healthcare professionals want to leave research to others. However, at a minimum, healthcare professionals must be able to interpret and apply research as steps in patient care. As some healthcare professionals become more involved and invested in their careers and practices, they may find roles and responsibilities in the research arena. Society expects healthcare professionals to understand healthcare research and apply it to the needs of the individual patient.

RESEARCH TAKES MANY FORMS

Research takes many different forms (**Table 1-1**). Research can be categorized in various ways, including pure research, experimental research, clinical research, applied research, descriptive research, laboratory research,[1] and outcomes research. These forms depend on many factors.

Table 1-1 Types of Research

Type	Description	Example(s)
Pure	Abstract and general, concerned with generating new theory and gaining new knowledge for knowledge sake	Theory development
Experimental	Manipulation of one variable to see its effect on another variable, while controlling for as many other variables as possible and randomly assigning subjects to groups	Double-blind random assignment control groups, response to an intervention
Clinical	Performed in the clinical setting where control over variables is quite difficult	Drug trials, therapeutic results
Applied	Designed to answer a practical question, to help people do their jobs better	Time use studies, evaluation of different types of interventions with the same purpose
Descriptive	Describing a group, a situation, or an individual to gain knowledge that may be applied to further groups or situations, as in case studies or trend analyses	Surveys, qualitative research, measurement of characteristics, response to phenomena
Laboratory	Performed in laboratory surroundings that are tightly controlled	Basic science research

Reproduced from: Bailey DM. *Research for the Health Professional: A Practical Guide.* 2nd ed. Philadelphia, PA: FA Davis;1997:xxii.

The design of a research study is an important factor that confuses many beginning investigators.[2] Some research can be done without any special knowledge or skills, such as counting how many patients have a particular diagnosis. Some research requires specialized skills and must follow an exact methodology, such as clinical drug trials. Research has a language of its own that must be learned. The recording of experimental results and writing of research have unique requirements that must be learned, practiced, and perfected. For most, research is about phenomena (something that can be perceived) that affect what is done and what needs to be known. Research is about observation and interpretation of what is learned in order to answer the questions posed.

Research can be challenging and difficult. It also can be enjoyable and rewarding. At every level and in every format and design, research should add to knowledge. It is unlikely that any single piece of research will make headlines. However, answering questions and making small contributions to the larger body of medical knowledge are very satisfying. Health care at every level continually creates questions that need answers. Society has questions that need answers. When healthcare professionals accept the challenge of answering those questions, a basic understanding of research and how to apply it is necessary. Learning the research process offers the greatest likelihood of finding those answers. One does not have to be a genius to do research. One does not have to be mathematically gifted. One must only have an interest. Research and its results can be used in the classroom, laboratory, or clinic. It is a process to be learned and used to help healthcare practitioners, patients, students, and others.

DEVELOPING A RESEARCH PROJECT

If a research project is part of education and training, it may take many forms. Choosing a project and developing its design depend on a number of factors. The first is to understand exactly what is expected. Schools or institutions may have specific guidelines. These parameters must be known before beginning any project. Many organizations prescribe a scientific writing format. Student investigators must know which style and style manual is required and should obtain a copy.

Schools or institutions may assign research topics and/or a specific design to follow. Development of a research project depends on many factors. Some introspection and consideration are required with regard to time, effort, cost, resources, and ability needed for any project. This introspection must include an assessment of personal attributes, interests, resources, and expectations of self (Jones PE, personal communication, 2004). Part of this assessment must consider strengths as a researcher and abilities to accomplish the project. One cannot do quantum physics without the education and skills necessary, no matter how interested one may be in quantum physics. Students and inexperienced investigators must be able to concentrate their research efforts to develop or use their expertise to the maximum benefit. It is better to be an expert in one small area than somewhat of an expert in several. Every beginning researcher needs mentors and collaborators. Students and beginning investigators should seek out people who have skills in their area of interest and ask for their help. They should explore the possibilities of collaborating with someone on their research as a learning activity. Another key element to a successful research effort is the allotment of adequate time for investigations. For students, time may be very limited by schedules, class obligations, planned graduation date, and the like. A timeline for a research project should be created and followed.

Research is a systematic, organized process that goes through a number of sequential (or near sequential steps (see **Figure 1–1**). The first step of developing a research project is brainstorming. This activity should be as expansive as possible by making a list (by hand or on the computer) of everything of interest. Once these ideas are recorded, a short break of a few minutes or a few days should be taken (the key is *not* to think about the project for a short while). Then the list can be refined; new items can be added, and those that do not seem important can be eliminated. This process may be repeated more than once before a project is defined. A student, for example, may have an assigned topic, but there may be many ways to approach the assigned project. Once a list of possibilities has been developed, the defining process can be done in this way:

1. Make a list of everything of interest or questions that need to be answered.
2. Prioritize the list in the order of interests.
3. Make a second ordered list (from the first) of the things that are within the capabilities of the investigator.
4. Make a third ordered list (from the first) of the things that are important to the effort.
5. Make a fourth ordered list (from the first) of the things that are important to society, or health, or the particular profession.
6. Compare the lists. Items that appear at the top of all four lists should be prioritized and merged into a single list.
7. Make decisions about what can and cannot be accomplished. Mark off the things that cannot be done. This includes financing the study. Financial support is just as important to the project's success as time and expertise.
8. The topic that survives or is central to the lists is the basis of the research project. This topic represents a process of summation that includes challenges that need to be researched; challenges to the capability of the researcher; and challenges that are important to the individual, the program, and the topic of interest. What could be better?
9. Develop a timeline for the study; set aside research time and plan the step-by-step process, and then . . .

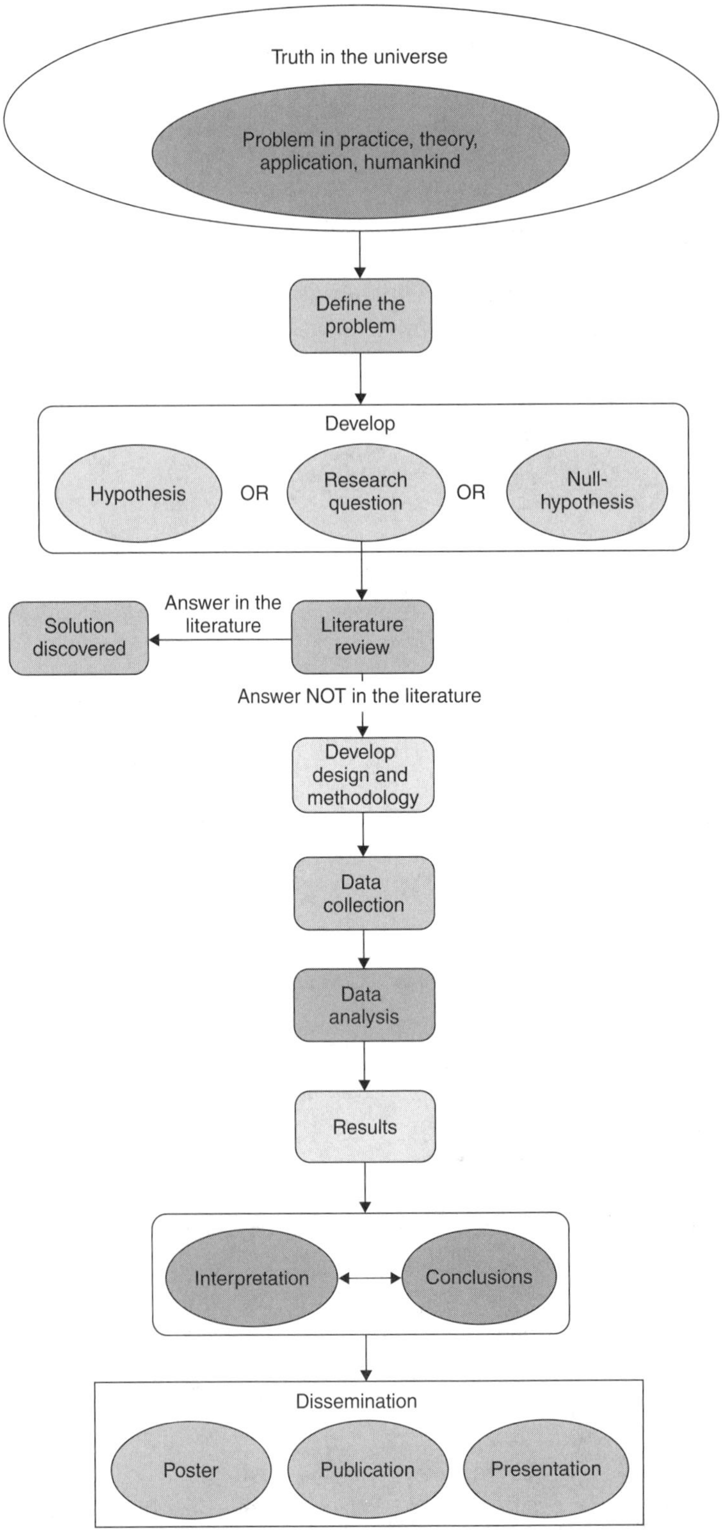

Figure 1–1 Outline of the scientific process.

10. *Get started.* A respected educator said, "Time goes by regardless of what you do. When it does, make sure you are not still waiting for the best time to begin" (Rahr RR, personal communication, 2004). A student may have a defined end date (e.g., project due date, end of semester, graduation, etc.). Do not hesitate to get started.

SUMMARY

Whether one loves it, hates it, or would rather not think about it, research is a part of professional life in a healthcare career. Research provides the basis for all that healthcare providers do. Individual research is unlikely to change the world or win a Nobel Prize; however, each small addition to our knowledge of the world and health care improves them both. Remember, research is not a dirty word; it is a powerful tool that every healthcare provider must learn to use and master in order to care for others.

REFERENCES

1. Campbell DT, Stanley JC. *Experimental and Quasi-Experimental Designs for Research.* Boston, MA: Houghton Mifflin; 1963:1.
2. Bailey DM. *Research for the Health Professional: A Practical Guide.* 2nd ed. Philadelphia, PA: FA Davis; 1997:xxii.

CHAPTER 2

Regulatory Protection of Human Subjects in Research

Rhonda Oilepo, MS, CIP
Kimberly K. Summers, PharmD
Joseph O. Schmelz, PhD, RN, CIP, FAAN

CHAPTER OVERVIEW

The protection of human subjects in research is paramount to any research effort. Research that involves human subjects is highly regulated by federal, state, and institutional policies and requirements. Protection is extended to almost every type of research that involves people, even survey research. The purpose of this chapter is to explain the federal regulations that govern research involving humans, to clarify the authority of the institutional review board (IRB), and to address the responsibilities of investigators conducting research using human subjects.

Learning Objectives

- Describe, discuss, and define the history of protection of human subjects.
- Describe and discuss the need for protection of human subjects.
- Outline and discuss the Belmont Principles.
- Describe the functions of the institutional review board.
- List the elements of informed consent.

INTRODUCTION

It is common for health professionals to perform projects or other activities that involve data collection, analysis, and interpretation. The use of data for the purpose of drawing conclusions and solving problems is usually defined as research; however, many activities considered to be research (e.g., quality improvement,[1] program evaluation, etc.) may not qualify as "regulated research" that requires the approval of an institutional review board (IRB). Although these activities share many of the data collection and analysis methods used by researchers, the outcomes serve different purposes. For example, nonregulated research activities (i.e., quality improvement, program evaluation, or community outreach) produce results to be used internally or locally to influence immediate change. In contrast, regulated research (i.e., clinical trials) results are widely applicable and generally not used to influence immediate change to the local organization or community. Health professionals may find it difficult to determine whether a particular activity is regulated research and whether it requires the approval of the IRB. After reading this chapter, the reader should have a basic understanding of human (regulated) research, how such research is regulated, and what responsibilities the researcher has when conducting a regulated research project.

Table 2–1 Belmont Principles

Respect for Persons
- Treat individuals as autonomous agents capable of making informed choices and acting on them.
- Individuals with diminished autonomy are entitled to protection.

Beneficence
- Maximize possible benefits and minimize possible harms

Justice
- Fairness in distribution of the benefits and burdens

HOW IS RESEARCH APPROVED?

Before involving living individuals in regulated research, the project and the protections provided by the investigator must be reviewed by the institution's committee designated to oversee such research. This committee is commonly referred to as the institutional review board (IRB). The IRB is composed of scientists, nonscientists, and individuals who are not affiliated with the institution (sometimes referred to as community members). Members of the IRB are selected based on their expertise in the types of research typically reviewed by the board or on the diversity of their background or experience. The goal of the IRB review is to ensure the individuals participating in the research are adequately protected. To achieve this goal, the IRB reviews the written plan for conducting the research and the safeguards that will be provided to protect participants. The IRB must conclude that the research fulfills the basic principles for conducting ethical research established by the National Commission for the Protection of Human Subjects in Biomedical and Behavioral Research.[2]

In 1979, the National Commission released the Belmont Report, which established three basic ethical principles for conducting research involving humans.[2] (See **Table 2–1**.) The Belmont principles are respect for persons (autonomy), beneficence, and justice. Application of the general principles led to the development of the following requirements: informed consent, assessment of risks and benefits, and equitable selection of subjects. The National Commission was established by Congress in the National Research Act of 1974. The act requires researchers funded by the U.S. Department of Health, Education, and Welfare (now the U.S. Department of Health and Human Services [HHS]) to obtain IRB approval and informed consent. This regulation, 45 CFR Part 46, Subpart A,[3] became known as the Common Rule when it was adopted by 15 federal agencies in 1991.[4] In addition to the Common Rule, the Food and Drug Administration's (FDA) regulations[5,6] for the protection of human subjects (21 CFR Parts 50 and 56) require IRB approval and informed consent for research involving drugs, devices, or biologics, regardless of the funding source. Finally, the Privacy Rule (45 CFR Part 164)[7] requires additional approval by a privacy board when research involves identifiable health information held by health-related entities, regardless of the funding source or whether the research uses a drug, device, or biologic. See **Figure 2–1**.

WHEN IS IRB APPROVAL REQUIRED?

IRB approval is needed whenever a project meets the regulatory definitions of human-subjects research provided in either the Common Rule[3]

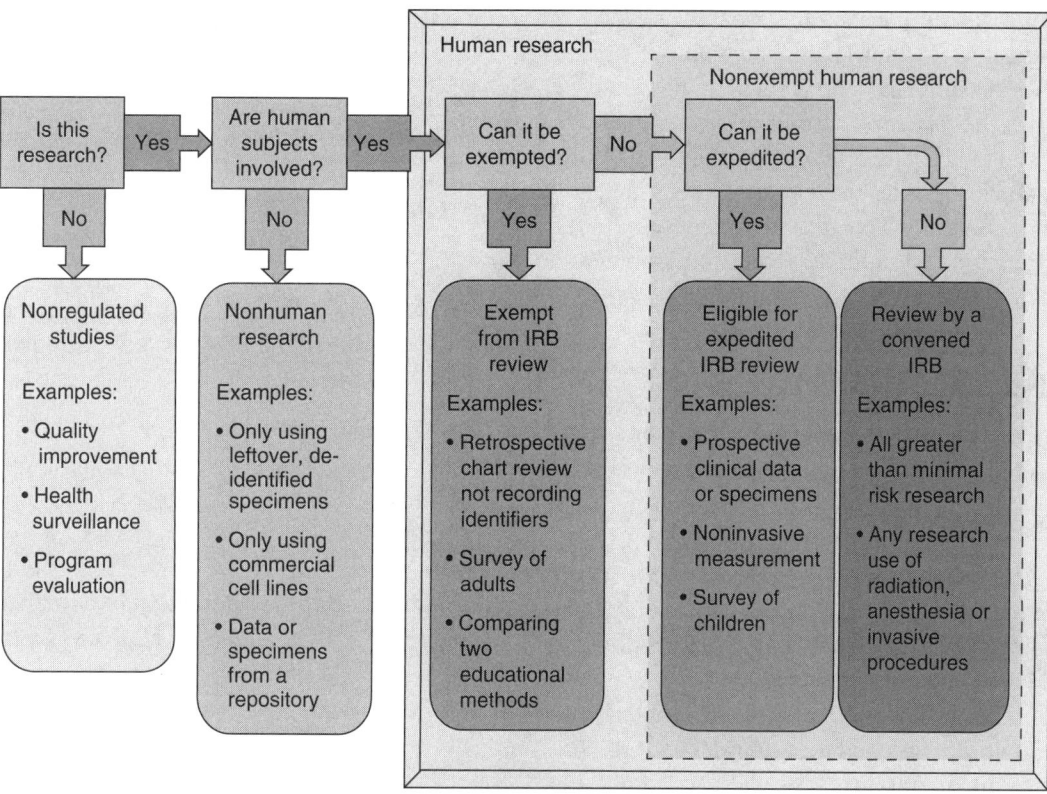

Figure 2-1 Determining whether human subjects are involved in research.

or the FDA regulations.[5,6] The Common Rule is generally applicable to most research conducted by healthcare professionals. Although the Common Rule is technically only applicable to federally funded or supported research, most institutions apply it to all research, regardless of the funding source. The Common Rule requires IRB approval of all "human-subjects research." Two questions help identify activities as human-subjects research: Is this regulated research? and Are human subjects involved?

Is This Regulated Research?

The Belmont Report noted that the distinction between research and practice (non-research) is blurred. The Common Rule defines research as "a systematic investigation, including research development, testing and evaluation, designed to develop or contribute to generalizable knowledge."[3]

Unfortunately, the two key concepts in the definition—"systematic investigation" and "generalizable knowledge"—are not clear. The definition is not particularly helpful in defining regulated research because many other activities such as patient satisfaction surveys and ward infection surveillance would be considered systematic investigations. Jeff Cooper (personal communication, May 2010) notes that a major problem with the definition of "[regulated] research" is the question, "What constitutes generalizable knowledge?" He suggests that "generalizable" should be interpreted as a matter of policy to mean "widely applicable." This interpretation has the advantage of meeting the common intuitive interpretation of "[regulated] research" and maximally carving out scholarly activities.[8]

In general, the purpose of research is to fill a gap in the current knowledge. The Belmont Report describes research as ". . . an activity designed to test a hypothesis, permit conclusions to be drawn."[2] (p4) If the conclusions drawn from the activity are widely applicable, one could say the results are generalizable. Research activities that meet both parts of the definition (systematic and generalizable) are considered to be regulated research.

Are Human Subjects Involved?

When it has been determined that an activity meets the regulatory definition of research, the next step is to decide whether the research involves human subjects. Regulated research involves human subjects if the researcher either obtains data through interacting or intervening with a living individual or obtains private identifiable information about a living individual. Interacting means the researcher communicates or has interpersonal contact with the individual (e.g., makes phone contact for recruitment or obtains consent to participate). Intervening includes physical procedures (e.g., obtaining blood), manipulating the individual (e.g., providing a treatment), or manipulating the individual's environment (e.g., changing room temperature). Information is considered private when it is provided for a specific purpose by an individual and the individual can expect it will not be made public. Private information is considered individually identifiable if the identity of the individual may be ascertained by the investigator or associated with the information. Whether or not an activity meets these criteria, it is still necessary when considering whether it is research under the FDA human protections regulations.[5]

Is This FDA-Regulated Research?

Although it is uncommon for students and practicing professionals in healthcare professions to conduct research that is FDA regulated, FDA regulations should be considered to determine if IRB approval and informed consent are required. The FDA often uses the term *clinical investigation* to indicate research. FDA-regulated research includes the following[9]:

- Use of an unapproved drug or biologic
- Use of an FDA-approved drug other than the use of a marketed drug in the course of medical practice
- Use of a device to evaluate safety or effectiveness of that device
- Submission of data from the use of a drug or device to the FDA for advertising or a change in labeling.

If a study involves any of these, the IRB should be contacted for guidance. Not only will IRB approval and informed consent be required, but additional FDA permissions may be necessary before the research can begin. If the activity meets either the Common Rule or FDA definition of human subject research, it will generally be reviewed by the IRB unless it qualifies for an exemption to the Common Rule.

Can It Be Exempted?

If a regulated human-subjects research project is not subject to the FDA human protection regulations (as described previously) and does not involve incarcerated individuals (i.e., prisoners), it may qualify for exemption from the Common Rule.

Certain regulated human research studies that involve very little or no risk and fall completely within one or more specific exemption categories (as defined in the regulations) may qualify for exempt status. This means that the institution is not required to follow the Common Rule with respect to the research (e.g., obtain IRB approval).[10] However, other rules may be applicable to an exempt study. In general, the institution or a higher authority establishes policy for approving/overseeing exempt human research. For example, because IRB approval is not required, most institutions designate an office or official to make a determination that the research is exempt. Currently, the Office for Human Research Protections (OHRP, a subdivision of HHS) does not recommend that investigators be given the authority to make an independent judgment. Most local policies applicable to exempt research are based on the Belmont Principles. (IRBs should be consulted for specific guidance.)

Examples of the most common types of research that can be exempted include (1) educational research involving normal educational practices such as comparing different curricula or instructional techniques, (2) surveys (not involving children) that collect information that would not likely pose a risk to those completing the survey if their answers were released (either because the information is not sensitive in nature or because it cannot be traced back to the individual), or (3) chart reviews of health information that is both preexisting and not traceable back to the individual. An institution's IRB generally provides the complete list of exemptions from the Common Rule.

If a research project does not meet the criteria for exemption (nonexempt regulated human-subjects research), it must be reviewed by the IRB. In reviewing nonexempt regulated research, the IRB can use one of two review processes: (1) expedited review or (2) review by a meeting of the IRB.

Can It Be Expedited?

Some nonexempt studies that involve only minimal risk to participants and fall completely within one or more specific expedited categories may be eligible for an expedited review procedure. The IRB chairperson or one or more experienced members of the IRB may carry out an expedited review instead of the study being reviewed by the convened board. It is necessary to understand the concept of risk when determining if a study is eligible for expedited review.[3] Risk is a measure of harm. It refers to both the likelihood (i.e., probability) that harm may occur and the magnitude of possible harm. Although investigators often focus on physical harms when developing their IRB application, the IRB views harm more broadly. Harm can be categorized as physical (e.g., injury or pain), psychological (e.g., anxiety or shame), social (e.g., adverse effect on relationships), economic (e.g., financial costs), legal (e.g., arrest or lawsuits), or dignitary (e.g., violates personal values).[4]

Like the regulatory definition of human-subjects research discussed earlier, the meaning of minimal risk is a source for debate and may be defined differently by different IRBs. In general, minimal risk means the risks from research activities are not greater than those ordinarily encountered in daily life. Recognizing the debate over whether daily life should be taken to refer to an absolute (i.e., daily life of healthy individuals) or relative (i.e., daily life of participants of the research), many IRBs consider any activities outside those conducted during a routine physical or psychological examination as carrying more than minimal risk.[3,5] Examples of minimal-risk procedures that meet this definition include simple venipuncture, physical examinations, magnetic resonance imaging [MRI] procedures (not involving contrast), surveys or interviews, and the like. If the risk is no more than minimal, the next step in determining whether the study is eligible for expedited review can be undertaken. The list of planned research activities is then compared with the expedited review categories.

The categories of research eligible for expedited review include the following[3,6]: research on approved devices that will be used in their approved manner; the study of approved drugs in a manner that does not increase the risk or decrease the acceptability of the risk associated with the use; collection of blood in limited quantities over specific time periods; noninvasive collection of biological specimens (e.g., urine, leftover specimens collected for other purposes); noninvasive data collected routinely in clinical practice that do not involve x-rays, general anesthesia, or sedation (e.g., MRI, weight, blood pressure); use of information or specimens that have already been collected for any purpose; use of information or specimens that will be collected solely for nonresearch purposes (e.g., medical record reviews); recordings (e.g., voice recordings, digital images); and surveys, focus groups, or interviews.

It is important to remember that the study cannot include any procedures that are more than minimal risk and that all research procedures must fall into one or more of the expedited categories. An example of a research study that may involve minimal risk but does not fall completely within the expedited review categories is a study involving the use of health information normally collected as part of routine dental care and a dental x-ray being completed for research purposes. The risk of all the research procedures may be categorized as no more than minimal risk. However, the dental x-ray procedure does not fit any of the expedited review categories (i.e., noninvasive data collection is not appropriate because this procedure involves x-rays). Therefore, although the risk to the participants may be minimal, the research study is not eligible for expedited review (at least initially) and would be reviewed by the convened IRB. If the convened IRB determines the study involves no more than minimal risk, future IRB reviews of the study may be completed using the expedited review procedure.

What If a Research Project Is Not Eligible for Expedited Review?

Regulated research that does not meet criteria as either exempt or expedited must be reviewed by the convened IRB (i.e., the full committee). A convened IRB is a committee of at least five members, each with varying expertise (scientific and nonscientific) and affiliations (both affiliated and not affiliated with the institution).[3,6] Notably, the IRB uses the same criteria for evaluating a study regardless of whether it is reviewed by expedited review or the convened IRB. The Common Rule and the FDA human-protection regulations impose specific criteria for approval of regulated research. Investigators should develop the study plan with the specific criteria in mind. Many investigators assume their scientific plan is the only information the IRB needs to approve their research. Although there are significant overlaps, they are not the same. In general, the IRB application calls for additional information not commonly found in the grant application or academic degree proposal. The criteria used by the IRB to approve regulated research are presented in **Figure 2-2**.

How Will the IRB Review a Regulated Research Project?

For the IRB to approve research, it must determine the following:

The risks to the participants have been minimized. In other words, the probability and magnitude of the reasonably expected research harms have been minimized. However, the nature of the study may limit the extent to which risks can be minimized. Some ways researchers can minimize risks are by choosing a procedure that would pose less risk to the participants over another or designing the study to use procedures that would be performed regardless of whether the individual was enrolled in the research.

The risks are reasonable in relation to anticipated benefits. Once the risks have been minimized, the possible benefits associated with the research are considered. In general, research can potentially benefit individual participants (direct benefit) and/or society (important knowledge gained). An assessment of risks to potential benefits is often referred to as a risk–benefit ratio. The IRB will approve only research where the probability of a benefit outweighs the risks of participating in the research.

The selection of subjects is equitable. With a clear understanding of the risks and potential benefits in the study, consider whether the selected population fairly distributes the burdens and benefits of the research. In making this determination, the IRB considers whether the study targets individuals who will likely benefit from the outcome of the research. For example, the board may ask whether there are participants who may benefit more from the study.

Informed consent will be sought from each prospective subject or the subject's legally authorized representative. Because informed consent is one of the three basic protections provided by the Common Rule, the IRB will require it in most cases. The human-protection regulations define the basic information that must be provided while obtaining informed consent (see **Table 2-2**). In some cases, a request may be made that some or all of the elements of consent be waived by the IRB. For example, a waiver of all elements of consent may be appropriate

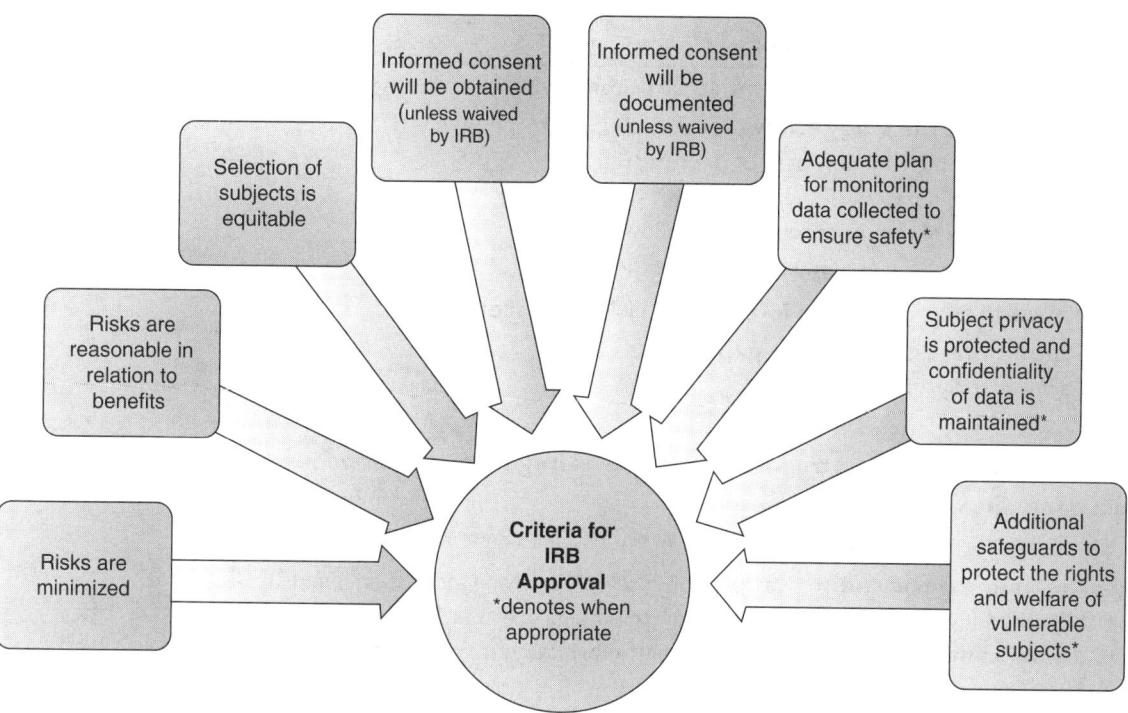

Figure 2–2 Criteria for IRB approval of nonexempt regulated research.

for a study using existing health information that was collected for clinical purposes where it is not feasible to obtain consent from the individual patients. An example of an alteration of informed consent (omitting some elements) would include a study where some of the required information is not appropriate for the research. In this case, the investigator can request an alteration in consent if the study meets the criteria for alteration of consent. In addition to the information provided during the consent process, the IRB also evaluates the researchers' plan for obtaining informed consent. A recruitment plan should provide ample opportunity for prospective participants (or their legally authorized representative) to make an informed choice. Considerations include the study setting, how and by whom the consent interview will be conducted, and timing for obtaining consent (to minimize the possibility that prospective participants may perceive undue pressure to enroll or feel coerced).

The informed consent will be appropriately documented. The investigator must have clear plans for obtaining appropriate signatures of participants (or their legally authorized representative) to document the informed consent process. Most IRBs provide a consent document template that provides the basic elements of consent. If this documentation is not possible (e.g., telephone surveys), the investigator may request a waiver of documentation of informed consent, which must be approved by the IRB. In these situations, the researcher must make a note in the research record that all of the required information (see Table 2–2) about the study was presented to the participant and the participant willingly agreed (consented) to participate in the research.

The research plan makes adequate provision for monitoring the data collected to ensure the safety of subjects (when appropriate). When required, a plan for monitoring the safety of the study using the data collected should be developed. This plan should include (1) how often safety data are compiled and reviewed, (2) by whom (an individual or committee), and (3) whether limits are needed for stopping the research procedures to ensure safety of the participants. A formal

Table 2–2 Elements of Informed Consent

Basic elements of informed consent provide participants with the following information:

A statement that the study involves research
- An explanation of the purposes of the research
- The expected duration of the participant's participation
- A description of the procedures to be followed
- Identification of any procedures that are experimental

Description of any reasonably foreseeable risks or discomforts

Benefits that may reasonably be expected
- To the participants (if applicable)
- To others

Alternative procedures or treatment, if any, that might be advantageous to the participant

Confidentiality of records
- The extent, if any, to which confidentiality will be maintained

Injury-related care or compensation (for research involving more than minimal risk)
- Whether any compensation and medical treatments are available if injury occurs
- If so, what they consist of, or where further information may be obtained

Contact information: whom to contact
- For answers to pertinent questions about the research and participants' rights
- In the event of a research-related injury to the participant

Participation remains voluntary—no penalty or loss of entitled benefits
- By refusing to participate
- By discontinuing participation at any time

Additional information when determined to be appropriate by the IRB
- A statement that the particular treatment or procedure may involve unforeseeable risks
- Anticipated circumstances under which the participant's participation may be terminated by the investigator without regard to the participant's consent
- Any additional costs to the participant that may result from participation in the research
- The consequences of a participant's decision to withdraw from the research and procedures for orderly termination of participation by the subject
- A statement that significant new findings developed during the course of the research that may relate to the participant's willingness to continue participation will be provided to the subject
- The approximate number of participants involved in the study

monitoring plan is usually required for FDA-regulated clinical trials, all National Institutes of Health (NIH) funded research, and more than minimal risk research.

There are adequate provisions to protect the privacy of subjects and to maintain the confidentiality of data (when appropriate).[11] For example, assigning study codes to participants rather than using names and storing the key to decipher the codes in a separate, secure location accessible only to the investigators is a way of demonstrating this type of protection.

In addition to the seven determinations just listed, if a study involves populations vulnerable to coercion or undue influence, such as children, prisoners, pregnant women, or mentally disabled (decisionally impaired) people, the IRB will evaluate whether the study provides safeguards capable of protecting the rights and welfare of those individuals.

In preparing a research project for review by the IRB, the study plan should be designed with the required IRB determinations in mind. Although it is the IRB's responsibility to determine whether these requirements for approval are met, it is the investigator's responsibility to design and carry out the study plan in such a way that the criteria for approval are met. This is one of several responsibilities assumed by the investigator responsible for the research.

WHAT ARE THE INVESTIGATOR'S RESPONSIBILITIES?

Obtaining IRB approval for a new project is only the first of many responsibilities for the principal investigator (PI).[12] During the conduct of the study, the PI must ensure the study continues to meet the criteria used by the IRB for the initial approval (e.g., the risks continue to be minimized, informed consent continues to be obtained and documented, safety data are collected and monitored, etc.).[13] The PI is also responsible for communicating regularly with the IRB under certain circumstances such as those described in the following sections.

Continuing Review

Many investigators do not realize that the approval they get when a study is first reviewed by the IRB has a time limit that cannot exceed 1 year. To request reapproval so that the research can continue uninterrupted, the PI must submit a status report to the IRB before the approval period expires. The report must include information about the number of participants accrued (if any); a description of any adverse events, unanticipated problems, participant withdrawals, or complaints; a summary of relevant new information (either published or learned in the research); and a copy of the current consent document(s) being used. The IRB reviews the status report, including any other new information, and reconsiders the required determinations for approval of research (e.g., risks continue to be minimized, risks continue to be reasonable in relation to the benefits, informed consent continues to be obtained and appropriately documented, etc.). If the study continues to meet the criteria for approval, the IRB will reapprove the study for up to one additional year.

Sometimes the IRB may decide to issue an approval for less than a year (e.g., for particularly high risk studies the IRB may approve the study for only a few months). It is the responsibility of the investigator to contact the IRB to request reapproval prior to the expiration of the original IRB approval.[12] If the IRB has not reapproved the study before the current approval period expires, research procedures (including analysis of identifiable data) may not be performed.

Modifications

When changes to a research study are needed, IRB approval must first be obtained before the modification is implemented.[12] Changes may be made to a study without prior IRB approval only when the modification is necessary to eliminate an immediate hazard to the participants. Examples of changes that must be approved by the IRB are changes in the number of participants needed to enroll; changes to the study design, methods, or procedures; changes to study sites or locations; changes in consent procedures and/or consent document; changes in recruitment materials; and changes in compensation amounts. Each IRB establishes a mechanism for requesting approval of modifications. Like new studies, the IRB may use expedited or full-committee review procedures. Minor changes to already approved studies are generally eligible for expedited review.

Tracking Adverse Events and Reporting UPIRSOs

Adverse events can be expected in research. A good data safety monitoring plan allows investigators to track adverse events that occur during a research study and to continuously monitor them to determine whether changes should be made to the research plan to minimize risks to participants.[14] Although adverse events should be tracked, not all occurrences must be reported to the IRB immediately.

Only adverse events that meet the criteria of an UPIRSO (Unanticipated Problem Involving Risks to Subjects or Others) must be reported immediately to the IRB. A UPIRSO is any incident, experience, or outcome that meets *all* of the following criteria[14]:

1. Unexpected (in terms of nature, severity, or frequency), *and*
2. Related or possibly related to participation in the research, *and*
3. Suggests that the research places participants (or others) at a greater risk of harm (including physical, psychological, economic, or social harm) than was previously known or recognized.

Although some UPIRSOs are also adverse events, keep in mind that not all UPIRSOs are adverse events. UPIRSOs may result from other problems such as the unintentional loss of identifiable private information that represents increased likelihood of harm, rather than actual harm. The IRB will review the UPIRSO and determine whether the research should continue and whether modifications should be made to the research to offer additional protection to the participants or others.

Reporting Noncompliance

Instances of noncompliance should be reported by the PI to the IRB. Noncompliance is an action by the investigator or member of the research team that disregards or violates federal regulations, IRB requirements and determinations, or institutional policies and procedures.[12] When noncompliance is discovered, the IRB reviews the events surrounding the incident; the seriousness of the event and whether it has occurred before; and the event's effect on the participants' rights, welfare, and safety. The IRB often requires a written report from the investigator that includes a corrective action plan. The IRB may decide that additional actions are necessary to address the noncompliance; such actions may range from retraining the PI or study staff to suspension or termination of the research (depending upon the severity of the event). If the IRB determines the noncompliance is either serious or continuing, the event is reported to the OHRP (for research funded by HHS) and/or the FDA (for certain FDA-regulated research).[3]

Inactivation

The investigator should notify the IRB when the study has concluded or when the IRB approval is no longer necessary. An IRB approval may be inactivated if *all* of the following are true:

- Enrollment is permanently closed to new participants.
- Data, private information, and/or specimens are no longer being collected for research purposes (including long-term follow-up).
- Participants are no longer being treated under the research protocol and there are no plans for future research treatment.
- Research assessments or procedures are no longer being performed and there are no plans for future research procedures.
- Data or specimen analysis has been completed, or if analysis continues, the materials undergoing analysis will be deidentified.
- Federal research funding for the study is closed (if applicable).
- The study is closed at all participating sites that are under the investigator's supervision.

The investigator notifies the IRB of the intent to inactivate the IRB approval by providing a final status report to the IRB. The IRB reviews the status of the study and determines whether inactivating the approval is appropriate.

Additional Responsibilities

In addition to the responsibilities of the investigator to the IRB as outlined in the previous sections, the following additional responsibilities are expected of PIs[15,16]:

- Complete and maintain training on human-subjects protection. Each institution has its own training requirements. (Several courses are available on the Internet. As a public service, the NIH Office of Extramural Research offers a free tutorial on "Protecting Human Research Participants" that institutions may elect to use to meet the human-subjects protections education requirement.)
- Follow the IRB-approved protocol and the regulations and policies related to research and privacy.
- Supervise everyone working on the project to ensure they follow the protocol and rules that govern research.
- Place the protection of research participants first.
- Verify IRB approval before allowing research to begin or before implementing changes.
- Keep participants informed and ensure they are willing to continue participating. Informed consent occurs at the beginning of research participation and should continue throughout a participant's involvement in the research.
- Regularly collect and assess information about safety or unexpected problems. This includes conducting regular literature reviews for new information that may affect the study or the study participants.
- Ensure those working on the project are qualified and are authorized to perform delegated tasks. This includes education, training, experience, and certifications.
- Provide ongoing communication with study staff. This communication allows the PI to assess problems as they arise and to make swift changes as necessary.
- Confirm that the data collected are accurate.
- Maintain organized records.

By following these guidelines, the PI protects research participants and improves the quality of the research conducted.

SUMMARY

In conclusion, a number of complex federal regulations govern research involving human subjects. This chapter provided a brief introduction to the major concepts involved in complying with the regulations. Understanding these concepts is essential for health professionals who must understand the basic ethical principles that guide research and their responsibilities to comply with the rules and regulations applicable to the type of research they may conduct. Investigators and their IRBs must work together to ensure that research is conducted safely and in an ethical manner. When any regulated human-subjects research project is planned, the local IRB should be contacted for assistance.

REFERENCES

1. Tolleson-Rinehart S. A collision of noble goals: Protecting human subjects, improving health care, and a research agenda for political science. *PS*. 2008;41:507–511.
2. National Commission for the Protection of Human Subjects of Biomedical and Behavioral Research. The Belmont Report: Ethical principles and guidelines for the protection of human subjects of research. 1979. Available at: http://www.hhs.gov/ohrp/humansubjects/guidance/belmont.html. Accessed September 6, 2014.
3. US Department of Health and Human Services, National Institutes of Health, Office for Human Research Protections. The common rule, title 45 public welfare, Department of Health and Human Services, part 46 protection of human subjects. 1991, 2009. Available at: http://www.hhs.gov/ohrp/humansubjects/guidance/45cfr46.html. Accessed February 25, 2011.
4. National Bioethics Advisory Commission. *Ethical and Policy Issues in Research Involving Human Participants*. Bethesda, MD. 2001. Available at: http://bioethics.georgetown.edu/pcbe/reports/past_commissions/nbac_human_part.pdf. Accessed March 4, 2011.
5. US Department of Health and Human Services, Food and Drug Administration. CFR—Code of Federal Regulations title 21, part 50. 1981. Available at: http://www.accessdata.fda.gov/scripts/cdrh/cfdocs/cfCFR/CFRSearch.cfm?CFRPart50. Accessed February 25, 2011.

6. US Department of Health and Human Services, Food and Drug Administration. CFR—Code of Federal Regulations title 21, part 56. 1981. Available at: http://www.accessdata.fda.gov/scripts/cdrh/cfdocs/cfCFR/CFRSearch.cfm?CFRPart56. Accessed March 2, 2011.
7. US Department of Health and Human Services. Title 45 (Public Welfare), Code of Federal Regulations, part 164 (security and privacy). 2003. Available at: http://www.ecfr.gov/cgi-bin/text-idx?tpl = /ecfrbrowse/Title45/45cfr164_main_02.tpl. Accessed September 6, 2014.
8. Cooper JA. Responsible conduct of radiology research. IV. The boundary of research and practice. *Radiology.* 2005;237:383–384.
9. Food and Drug Administration. Protection of human subjects: Standards for institutional review boards for clinical investigations 21 CFR parts 16 and 56 [Docket No. 77N-0350] 46 FR 8958. 1981. Available at: http://www.fda.gov/ScienceResearch/SpecialTopics/RunningClinicalTrials/ucm118296.htm. Accessed February 26, 2011.
10. Bankurt EA, Amdur RJ. *Institutional Review Board: Management and Function.* 2nd ed. Sudbury, MA: Jones and Bartlett; 2006.
11. Shaughnessy M, Beidler SM, Gibbs K, Michael K. Confidentiality challenges and good clinical practices in human subjects research: Striking a balance. *Top Stroke Rehabil.* 2007;14(2):1–4.
12. US Department of Health and Human Services, Office for Human Research Protections. Investigator responsibilities, FAQs: What are investigators' responsibilities during the conduct of an approved research study? January 20, 2011. Available at: http://answers.hhs.gov/ohrp/questions/7216. Accessed February 26, 2011.
13. Emanuel EJ, Wendler D, Grady C. What makes clinical research ethical? *JAMA.* 2000; 283:2701–2711.
14. US Department of Health and Human Services, Office for Human Research Protections. Guidance on reviewing and reporting unanticipated problems involving risks to subjects or others and adverse events. 2007. Available at: http://www.hhs.gov/ohrp/policy/advevntguid.html. Accessed February 26, 2011.
15. US Department of Health and Human Services, Office for Human Research Protections. Investigator responsibilities—FAQs. January 20, 2011. Available at: http://answers.hhs.gov/ohrp/categories/1567. Accessed February 26, 2011.
16. Merritt MW, Labrique AB, Katz J, Rashid M, West KP Jr, Pettit J. A field training guide for human subjects research ethics. *PLoS Med.* 2010;7(10):1–4.

CHAPTER 3

The Research Problem

Salah Ayachi, PhD, PA-C
J. Dennis Blessing, PhD, PA

CHAPTER OVERVIEW

This chapter discusses the development and refinement of the research problem. Developing a research question, hypothesis, or null hypothesis is not automatic and sometimes is not easy. Identification of the research problem and defining it in terms that can be investigated, studied, and researched is a critical step in the research and scientific process. Sound methodology can be developed only when the research problem is well defined in a format that can be investigated. Defining the research problem and developing a research question, hypothesis, or null hypothesis requires effort and time. Students in healthcare professions must be able to define research projects by formulating a research question, hypothesis, or null hypothesis. The way the research problem is defined depends on how the problem is framed and, ultimately, how it is investigated. This can present a challenge.

Learning Objectives

- Describe where research problems originate.
- Define what constitutes a research problem.
- Develop a research problem list.
- Identify a research problem.
- Define and describe the need to study a research problem.
- Develop a research question, hypothesis, or null hypothesis for a research problem.

INTRODUCTION

Research provides a systematic process for uncovering answers to clinical and other questions. Research also expands on current knowledge that can be applied to education, to clinical practice, and for the benefit of society. Although some problems may be evident, others are not as easily recognized or defined. When a problem or question is identified that requires study, that problem must be defined in a format that allows for successful study. To the novice this may be the most difficult step.[1]

So, how does a healthcare professional go about identifying the problem for research? The process involves more than just asking or writing down a question; it involves a mental exercise that requires moving stepwise from general to more specific concepts, thereby focusing on and defining the question as specifically as possible.[2] This skill or mental exercise needs to be learned, developed, and honed, just like any other.

Why go through the mental exercise and invest time before beginning a research project? Because determining the right researchable question or statement will define the problem effectively and accurately (i.e., clarify it), thus setting the tone for the entire exploratory process and subsequent work. Generally, healthcare professionals investigate problems that interest them or impact their work and clinical care. Therefore, any question in practice, specialty, or interest is worth researching.

Identifying the research problem is not always a simple task because every problem has compounding factors that can interfere with what needs to be studied. This challenge is particularly true for those who are new to research. For many investigators, getting to the exact problem that needs to be studied is like looking through foggy glasses or a smudged windshield. Without a clear focus (that is, a well-defined research question) the process is confusing, frustrating, time consuming, and wasteful. In fact, failure to develop a clear, concise, and defined research problem can lead to unsuccessful research. Think of the research problem as the guiding light that points the investigator in the right direction. Until the fog has dissipated, or the windshield has been cleaned, the view remains unclear.

THE PROCESS

How are topics selected? Generally, the topics of interest come from the environment, work, or interest in a particular subject or problem.[1] Sometimes the literature creates a topic that needs further investigation; some research articles generate more questions than they answer. This provides healthcare professionals a chance to take a study a step further to answer some of those questions. For example, when a study indicates that one healthcare profession spends more time with patients than other healthcare professions, a natural follow-up question would be: What component of care allows or causes that particular group of healthcare professionals to spend more time with patients? Anyone interested in the subject recognizes that a research problem has been identified for further investigation.

Study replication (doing the same investigation to confirm or refute findings) can be an exciting adventure and may lead to confirmation of findings or perhaps new findings. Published work may lead an investigator to research a similar problem in a group or area not covered by the first study. Questions about study methodology or an author's conclusions can lead to new studies and research replication. Replication is a good way to determine whether findings are applicable in a different clinical setting or practice. Replication can confirm or repudiate study findings or redefine previous study results or conclusions.

In general, existing knowledge or prior experience in a specific field is necessary to discern what research needs to be done. Researchers must be sufficiently knowledgeable about what has been accomplished, where current knowledge stands, and where to go from there. A preliminary literature review and search is conducted to examine current information and to help further define the problem or research question. Otherwise, the problem will remain unclear as long as there is uncertainty about the nature of the issue or problem. Knowledge of previous research is key to developing a project that will truly explore a problem. New understanding or knowledge must be built on what has gone before. Researchers who do not consider what has been done before may repeat what has been done and add nothing to the fund of knowledge. Research done without awareness of previous studies and existing data is a waste of time and effort. The research problem needs to be defined by a literature search that explores what is known and aids in defining what is not known.

WHAT CONSTITUTES A RESEARCH PROBLEM?

A research problem may be viewed as a situation that begs resolution or needs improvement, modification, or an answer. In other words, it is a situation that warrants examination and study, whether for the purpose of doing things more effectively and efficiently or to validate observations made in the classroom, clinic, or another setting. Alternatively the research problem could be something in which a healthcare professional is curious or interested.

An example of a research problem that is often studied in the healthcare professions is the identification of factors that determine patient satisfaction with care provided by a healthcare professional. This satisfaction might deal with a particular profession or satisfaction within a specific practice or setting. A similar and related problem of interest is the contrast among patient satisfaction with care provided by different types of providers. Another example of a research problem is identifying the factors that affect patient adherence to treatment regimens. These influences could be religious beliefs, cultural beliefs and ethnic standards, socioeconomic factors, or the like. These problems are interesting to others, both within and outside the healthcare environment. For the researcher, the results are the results. Results are accepted, even if they do not reflect what the investigator believes or thinks.

Table 3–1 summarizes the various origins of research topics.

GETTING STARTED

One way to get started on a research endeavor is to take a few moments to list some problems or questions for which solutions or answers are needed. **Box 3-1** offers one way to prioritize the questions. Keep in mind that substantive research is not accomplished overnight. Research can be a lengthy process and has the potential to become tedious and frustrating. Investigators sometimes have to work to maintain enthusiasm for their research, but without continued enthusiasm, goals are not likely to be met.

Table 3–1 The Origin of Research Topics

- Work environment (clinical observations, problems, or challenges)
- Personal interest (medical condition of self, family member, or acquaintance)
- Prior studies (journal articles or reports in medical and lay literature)
- Mentor, preceptor, or teacher interest
- Literature review
- Studies by others
- Graduation requirements

HOW TO IDENTIFY A RESEARCH PROBLEM

Identifying the research problem is the first step in conducting research. It begins by asking: What is the question to be answered? It is a good idea to write down questions to begin the recordkeeping for a study. Every researcher must be able to manage problems, because having a large number of problems in a single study can hinder its success. Remember, "keep it simple." It is best to identify a problem in its basic form and to do a thorough investigation of that problem rather than tackle a large number of problems. This aspect is analogous to a predator that becomes successful only after it has learned to identify and focus on the appropriate

---

Box 3-1 Prioritizing Research Questions

Exercise: List five research problems of interest (see Table 3–1). Rank the degree of interest in each (most interesting = 5; least interesting = 1).

Problem	Rating
1. _____	_____
2. _____	_____
3. _____	_____
4. _____	_____
5. _____	_____

prey. A successful predator chases one prey, not the whole herd. Otherwise, the negative outcome of the chase is a foregone conclusion, and the predator is left hungry. The same is true for identifying research problems. One well-identified and well-defined problem is much better than a number of ill-defined or general problems. It is worth remembering that it is unlikely that an earth-shattering discovery will be made, but each investigation can add a small piece to the larger body of knowledge.

A healthcare professional determined to investigate a problem must be able to focus on what needs to be done to resolve the problem (or situation) at hand. To further define the problem, several useful questions can be posed along the following lines:

- Given a problem, what can be done or what approach should be taken to improve it?
- What is known (what does the literature say) about the problem?
- What is not known about the problem (the literature gap)?
- What information or data are needed to improve the situation?

Based on answers to these and other questions, the problem(s) should become better defined.

Consider the following as examples of a process for development of a problem and study:

Scenario 1. A respiratory therapist (RT) is keeping a log of patients who are on ventilators. She notes an unusual number of postoperative infections in patients needing postoperative ventilation. The RT discusses this observation with the chief of pulmonology. After perusing several patient charts, the two concur that the problem is real and decide "someone should look into it" to determine the reason for these infections and ultimately minimize the number of cases of postoperative infections. In this case, determining the reason for the infections is the purpose of the study, and minimizing the number of postoperative infections is the goal of the study. Other reasons for performing the study include reducing morbidity and mortality, reducing the costs of care, and other equally important goals, such as improved patient outcomes and, maybe, patient satisfaction.

The RT and the pulmonologist then devote time deciding what to do (brainstorming), and they formulate questions to narrow the focus, determine the importance of the study, and decide the degree to which an investigation can be done. They consider, among others, the following questions:

- What information needs to be gathered?
- Where can the information be accessed?
- Will the investigators rely only on medical records or will they include survey data from patients, nursing staff, or others?
- What, if any, consents need to be obtained from patients and the institutional review board (IRB)?
- Will the investigators recruit a consultant to help design the study or analyze the data? If so, whom?
- Should the results be published, and if so, in what medium (i.e., how should the information be disseminated)?
- What are the ethical issues, and how will they be addressed?
- Where can the investigators find financial support to perform the study?

Figure 3-1 is a schematic of the process of developing a hypothesis from an observation based on this scenario.

Some examples of possible research questions for this particular scenario include the following:

- Are there procedural differences between infected patients and noninfected patients?
- Are there demographic differences between infected and noninfected patients?
- Are there care differences between infected and noninfected patients?

Using the null-hypothesis format, these questions would be considered with regard to the following statements:

- There are no procedural differences between infected and noninfected patients.
- There are no demographic differences between infected and noninfected patients.
- There are no care differences between infected and noninfected patients.

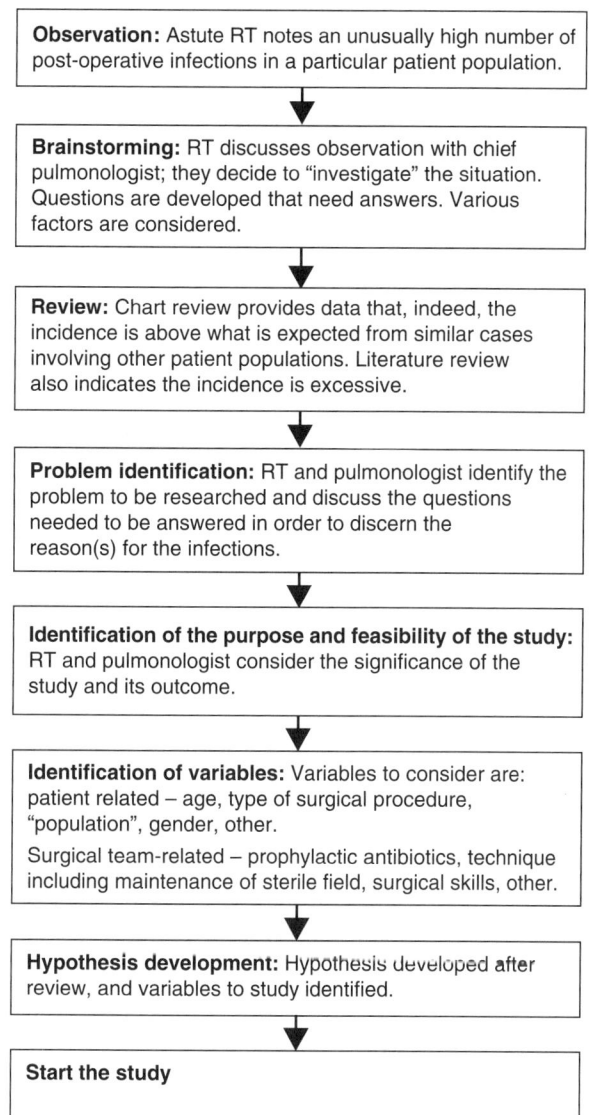

Figure 3–1 Schematic diagram of developing a hypothesis from an observation.

Using the hypothesis format, these questions would be considered with regard to the following statements:

- There are procedural differences between infected and noninfected patients.
- There are demographic differences between infected and noninfected patients.
- There are care differences between infected and noninfected patients.

Using a research question format, these questions would be considered with regard to the following statements:

- What are the procedural differences between infected and noninfected patients?
- What are the demographic differences between infected and noninfected patients?
- What are the care differences between infected and noninfected patients?

Which format should be used? Certainly, the research question is broad and can be used for almost any study. However, the null-hypothesis and hypothesis formats are stronger in their specificity and better define the relationship between two or more variables. Hypotheses are predictive statements. Null hypotheses can be thought of as a "no difference" contention. Often hypotheses deal with probability. Null hypotheses deal with differences or change caused by some action or intervention. The choice of format can influence the approach to the problem as well as the statistical analysis of data collected.

All variables need to be identified as a study design is developed. Statistical analyses will determine the answers to the research questions, indicate whether null hypotheses should be retained or rejected, or prove the hypotheses. (See **Box 3-2** for work practice.)

Scenario 2. A group of three students in a healthcare profession are required to identify a research problem and conduct a project as part of the curriculum. They choose to study the effectiveness of a new postoperative method for managing pain in surgical patients with herniated disks. They discuss the idea with their mentor, and they decide it is a worthwhile endeavor to determine whether the new method is "better" than the older methods. They discuss the following

---

Box 3-2   Revising a Topic from General to More Specific

Exercise: Consider the top choice problem (from Scenario 1). Work from general to specific in the manner outlined in the previous example.

Problem statement:
_____
_____
_____

Question:
_____
_____
_____

Aim/purpose:
_____
_____
_____

Objective(s):

1._____
_____

2._____
_____

3._____
_____

4._____
_____

5._____
_____

6._____
_____

7._____

aspects of the study (suggested answers are given in parentheses):

- What information to gather (patient satisfaction, pain scales, etc.)
- Where to access the information (surgical practice)
- Whether to rely solely on subjective data (reported pain score) or to include objective data (type to be determined)
- What, if any, consents to obtain (patient and physician consent, approval from the IRB)
- Whether to recruit a consultant to help design the study or analyze the data after they are collected (perhaps a faculty member who is savvy in statistical methods)
- Whether the results should be published and in what medium (i.e., how the information should be disseminated)
- What the ethical issues are and how to address them (patient consent, confidentiality, etc.)
- Where to find financial support for the study (or could this be accomplished without incurring financial expenses?)

Research questions related to Scenario 2 include the following:

- How safe is the new method?
- What is the cost of the new method?
- What are the morbidity and mortality rates of the new method (compared to older methods)?
- What is the degree of patient satisfaction with the new method?
- How many work days (days for patient return to normal activities) are saved using the new method (compared to established methods)?

As an exercise, the null hypothesis is used to develop the appropriate hypotheses:

- There are no differences in patient satisfaction between new and older methods.
- There are no differences in morbidity and mortality between patients undergoing the new vs. older methods of pain management.
- There are no differences in outcomes between the two methods.

NARROWING THE FOCUS OF THE QUESTION

To achieve the focus necessary, investigators must be systematic in the approach to honing and defining problems and questions. Generally, the research concept begins broad and becomes more specific.[2] Here is an example of one approach; an outline version is provided in **Table 3-2**.

Problem statement: There is no information on how many people, trained and educated as healthcare professionals, never practice clinically following successful completion of a program.

Question (problem converted into a question that can be answered): How many healthcare professionals do not practice clinically following successful completion of an educational program?

Aim (or purpose) of the research project: To determine how many students in healthcare professions do not practice clinically following successful completion of their particular program.

Objective(s) (more specific than the aim): What the researcher is going to do to answer the question:

- Collect information on the number of graduates in healthcare professions who do not practice clinically
- Determine how many are males and how many are females
- Determine the age distribution of these graduates
- Determine how many practiced initially then stopped and how many never practiced

Table 3-2 Going from Broad to Specific

- Problem statement
- Question (problem converted into a question that can be answered)
- Aim/purpose
- Objective(s) (what the researcher(s) will do to answer the question)

- Identify the reasons provided for not practicing clinically
- Determine whether the type of healthcare professional has any impact on the decision not to practice
- Determine the impact on the decision of personal, marital, financial, or other reasons

Here is a second (reverse) approach using a different problem. A group of public health nurses are interested in the subject of hyaline membrane disease, but they are not quite sure what to study and/or research. Moving from general to more specific, they take this approach:

1. Incidence of hyaline membrane disease (too broad)
2. Incidence of hyaline membrane disease in African American neonates (better)
3. Incidence of hyaline membrane disease in female African American neonates (even better)
4. Incidence of hyaline membrane disease in female African American neonates born to teen mothers (even more specific)
5. Incidence of hyaline membrane disease in female African American neonates born to teen mothers between 2000 and 2010 (getting even more specific)
6. Incidence of hyaline membrane disease in female African American neonates born to teen mothers between 2000 and 2010 in Bexar County, Texas (very specific)

The nurses have identified a research problem aimed at determining the incidence of hyaline membrane disease in a specific population. Is such a project feasible? Theoretically, yes it is; however, other issues have to be addressed and other factors must be considered, including costs and available resources, before the study can be performed successfully. As a cautionary point, if a study is too narrow in it subjects or demographics there may be difficulty extrapolating findings to the general population. The final topic (number 6 in the previous list) is an example of a focus that may be too narrow.

SOURCES OF IDEAS FOR RESEARCH PROBLEMS

Some topics that are certainly in the realm of possibility for any healthcare professional or student to research or, at least, explore for a research project include the following:

- The role of the healthcare professional in health promotion
- Learning styles of students in the healthcare professions
- Patient attitudes toward healthcare professionals
- Cost-effectiveness of healthcare professionals
- Best healthcare profession to provide a service
- Attitudes of healthcare professionals toward specific patient populations (e.g., people with HIV/AIDS, minorities, gays and lesbians)
- Impact of healthcare professionals on health care in medically underserved areas
- Any type of clinical investigation
- Does the degree level of the healthcare professional improve the quality of patient care? (Do higher degreed professionals provide better care?)
- Does research training in a program have an effect on practice?
- The healthcare professional's niche in research
- Differences in professional healthcare practice by site (e.g., hospital, clinic, nursing home, etc.)
- Economic impact of a professional healthcare practice on a community
- Professional healthcare malpractice and liability
- What is the effect(s) of the Patient Protection and Affordable Care Act in a number of areas, such as access, delivery, demand, and the like?

Healthcare professionals, especially those new to research, may glean research ideas from various sources, including clinical practice (as in the scenario described earlier), literature review, interaction with other students in didactic and clinical settings, interactions with colleagues at meetings, interaction with supervisors, or published work where authors point out aspects that need to be explored further. Ideas can also be obtained from government, private, and public organizations (e.g., requests for proposals [RFPs]) that seek information and data on or about a particular subject or point of interest. These types of requests are distributed by government agencies or private foundations, and often are formulated by experts and specialty groups.[3]

Need for the Study

As alluded to previously, the need for studying a particular problem is determined by many factors such as the following:

- Significance in medical, legal, and socioeconomic terms[3]
- Whether the issue has already been addressed (i.e., its novelty)
- Acuity or seriousness
- Human, time, and financial costs
- Contribution to knowledge

A survey of nurse researchers indicated that focus on "real-world concerns" and soundness of methodology are the criteria of greatest significance in research projects, and that focus on timely or current concerns was less important.[3] On the other hand, personal interest in a particular problem may be the most important driving force.

Must a Study Be Original?

Although some researchers view replication studies as less scholarly and less valuable than original studies (an attitude that is more pervasive in some disciplines than in others), the fact remains that there are many instances where replication may be indicated, valuable, and needed. Some of the reasons studies are replicated include extending the generalizations of the findings, establishing credibility, reducing errors (types I and II), and providing support for developing theories.[4] For novice researchers who might find identifying research topics and problems confusing and overwhelming, replication studies may actually be a good place to begin their first efforts.

Stating the Research Question

A good research question is one that can be answered using observable data or phenomena (something that can be observed and measured), includes the relationship between two or more variables, and is logical.[5] According to Sutherland et al.,[4] the three most frequently identified indices of the merit of a research question are potential impact, justification, and feasibility. These terms should be considered as research questions are developed. The questions should be posed in a straightforward way, regardless of structure or format. Only one variable per research question should be addressed, if possible. Questions should be developed to fully explore the problem being investigated. One question answered well with sound methodology is better than many questions not answered well.

There are three ways to frame the research subject/question/project:

Null hypothesis: A statement of no relationship or difference between two variables. Example: There is no difference in outcomes between patients with acute otitis media treated with "watchful waiting" and those treated with antibiotics.

Hypothesis: A statement of prediction/observation that can be evaluated, measured, or analyzed. Example: Patients with acute otitis media treated with antibiotics have better outcomes than patients treated with "watchful waiting."

Research question: A question that needs to be answered through systematic testing/evaluation/analysis. Example: Is there a difference in outcomes between patients with acute otitis media treated with antibiotics versus watchful waiting?

> **Exhibit 3-1 Pearls**
>
> 1. Carry a pocket notebook or piece of paper and write down research ideas when they occur.
> 2. Define the research problem in the simplest format.
> 3. Learn what is known or has been done about the problem or related issues.
> 4. Be able to define goals, objectives, and purposes.
> 5. Be able to describe the significance of research and why it can be the solution or part of the solution to the problem.
> 6. Be able to answer the question of why a project is important to society, health care, and your profession.

SUMMARY

The first step in any research effort is to identify the problem(s). Each problem is then put into a research question, hypothesis, or null-hypothesis format. These statements should be concise and should deal with only one variable or subject. Each statement must be in a form that allows investigation. In developing questions, a manageable number of questions or variables should be adopted. Small steps are best; some helpful tips are listed in **Exhibit 3-1**.

REFERENCES

1. Bailey DM. *Research for the Health Professional—A Practical Guide.* 2nd ed. Philadelphia, PA: FA Davis; 1997:1–4.
2. Jenkins S, Price CJ, Straker L. *The Researching Therapist: A Practical Guide to Planning, Performing and Communicating Research.* London: Churchill Livingstone; 1998:21–26.
3. Lindeman CA, Schantz D. The research question. *J Nursing Admin.* 1982;12(1):6–10.
4. Sutherland HJ, Meslin EM, Cunha DA, Till, JE. Judging clinical research questions: What criteria are used? *Soc Sci Med.* 1993;37(12):1427–1430.
5. Moody L, Vera H, Blanks C, Visscher M. Developing questions of substance for nursing science. *West J Nurs Res.* 1989;11(4):393–404.
6. Beck CT. Replication studies for nursing research. *Image J Nurs Sch.* 1994;26(3):191–194.

CHAPTER 4

Review of the Literature

Linda Levy, MSW, MLS, AHIP
J. Dennis Blessing, PhD, PA
Richard Dehn, MPA, PA-C

CHAPTER OVERVIEW

No research project begins in a vacuum. There is always something that has gone before. For any project to advance knowledge, what has occurred must be known and understood. A thorough and expansive literature review and search is the key foundation to every research effort. This chapter provides an overview and guide to the literature review.

Learning Objectives

- Define and discuss why the review of the literature is important.
- List the elements of a successful literature review.
- Create a list of searchable databases.
- Develop keywords for a literature search.
- Write a literature review.
- Write a clinical review from a literature review.

INTRODUCTION

One of the most important steps in performing research is the review of the literature that has already been published on the study topic. The review should be as comprehensive as possible and should cover relevant journal articles, books or book chapters, dissertations, meeting presentations, government documents, resources, and pertinent personal communications like emails. The format of the review is determined by the objective of the research, so the literature review and a summary of the research or an annotated bibliography may be the final product. More commonly, however, the literature review will be used to formulate a summary of what is known in the research area, the strengths and weaknesses of existing research, and a discussion of the purpose of the new research interest in terms of what is yet unknown.

This chapter is designed as a guide through the systematic process of the literature review, including designing a research strategy, selecting the appropriate sources to search, performing effective and efficient searches, and critically analyzing search results.

A successful literature review should:

- Provide an overview of the available literature on the study topic
- Help to determine what is known and what is not known about the study topic based on the relevance of the search results
- Identify areas of controversy
- Identify weaknesses in the existing research
- Help to formulate questions requiring further research

A review may also provide research tools such as instruments that have already been validated, studies that can be replicated, and data that can be useful for research design or correlation.

A review of the literature is typically a large and well-referenced section of a thesis, dissertation, or manuscript. The literature review should provide a solid basis for evaluating and understanding the depth and breadth of the research investigation and its significance. A good review also provides information with which the reader can contrast the results and conclusions of the current research with what was known about the problem(s) being investigated.

WHERE DO I START?

It is important to carefully determine a study topic or research question *before* beginning the literature review. What information is needed? It may help to consider the research question in the form of a sentence instead of just words. Taking the time to develop a well-written, carefully defined, and focused research question helps the researcher choose the best resources for the literature search and the most appropriate keywords to use during the search process. A focused research question also avoids wasting time as the search is performed, because the results will be more precise.

For example, a research interest may involve the role of the physician assistant on the healthcare team. What does the researcher want to know specifically? Is there a particular interest in a specialty practice area such as pediatrics or orthopedics? Does the question relate to the acceptance of physician assistants by patients in general or patients of a specific age or ethnic population? Is there an economic advantage to integrating physician assistants into the healthcare team for in-office or in-hospital practice? What is the job satisfaction of physician assistants who are part of healthcare teams? The more specific the topic of inquiry, the better the resulting review will be.

SELECTING RESOURCES

Once a research question has been defined, the resources needed for the literature review can be considered. Resources such as printed books can help to define terms, establish the state of the science or practice at the time the book was written, and possibly identify authorities in specific fields. Because the publication of printed books requires time, however, the information published in books may not be current.

Although the literature review should include any resources that are relevant to the background of the research topic, the review normally focuses on resources that offer the most current *primary* information about original research, meaning that they directly discuss the original research done by the author(s). That information is usually published in scholarly, peer-reviewed professional journals, where research articles are reviewed and the research is critiqued by experts in the field before the articles are accepted for publication. (This process is sometimes called *refereeing*.) Citations relevant to the research topic from peer-reviewed journals are found by searching an online bibliographic database of discipline-specific information rather than by using a general Internet search engine like Google. Information published in magazines and newspapers does not go through the same rigorous review process. Instead, they are usually considered *secondary* sources that discuss the original research. (Information found in electronic databases generally is relatively recent, depending on the database. Prior to the development of these databases, biomedical information was categorized by subject and organized in print indexes. If the research interest involves human subjects, especially the use of drugs or other interventions, it is wise to investigate the older literature, as well. Librarians can help the researcher utilize the print indexes.)

Most bibliographic databases are subject specific, meaning that the information within a database is focused on a specific area of knowledge. Research information and study results presented at professional conferences are also considered primary information. Although many bibliographic databases do not include conference proceedings, some research information may also be available through a database that includes meeting abstracts or specifically covers conference content. Conference content is sometimes included on the conference sponsor's Internet site, as well. Theses and dissertations provide another resource for research information, and some bibliographic databases do include records for theses and dissertations. For example, Proquest's Dissertations & Theses database, which is available at many academic libraries, consists wholly of records for dissertations and theses, and the full text is often available.

Some databases are free to all, but access to the information in most professional-level databases depends upon a licensed subscription that is purchased by the library at an academic institution, a large public library, an organization, or a hospital or healthcare facility. When a database is licensed, access is usually restricted to people who are affiliated with the purchasing organization. In some cases, the academic institution or organization allows unaffiliated people to use the database at their site.

Another helpful way to locate comprehensive information is by taking advantage of citation information included in many databases. This step can lead to experts in the research area of interest and reveal the bibliographies of articles (and other sources) that they consulted. Sometimes it is possible to determine who has cited these experts in subsequent publications. This method provides a means to track research progress. If the information is not included in the database, the bibliography of cited references will be available as part of the research article.

There are *many* different databases and other types of information resources. Talking to a librarian or to a professional in your field before starting a literature search can help determine which resources will be most appropriate for the research.

Once the best resources have been located, it is always wise to spend some time learning to use them effectively and efficiently, especially when online academic or professional databases are involved. Read (or listen to) the available tutorials, Q&A sections, FAQs, and use the Help options. Students and those associated with an academic institution or a hospital with a librarian on staff can take advantage of any database classes that are taught through the library. Hospital or academic librarians are excellent resources for additional help. Time spent deciding which resources are pertinent for the needs of the project and learning to use those resources well ultimately saves time and leads to a better literature review. Even the databases that are designed with "user-friendly" interfaces can usually be searched more thoroughly and yield better results when the advanced features like a "controlled vocabulary" or special search limits are utilized.

If the research question relates to a biomedical or social science topic, some online databases to consider for a literature search are described in the sections that follow. A single resource is usually not adequate for a comprehensive literature search.

MEDLINE

MEDLINE is a very large electronic database with records of journal articles dating back to 1948. MEDLINE provides links to biomedical information in professional journals in the subject areas of medicine, dentistry, nursing, allied health, veterinary medicine, and the biomedical sciences.

MEDLINE, which is produced by the National Library of Medicine, is free to all as part of the content of a user-friendly interface called PubMed (http://pubmed.gov). Many academic institutions also buy access to MEDLINE through proprietary interfaces like OvidSP or EBSCO.

How Do I Search?

The MEDLINE database has a very useful feature called a *controlled vocabulary*, which is a carefully selected thesaurus or list of words and phrases that are used to describe subject concepts. Controlled vocabulary terms (often called *keywords*) are added as part of the article record before the record is added to the database. Assigning controlled vocabulary keywords is a way of uniformly indexing articles by subject. Taking advantage of a controlled vocabulary means that synonyms or other issues of natural language are avoided. The system often can automatically determine the necessary keyword based on the term or terms that have been entered. The controlled vocabulary of MEDLINE is called *MeSH* (Medical Subject Headings). Using our previous example of the role of physician assistants and patient care teams, the MeSH heading would be "physician assistants" and "patient care teams." MeSH terms can be combined with AND or OR to achieve precise results.

Whatever interface is selected to search MEDLINE, it will probably use MeSH to retrieve the most relevant citations for your research interest, even if that is not obvious. The tutorials or search guides associated with the interface are useful for learning more about using MeSH effectively.

For expert authors in the field, authors' names can be searched to retrieve articles published in the professional journals included in MEDLINE. For specific articles, the citation-matching feature can be used to retrieve them. Non-MeSH terms for concepts that are not included as part of the MeSH vocabulary can also be used in searches when necessary. Limits are available, so searches may be limited to a specific range of years, by English or other language, by age groups, or by publication types.

How Do I Find the Articles?

Searching MEDLINE through PubMed yields some citations that have links to the full articles available for free or via "open access" in a separate database called PubMed Central (PMC). Free and open-access articles are selected from a range of journals and are deposited there by publishers for free access. PMC also has the author-prepared manuscripts of articles published by National Institutes of Health (NIH)–funded researchers in other journals not available through PMC. PMC can be searched directly at http://pubmedcentral.gov.

An open access publisher called Biomed Central (http://www.biomedcentral.com) provides access to over 250 peer-reviewed open access journals in science, technology, and medicine. Articles in these journals are linked through their citations in PubMed.

Other than the journal articles available through PubMed Central and Biomed Central, access to articles published in most professional journals is not free. An academic library that subscribes to the journal can provide access to them, or articles may be ordered through interlibrary loan at a hospital library or public library.

CINAHL

CINAHL (Cumulative Index to Nursing and Allied Health Literature) is a database that covers content in the subject areas of nursing and allied health. CINAHL is available only through an interface with the database vendor EBSCO. Many academic libraries, hospitals, and even some public libraries purchase access to CINAHL. Whereas MEDLINE includes records of only journal articles, CINAHL includes other formats such as dissertations, tests and evaluation instruments, and patient education materials.

How Do I Search?

Like MEDLINE, the CINAHL database includes a controlled vocabulary of subject headings.

Depending on where CINAHL is used, the interface may be set to default to searching the CINAHL vocabulary. If that is not the case, the controlled vocabulary can be used to combine heading terms. The "Help" link in the CINAHL database is a useful tool, and librarians are invaluable resources, as well. CINAHL can also be used to search by author or to access articles from a specific journal or articles of a specific publication type. The subject content of CINAHL overlaps in some areas with the subject content of MEDLINE, so some of the same journal articles are present in both databases. It is important to search both databases, however, to achieve comprehensive results.

How Do I Find the Articles?

The basic CINAHL database includes very limited full-text information. At an academic or hospital library, the site may have purchased an expanded version of CINAHL that includes links to many full-text articles. Other full-text information may be accessible because the library provides links to articles in other subscription journals. If a particular article cannot be accessed, it may be possible to order it directly from the publisher or through interlibrary loan.

PsycINFO

PsycINFO, produced by the American Psychological Association (APA), is a database that covers content in the areas of behavioral science and mental health. PsycINFO is available through database vendors such as EBSCO, OvidSP, or ProQuest at institutions that subscribe to the database. Individual subscriptions are also available through the APA.

How Do I Search?

PsycINFO also uses a controlled vocabulary of keywords to help locate citations relevant to a search. The database can be searched by author, research area, or publication type.

How Do I Find the Articles?

Sites that support PsycINFO, such as an academic or hospital library, may have purchased an expanded version of the database that includes links to many full-text articles. Other full-text information may be accessible because the library provides links to articles in other subscribed journals. If a particular article cannot be accessed, it may be possible to order it directly from the publisher or through interlibrary loan.

GOOGLE SCHOLAR

Although we cautioned against using Google or another general Internet search engine to find information for research, Google Scholar (a subset of Google available at http://scholar.google.com) can be very helpful in finding scholarly literature across many disciplines and sources including journal articles, abstracts, and theses. Retrieval is "ranked" based on where the full-text article was published, who wrote it, and how often and how recently it has been cited in other scholarly literature.

Google Scholar also includes records of dissertations since 2007. Searches retrieve basic metadata for each graduate work (e.g., title, author, abstract, keywords, etc.) and provide links to ProQuest for purchase or access.

How Do I Search?

Google Scholar has both a friendly "Google-like" option and an advanced feature, which increases the accuracy and effectiveness of the search. Although controlled vocabulary is not used in Google Scholar, the advanced feature supports the specification of words or phrases that must (or must not) appear in the article. Searches can be limited by author, source, date, and PDF format, and by broad subject area such as medicine, pharmacology, and veterinary science.

How Do I Find the Articles?

Some articles may be available for free, depending on the source. Otherwise, a library that subscribes to the journal can provide access to specific articles, which may also be purchased from the publisher or ordered through interlibrary loan.

WEB OF SCIENCE

Web of Science contains information gathered from thousands of scholarly journals in all areas of research. Web of Science is available only through access to the ISI Web of Knowledge set of database resources. Many, if not most, academic libraries subscribe to the Web of Knowledge.

How Do I Search?

Web of Science can be searched by subject topic using a word or phrase or by author; however, the strength of this resource is in searching for cited references. The citations include references cited by authors of the original articles. Once a relevant article is located through searches of MEDLINE or another database, a cited reference search can find subsequent articles that cite this article.

How Do I Find the Articles?

Web of Science includes only citations to articles. Access to the full text of an article depends on the subscriptions purchased by the library or institution where the database is used. Articles from journals that are not available can sometimes be purchased from the publisher, or they can be ordered through interlibrary loan.

Other databases should be considered depending on the subject of the search question. **Table 4–1** summarizes the information about the databases described here and also includes additional databases that could be useful for you.

DATABASE SEARCH HINTS

Databases can be searched in a variety of ways. For subject searching, a controlled vocabulary (if there is one) limits the search to information relevant to the research without worrying about issues of natural language, alternate terms, synonyms, and so on. Searches for words or phrases can also be achieved if the controlled vocabulary does not provide a satisfactory result or if there is no controlled vocabulary for the database being searched. Searching by author, journal title, publication type, research type, questionnaire, and many other indexed fields of the record can also be productive, but the available fields vary among databases.

The best approach to searching for subject terms is to search for each term separately and then to combine them. Subjects can be combined with an author's name; an author's name can be combined with a journal title; a word or phrase search can be combined with a questionnaire name, and so on. In most databases, at least two options for combining sets are available: OR or AND. When using OR, the retrieval from two (or more) sets is pooled. Thus, the number of retrieved items is larger than any of the individual sets. When using AND, the combined set containing each individual item must be present. Thus, the number of retrieved items is smaller than any of the individual sets. Any number of search terms can be combined, but when using AND, the more items that are combined, the smaller the number of items retrieved.

The OR and AND operators are often illustrated using Venn diagrams as shown in **Figure 4–1**.

RESULTS OF THE SEARCH

Some preliminary criteria should be considered as the search is performed. Questions to address might include the following:

- Who is the author and what is the author's area of expertise?
- What is the type of publication in which you found the information: a scholarly journal, a website, an academic textbook?
- What is the date of publication? How current is the information?
- Is the content of the material relevant to your research topic?
- Are other authors citing this material? If so, how frequently?

Table 4–1 Summary of Databases

Database	Coverage	Free Access	Subscription Vendors	Citation Information (for tracking research)	Free Full-Text Articles
MEDLINE (www.pubmed.gov)	Medicine, nursing, allied health sciences, dentistry, biomedical sciences	Internet: PubMed interface; other Internet sites	OvidSP, EBSCO		Some through PubMed links to PubMed Central
CINAHL	Nursing, allied health sciences	No	EBSCO	Yes	Depends on subscription
PsycINFO	Psychology, psychiatry, social sciences	No	OvidSP, EBSCO, DIALOG, ProQuest		Depends on subscription
Google Scholar (scholar.google.com)	Scholarly literature	Google		Yes	Some
Web of Science	Science, medicine, social science	No	ISI of Knowledge	Yes	none
ERIC (www.eric.ed.gov)	Education	Internet: Education Resources Information Center (ERIC)	EBSCO		Some
SCOPUS	Science, medicine, social science	No	SciVerse	Yes	Depends on subscription
Digital Dissertation & Theses	Dissertations from U.S. universities	No	ProQuest, DIALOG		Available with subscription

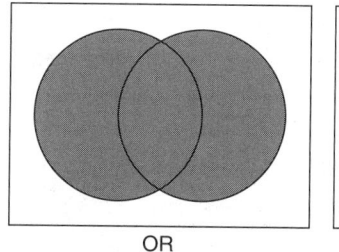 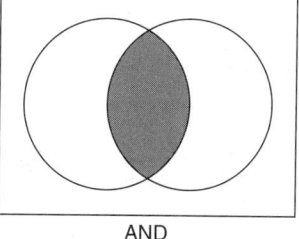

Figure 4–1 OR and AND operators.

- When an article discusses original research, how extensive was the research and how large was the research population?

Articles published in professional journals can include original (primary) research such as cohort studies, clinical trial results, and results of large randomized studies. Journals may also include secondary information such as narrative review articles on a single subject or comprehensive systematic reviews and meta-analyses, which represent literature reviews focused on a single question that try to identify, appraise, select, and carefully synthesize all high-quality research evidence relevant to that question. Sorting articles that have been retrieved by recognizing and evaluating differences in the process of conducting research helps to determine the current state of research regarding the study question and to identify gaps in knowledge. Articles can be graphically represented by a pyramid (**Figure 4–2**) where the top of the pyramid represents articles that discuss the types of research that are most time-consuming, objective, and clinically relevant.

CITATION TOOLS

Before citations are gathered, it is helpful to consider the use of reference management tools. These tools allow the researcher to gather citations from database searches and to add additional references manually. Not only can citations be gathered in an easily accessible way and be used to keep track of the information that has been found, but with some tools, citations may be organized into folders, and the citations that have been saved may then be searched. When the research

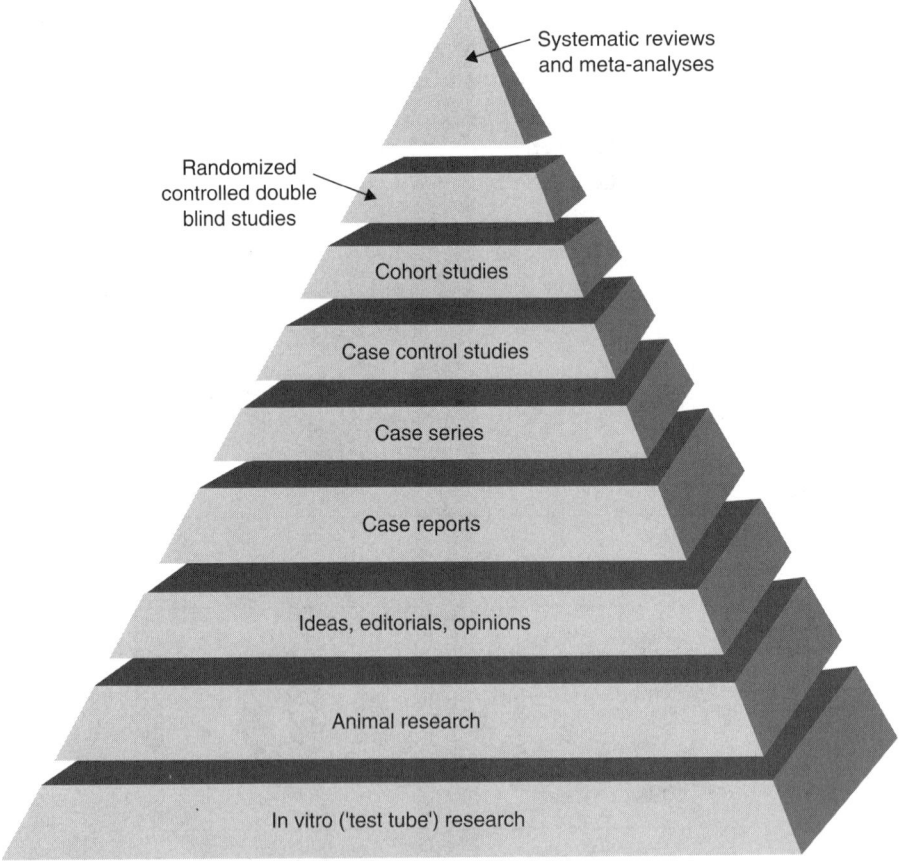

Figure 4–2 The evidence pyramid.

has been completed and the writing stage begins, the tool formats in-text citations and the bibliography in the preferred output style, such as APA or Vancouver. If the review is being written for publication, the more sophisticated management tools also "know" the formatting styles required by most professional journals; they accurately format the paper automatically. If the literature review itself and a summary of the research are to be the final products, citation tools can also produce a bibliography to be annotated. When the review is to be formatted in the APA style, which is often used in the sciences and social sciences, excellent help is available through the American Psychological Association (http://www.apastyle.org) and through the Online Writing Lab (OWL) at Purdue University (https://owl.english.purdue.edu/owl/resource/560/01/).

Students or researchers at an academic institution may use the resources purchased by their institution, such as management tools like RefWorks or Noodlebib that require a subscription. Software programs can also be installed on a personal computer. Available programs include Reference Manager (http://www.refman.com) and EndNote (http://www.endnote.com), both of which are powerful tools from Thomson Reuters. Because the software is personally proprietary, its use is not dependent on any institutional affiliation.

Some free Internet-based resources are also available. These include Easy Bib, BibMe, RefBase, and Zotero. Some are completely free; others are free for basic use. When deciding which tool most closely fits the research need, considerations include ease of downloading citations or manual addition of citations into the resources as well as the process of adding in-text citations and formatting a bibliography in the required style. Free resources usually provide a basic set of reference styles, so for research that is potentially going to be published, it may be worth investing in one of the software programs. Worthwhile reviews and comments by other users are available for many of these programs.

Some word-processing programs include a citation feature. Although these allow the addition of citations at the writing stage, citations cannot be stored for another use, nor are the features as powerful as those available through resources designed for this specific purpose.

WRITING THE LITERATURE REVIEW

Once all of the information is gathered, a literature review can be written as a summary of what is known (and not known) in the research topic area. This review is a discussion of previous research, not a list of references, so it is important to plan and organize the review carefully, whether it is organized chronologically or by research method or research trends. Literature reviews begin with a brief introduction summarizing the research question, the resources used for the literature review, and the search strategies. Then the results of the review are summarized. Be sure to discuss key points, reference quoted information, and include gaps in the existing research as well as areas of weakness or controversy. The reader should be made aware of the pertinent points of your research question and the research history on which they are built. Before the conclusion, readers should understand why answering this research question is important.

Additional hints for writing a good literature review are available on the Internet from writing centers at many academic institutions. Research in professional journals also provides valuable examples of literature reviews in terms of their content and how they are written.

CLINICAL REVIEWS

The literature review is a major part of a research project. If the research project is on a clinical problem, the literature review can be used to develop a clinical review. Clinical reviews are one of the most common types of articles in professional journals that target clinical practice. A clinical review is a summary of the presentation, evaluation, diagnosis, and treatment of a clinical problem. The intent of the clinical review is to refresh knowledge about or inform the reader of updates for a clinical entity or problem. Basically, the clinical review is an update for practitioners about something they will encounter in practice.

Clinical reviews are relatively short, 1500 to 3000 words. The length will vary among journals and publication sources. The review provides information from recent updates, within the past 1–3 years and probably not older than 5 years, on a clinical problem. Clinical reviews can be divided into three subcategories:

1. General review of a clinical topic
2. Systematic review of a specific topic
3. Case or case series report (based on a case encountered in practice)

Although there is some variety in the manuscript format for clinical reviews depending on where the review is to be published, the following sections are fairly common.

Introduction and Background

This section typically includes a definition of the disease, the historical background of the disease, and the disease prevalence. Here, the author tries to justify the importance of the topic to the practicing clinician as well as to pique interest. Thus, the beginning of a clinical review should be written in a way that convinces the reader to invest the time and effort to read the rest of the article.

Body of Manuscript

As stated previously, there are some differences in journal requirements for clinical reviews, but the following key points are likely to be universal.

Review of Anatomy, Physiology, and Pathophysiology

This section should review the basic anatomy, physiology, and pathophysiology as they apply to understanding the disease presented.

History and Physical Exam Findings

The signs and symptoms associated with the topic are reviewed. Risk factors and historical data commonly associated with the disease should be included. Any required physical examination techniques must be described and explained. Unique physical findings that allow differentiation of this particular disease or condition and that rule out competing diagnoses should also be discussed.

Laboratory and Diagnostic Testing

The selection and interpretation of appropriate studies are presented and discussed. A full explanation of study indications, cost-effectiveness, test sensitivity and specificity, and value to the assessment should be included.

Assessment and Differential Diagnosis

This includes a discussion of the reasoning processes that lead to the correct diagnosis of the disease or condition. This section often includes a broad differential diagnostic list. The reasons for selecting the correct diagnosis over other possible diagnoses should be explained in this section.

Treatment and Follow-up

This section includes the prioritization of the medical interventions necessary for treatment and emphasizes the need for referral, consultation, hospital admission, necessary emergent/acute care, and the reasoning by which decisions are made. Well-accepted treatments are emphasized here, as are potential complications, appropriate aftercare, pharmacotherapy, and drug–drug interactions. Finally, this section provides a follow-up plan and monitoring regimen that includes signs of relapse and treatment failure.

Prevention and Patient Education

This section provides patient education and disease prevention guidelines. It explains the common screening tests for the condition, including the relative value of each test. In today's society, patient education is a must and should be a part of the treatment plan for every disease condition.

Discussion/Conclusion

Some journals will want a discussion section that summarizes the important points of the review, particularly if something new or dramatically different from accepted dogma is presented. The conclusion section is brief and closes the manuscript.

A Good Clinical Review

The review should be written in a concise, easy to understand fashion. It should be direct and summarize current theory and application for the process. Proper references are a must to ensure that readers can do their own research and background work if they wish. References become more important in reviews that introduce new evaluation techniques, changes in disease etiology or presentation, or changes in treatment. The clinical review is intended to be an update on a disease entity and must reflect recent research. If radical changes in the aforementioned areas have occurred or the author is advocating changes that go against conventional wisdom, then the clinical review may not be the delivery format of choice.

A good clinical review is an excellent scholarly effort for students and health professionals who want to contribute to the literature, but do not have the time, skill, or opportunity to complete full research projects. The skills gained in doing a clinical review can lead to more advanced writing and scholarly work skills.

SUMMARY

The review of the literature is a key component of any research project. It is incumbent on the investigator to do a concise and comprehensive review. The review must provide information on what is known and allows the investigator to further define what needs to be known. Understanding and using literature databases are skills that must be mastered. Investigators must understand the content of different databases and use those related to the research project. Without a literature review, there can be no project.

For many students and clinicians, a good literature review can become a clinical review of a disease process. Clinical reviews are a common journal article format in professional journals. Clinical reviews are used to update clinicians on new treatments or new disease presentations, or as reviews for practice. A clinical review may be a good starting point for students and clinicians as they develop their research expertise.

CHAPTER 5

The Systematic Review

Margaret J. Foster, MS, MPH

CHAPTER OVERVIEW

This chapter provides an overview of the steps to complete a systematic review. A *systematic review* is a research method where studies are collected, assessed, and synthesized using rigorous and transparent methods to minimize bias. If the review includes combining data from many studies into one calculated outcome, it is called a *meta-analysis*. These reviews are becoming more common than literature reviews as the need for evidence-based guidelines and syntheses has increased. Systematic reviews perform an important role in evidence-based practices by providing practitioners with a concise view of a specific health issue.

Learning Objectives

- Identify the five main types of systematic reviews.
- Write a research question in PICO format.
- List the main steps used in a systematic review.
- Conduct a bibliographic database search.
- Define and discuss the concept of *gray literature*.
- Contrast the purpose and interpretation of a forest plot and a funnel plot.

THE SYSTEMATIC REVIEW

What Is a Systematic Review?

As the volume of health sciences information, such as published articles and data, has grown rapidly over the past decade, so has the need for evidence-based summaries that review studies in a particular area. The typical literature review does not meet this need because many are lacking in rigorous methods, cannot be properly evaluated due to poor reporting standards, and/or have conclusions that are subjective and biased.[1] This deficit led to the development of the systematic review as a more reliable method to gather, analyze, and synthesize studies to answer a specific research question using rigorous and transparent methods. Systematic reviews are a "powerful tool to help clinicians use evidence for patient care decisions"[2(p29)] when conducted using appropriate standards.

Role in Research and Evidence-Based Practice

Single, primary studies include a narrowly defined group of patients, measure few outcomes, and can contradict other studies' results.[3] Evidence-based practice calls for health practitioners to answer questions by gathering and analyzing data, but time constraints limit the amount of evidence that most practitioners can synthesize. By utilizing systematic reviews, practitioners receive a more comprehensive look at a situation than one individual study can provide and a clearer perspective of previous research. Without this understanding, new studies could be conducted that are unnecessary, inappropriate, or even unethical.[4] Authors of reviews can also identify gaps in current research and organize evidence for decision making. Gaps in the literature are those instances when a question has never been explored, has not been addressed with a particular population or intervention, or has been studied but with questionable/outdated methods. Researchers can then address these holes in the evidence by conducting new primary studies.

Organizations Leading Systematic Review Development

Several international and national organizations offer guidance, funding, and/or a forum for producing or disseminating systematic reviews. The most notable is the Cochrane Collaboration, which was founded in 1992 as a nonprofit international organization with the mission to "promote evidence-informed health decision-making by producing high-quality, relevant, accessible systematic reviews and other synthesized research evidence."[5] These reviews are usually conducted by a group of expert volunteers and focus on clinical questions, although recently reviews centering on other types of questions such as population health and public policy have been published. The procedures for conducting a Cochrane review are detailed in the *Cochrane Handbook*, which is available for free online.[6] Other leading organizations include the Agency for Healthcare Research and Quality (AHRQ), Joanna Briggs Institute (JBI), and Centre for Reviews and Dissemination (CRD).

Types of Reviews

More than 20 types of systematic reviews have been described, varying on the type of evidence included, the scope of the search, the depth of assessment, and the type of synthesis presented.[1,4,7] The general systematic review and meta-analysis have already been defined. Four other types include:

- *Integrative review:* A review that combines qualitative and quantitative studies on a similar issue
- *Qualitative review:* A review that includes qualitative studies only
- *Review of reviews:* A synthesis of systematic reviews
- *Scoping review:* A broad review, gathering studies on a single topic and providing some categorizing, without assessing methods

This introduction describes steps that all reviews should conduct, although the comprehensiveness of methods will vary.

STEPS OF THE REVIEW

Step 1: Define and Plan the Review

Defining the review involves determining the research question, ensuring that the research question is unique by locating/assessing related reviews, detailing the purpose of the review, and planning the management of the review.

Step 1a: Frame the Question and Define Criteria

One of the primary characteristics of a systematic review (SR) that makes it different from a literature review is that the main objective is to answer a research question. Framing that question is key to ensuring that the question is specific. The narrowness of the question should be strategically gauged in order to produce a useful review that will be generalizable yet applicable to many patient groups. If it is too vague, it will be difficult to answer the question, collect relevant studies, or synthesize the data. In most health-related reviews, the PICO format, which stands for Population, Intervention, Comparison, and

Table 5-1 Defining the Question and Criteria

PICO Format of Question	Study Criteria
Do the published studies show that reducing screen time reduces/prevents obesity in children? • *Population:* Children • *Intervention:* Reduce screen time • *Comparison:* No intervention • *Outcome:* Reduced weight or body mass index (BMI)	Study will be included if: • Participants are children 2–19 years old • It is a randomized controlled trial to reduce screen time • It reports weight or BMI • It is in English and published after 1990 • Its methods are appropriate according to the selected checklist

Outcome, is selected. The inclusion criteria are created as a list of characteristics required by a primary study to be included in the review. **Table 5-1** shows an example of a research question, PICO framework, and study criteria. This research question will serve as an example throughout this chapter.

Step 1b: Find and Appraise Relevant Reviews

Locating and analyzing relevant reviews is necessary to determine to what extent other authors have explored a similar topic. Three types of databases can be searched for relevant reviews: subject-specific, review, and dissertation databases. *Subject-specific databases* like MEDLINE, Embase, or CINAHL collect research on a particular topic (in this case, clinical medicine), and many provide an option to limit retrieved articles to systematic reviews. *Review databases* collect only systematic reviews, meta-analyses, and/or review protocols (see **Table 5-2** for an

Table 5-2 Free Review Databases

Provider	Database Name	Internet Address
Allied Health Evidence	Combination of four databases: Physiotherapy Evidence Database (PEDro); OTseeker (occupational therapy); speechBITE (Best Interventions and Treatment Efficacy; speech pathology); PsycBITE (Psychological Database for Brain Impairment Treatment Efficacy)	http://www.alliedhealthevidence.com
Cochrane Collaboration	Cochrane Database of Systematic Reviews	http://summaries.cochrane.org (subscription version also available)
Health Evidence	Database of reviews of health promotion interventions	http://www.healthevidence.org
PubMed Health	Includes systematic reviews from PubMed, Cochrane, and other resources starting from the year 2000	https://www.ncbi.nlm.nih.gov/pubmedhealth/
Evidence for Policy and Practice Information and Co-ordinating Centre (EPPI-Centre)	Includes three databases of health-related reviews: Bibliomap; Database of Promoting Health Effectiveness Reviews (DoPHER); Trials Register of Promoting Health Interventions (TRoPHI)	http://eppi.ioe.ac.uk

abbreviated list). Protocols describe the proposal for a systematic review and can be published and/or registered, similar to the idea of registering a clinical trial. Lastly, *dissertation databases* collect theses and dissertations.

When searching for related reviews, begin by finding reviews that are very close to the same subject, and then continue broadening the search until at least a few reviews are found. When evaluating a related review, record the research question, criteria, resources searched, years covered by the search, synthesis type, main conclusion, quality assessment, and validity of the findings, in order to easily compare the reviews. Several checklists have been developed for appraising the quality of systematic reviews, including the Critical Appraisal Skills Programme (CASP) Systematic Review Checklist and A Measurement Tool to Assess Systematic Reviews (AMSTAR).[8,9] All of the checklists evaluate these elements: appropriateness of the question and criteria, comprehensiveness of the search, rigor of the critical assessment, and quality of the synthesis and analysis. After examining the related reviews, the research question or criteria may need to be altered so that the review will be unique or, if not distinctive, an update of a previous review.

Step 1c: Define the Purpose of the Review

It is important to establish the main objective of the systematic review as well as its scope, final products, and appropriate standards. The main objective of the systematic review depends on its type. For example, scoping reviews aim to characterize the size of existing literature, qualitative reviews generally seek to generate or explore theory, and most traditional reviews try to test a hypothesis. The scale or scope of the review can vary between taking a representative approach (searching in just a few resources) or a comprehensive approach (conducting a wide sweeping search).[10] By defining the scope at the beginning of the review process, authors can prevent "scope creep"—the slow, and sometimes unrealized, adjustments that often occur to the study's goals, scale, or timeline.[7] The author(s) should determine the products of the review, which could include a protocol, a journal article, and/or an executive summary. For each of these outputs, authors can select from the several available appropriate standards. Many authors in clinical medicine rely on the *Cochrane Handbook* for systematic review procedures and on the Preferred Reporting Items for Systematic Reviews and Meta-Analyses (PRISMA) guidelines for the report of a protocol and/or completed review.[6,11]

Step 1d: Project Management

Systematic review developers should consider three main areas in managing the project—developing a team, setting a timeline, and choosing software. A systematic review team should include experts in the topic of the review as well as in searching, systematic review methods, and statistics (if appropriate). If the review will be done by a single author, the author should find experts to consult throughout the process. The Institute of Medicine's standard requires that systematic review searches be developed by expert searchers.[12] In addition to experts, some systematic review authors choose to include stakeholders at some point in the process to provide different perspectives and to increase the possibility that the review's findings will have wider-reaching effects.[4] The time investment in a systematic review is significant and essentially depends on the size of the evidence base and depth of the search and assessment. The *Cochrane Handbook* shows a timeline to complete a review within a year.[6] Software selection will include choosing tools for various activities: project management, file storage, collecting citations, coding text/data, and statistical calculations. Specialized software applications have been designed for conducting all or part of a systematic review. (See **Table 5-3** for examples.) Several factors will affect selection: accessibility of the software, customizability, number of functions it can perform, the ability of the software to accommodate multiple users, and cost.

Table 5-3 Examples of Software for Various Processes in the Review

Name	Organization
EPPI-Reviewer	Evidence for Policy and Practice Information and Co-ordinating Centre (EPPI-Centre)
Systematic Review Data Repository (SRDR)	Agency for Healthcare Research and Quality (AHRQ)
RevMan	Cochrane Collaboration
System for the Unified Management, Assessment and Review of Information (SUMARI)	Joanna Briggs Institute
NVivo	QSR International

Step 2: Bibliographic Database Searches (Part 1 of Search)

Performing an efficient and thorough search is important for three reasons: to endeavor to locate all relevant articles, to minimize bias in the review, and to minimize the number of irrelevant articles retrieved. Systematic review searches follow a sequence of four phases: develop the search, evaluate the search, save and document the final search, and de-duplicate and translate for other databases. At the end of the search all of the retrieved articles will be screened, labeled, and assessed. Enlist the assistance of a librarian to ensure that the appropriate resources for the topic are searched with a thorough list of search terms and phrases.

Step 2a: Develop the Search

First, list the databases to be searched, making sure to include databases that cover a wide range of disciplines likely to be interested in the review topic. The *Cochrane Handbook* suggests at least three databases be searched: MEDLINE, Embase, and Cochrane CENTRAL.[6] By searching more than one database, researchers ensure that the search has covered a broad range of biomedical journals.

Second, select those concepts from the inclusion criteria that are appropriate for the search. For most clinical reviews, those concepts are the designated population, health issue, and intervention. **Table 5-4** illustrates an example. List synonyms for each concept, including clinical and natural language terms as well as alternative endings and spellings for all terms. Collect search terms from those provided in previous reviews, by consultation with experts, and from any articles already located that will be included.

Next, select the most important database for the review topic, which is usually MEDLINE. The *Cochrane Handbook* calls for searching for concepts using keywords and thesaurus terms, such as MeSH terms for MEDLINE. MeSH stands for Medical Subject Headings and are a set list of terms arranged into hierarchal trees of subjects, branching from one overall concept to more specific concepts. (See **Figure 5-1** for an example of the MeSH *body weight* and its branches.) Searchers can select all of the terms along one branch by selecting "explode." For example, if the term *overweight* was selected and exploded, that would capture all of those terms marked with overweight and all of the terms down the branch. By combining keywords and MeSH terms, the search will retrieve more relevant articles than by using only one of these fields. See **Figure 5-2** for an example of combining these fields for the term *obesity*.

Step 2b: Evaluating the Search

The systematic reviews search will typically have many drafts, each undergoing careful assessment, with necessary changes incorporated before settling on the most effective search. When evaluating the first draft of the search, survey the first 50–100

Table 5-4 Developing a Search in Medline

1. Define concepts to be searched	Concept 1: Children Concept 2: Screen time Concept 3: Obesity
2. List synonyms	Concept 1: Children or adolescents or teenagers or youth or toddlers or preschool Concept 2: Screen time or screen media or video game or television or TV or computer Concept 3: Obesity or obese or overweight
3. Add truncations and alternate spellings	Concept 1: Child* or adolescen* or teen* or youth* or toddler* or preschool* Concept 2: Screen time* or screen media* or video game* or videogame* or television or TV or computer* Concept 3: Obes* or overweight*
4. Find MeSH terms for each concept	Concept 1: *exp child* or *exp adolescent* Concept 2: *exp video games* or *exp television* or *exp computer* Concept 3: *exp overweight*
5. Combine keywords with MeSH terms with OR; then combine all terms for each concept with AND	<child* or adolescen* or teen* or youth* or toddler* or preschool* or *exp child* or *exp adolescent*> AND <screen time* or screen media* or video game* or videogame* or television or tv or computer OR *exp video games* or *exp television* or *exp computer*> AND <obes* or overweight* or *exp overweight*>

MeSH are in italics.

* returns any records with words starting with search string (e.g. adolesc* returns adolescent, adolescents, adolescence)

exp stands for explode, will retrieve all studies labeled with this MeSH term and any MeSH terms under it in the hierarchy

Adapted from Foster M. Introduction to systematic reviews for healthcare design. *Health Env Res Design J.* 2013;7(1):143–154.

results and collect any article that matches all criteria. Review these articles for other keywords and MeSH terms that should be added to the search. It is also important to plan for a peer review of the search by another expert search to meet the standards for the Institute of Medicine.[12] The author(s) may consult one or more checklists to aid in search evaluation, such as the Peer Reviews Electronic Search Strategies (PRESS), created by the Canadian Agency for Drugs and Technologies in Health.[13] The PRESS list looks at translation of criteria into search terms, correct use of Boolean and proximity operators, appropriate use of index terms, inclusion of all important keywords and spelling variants, spelling/syntax errors, limits, and correct translation of the search into other databases.

Step 2c: Save and Document the Search

Whenever possible, save the search within the platform it was searched (i.e., NCBI [PubMed], EBSCO, Proquest, OvidSP) so that it can be easily rerun at a later date and/or altered as necessary. Also, the exact search should be copied and stored in a separate location. Other information to record: database name, platform, date of the search, years covered, limits applied, number of articles retrieved, and new articles added.[6]

Step 2d: De-duplicate and Translate for Other Databases

Translating the original search into other databases can be tricky, especially when moving to different

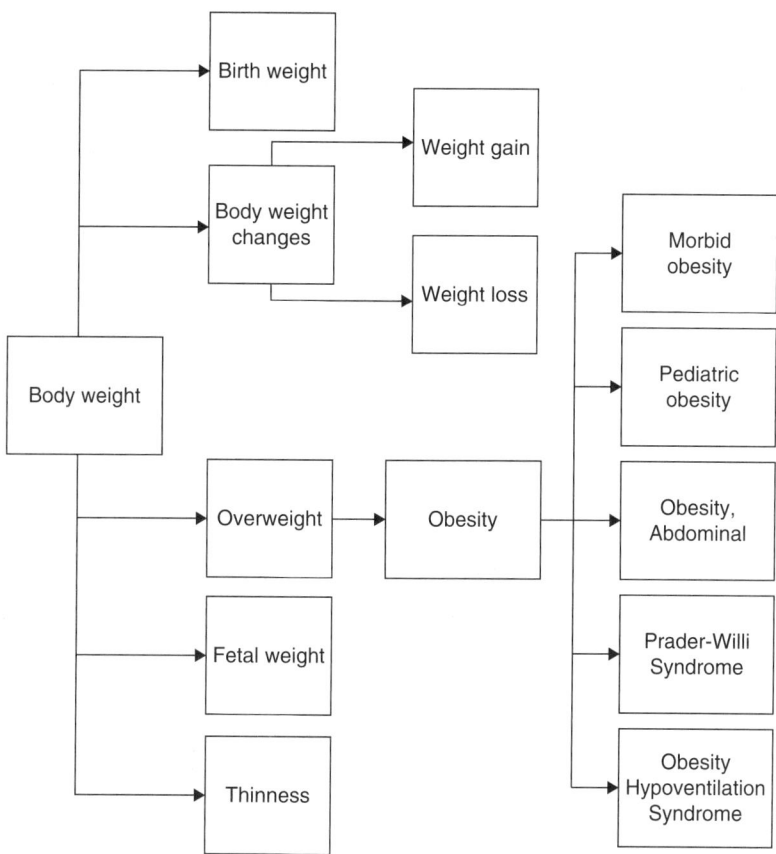

Figure 5–1 MeSH tree for *body weight*.

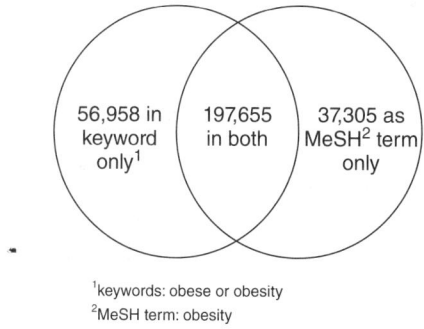

[1]keywords: obese or obesity
[2]MeSH term: obesity

Figure 5–2 Number of articles with obesity as a concept in various fields.

platforms. In addition, some resources have very limited options for searching, such as only offering browsing and lacking export options.

Step 3: Appraisal

The appraisal process involves narrowing down the retrieved articles to those studies that will be critically analyzed, coded, and ultimately synthesized. Screening is conducted in multiple steps, evaluating the articles increasingly in-depth as they pass through each step, by title, abstract, full text, and then appraisal of methods. Each part of the process should be tested and evaluated with a small group of articles.

Step 3a: Screening

In developing the screening process, decide on screening questions and labels, who will screen, how articles will be divided among the screeners, and software applications to be used. The

Table 5–5 Screening Questions

Question	Label
1. Is this article in English? 2. Is it published after 1989? 3. Is it about reducing screen time in children? 4. Does it include outcome measure—weight, BMI?	• *Included:* Yes to all questions. • *Maybe:* Unsure. • *No 1:* If no to question 1, stop screening. • *No 2:* If no to question 2, stop screening. • And so on.

screening questions are yes/no questions used to decide if a study described in an article will be included in the review. An example is shown in **Table 5–5** along with suggested labels. Except perhaps during title screening, the number of screeners should be at least two per article, and each excluded article should be labeled with a reason for exclusion.[6] There are various options for software to use during screening—some reviewers choose to do the screening within a citation software (e.g., Endnote, RefWorks) whereas others choose a spreadsheet.

Step 3b: Evaluating Screening

Authors should determine the procedure and should document the method of settling disagreements between screeners. Compare labels between authors, focusing especially on those where one screener labelled articles as "include" and the other labelled them as "exclude." The objective level of agreement between screening decisions can be calculated using Cohen's kappa, a measure of interrater reliability.[14]

Step 3c: Appraise Methods of Articles

Appraisal of the included articles focuses on the studies' methods; it is recommended that two people assess each article. Appraisal checklists are freely available for a variety of study types including randomized controlled trials, cohort, case control, survey, qualitative study, and others. Although the checklists will vary, all evaluate suitability of the study design to the research question, correctness of the sampling, appropriateness of the exposure/outcome measures, and validity, reliability, and significance of the results.[15]

Step 3d: Evaluation of Appraisal

Compare the appraisal answers for each article and resolve any disagreements. Document the procedure for the resolutions.

Step 4: Expanded Search Techniques (Part 2 of Search)

After screening the articles from the bibliographic database searches, a variety of expanded search strategies could be employed to further ensure that all relevant articles have been located. The main reason for expanding the search beyond bibliographic databases is to minimize publication bias, which is the known systematic tendency of commercial publishers to publish empirical research based on the nature and direction of the results.[16] Not all reviews will employ all of these strategies, but nearly all will include the citations search, and many will include some type of gray literature. All articles retrieved using any of these strategies will then go through the appraisal process.

Step 4a: Reference/Citation Searching

Create a list of all included articles, previous reviews, and highly related articles, and then browse the references of these articles and any articles that have cited them. There are three main resources for conducting these searches: Scopus, Web of Science, and Google Scholar. Each of these resources documents the resources citing each other, and each one indexes a different list of resources. Of the three, Scopus indexes the most journal titles, Web of Knowledge indexes the widest range of years, and Google Scholar includes a large amount of gray literature. Comparing the coverage of journal titles, Scopus indexes 19,809 titles (8,432 unique) whereas Web of Knowledge indexes 12,311 titles (934 unique). The journal titles indexed by Google Scholar are not provided by Google.[17] While browsing the cited and citing articles, retrieve all titles that may be relevant.

Step 4b: Gray Literature Search

Gray literature refers to any publications not published or indexed by commercial publishing companies. This includes preprints, government reports, white papers, conference papers/presentations, patents, technical reports, dissertations, theses, trial registries, grants, websites, open access journals, and blogs. Each of these resources is indexed in varying degrees by databases that often present few search options and are inefficient and/or retrieve thousands of irrelevant results. **Table 5–6** is an abbreviated list of gray literature databases.

Step 4c: Handsearching

The *Cochrane Handbook* suggests *handsearching* journals or conference proceedings that are included in major databases. Also, some sections in journals, such as supplements and conference abstracts, may not be well indexed. An expert searcher should determine which specific titles should be handsearched, because titles are very specific to the topic of the review. The Cochrane Collaboration offers guidance through a free online training manual.[18]

Step 4d: Request Studies

Posting a request in places likely to be seen by researchers in a review's topic area is a useful strategy. Requests could be posted in listservs, blogs, and professional organization websites' discussion areas, or sent directly to a selected list of authors. This activity can generate a list of studies that were unpublished, are nearing publication, or are otherwise hidden.

Step 5: Code and Synthesize

Synthesizing the studies requires first coding data/characteristics from each study and then combining the information in appropriate ways. There are dozens of methods for synthesis, and a review may use several. The most often utilized approaches are described here.

Step 5a: Coding

Coding, or data abstraction, involves creating a worksheet or form to complete for each study. The form is a tool to collect all important data needed to answer the research question and to conduct the appropriate synthesis type. Review authors may consult several good examples to get ideas for developing the codebook. The *Community Guide* and the *Cochrane Handbook* provide a list of data elements that should be included.[6,19] Data elements include study population characteristics, study design, details of the intervention(s), and measurements/outcomes. The codebook could be created in a variety of tools including review software, a database creator, or a spreadsheet.

Step 5b: Qualitative Synthesis

Qualitative synthesis is conducted by nearly all systematic reviews, even those that plan to conduct a meta-analysis. The most common approach is a

Table 5–6 Gray Literature Databases

Conference papers and abstracts	Biomed Central, PapersFirst (OCLC), COS Conference Papers Index, ProceedingsFirst, Conference Proceedings in ISI
Overall gray literature	Grey Literature Report; OpenGrey; WorldCat
Government documents	GOP access; LexisNexis, National Technical Information Service (NTIS)
Guidelines	National Guidelines Clearinghouse, NICE guidelines, TRIP
Trial registries	Clinical Trials, CenterWatch, TRoPHI

narrative synthesis, which combines results from different types of research by describing its scope and its strength, presented by text and tables. There are several potential uses for this approach: to develop, advance, or validate a theory; to examine relationships in the data; to describe and explain complex or contentious issues; and to highlight emerging topics. Other types of qualitative synthesis include *framework synthesis*, which compares results of collected research with a preselected framework, and *thematic synthesis*, which combines results from qualitative research into themes.[4]

Step 5c: Quantitative Synthesis (Meta-analysis)

A meta-analysis is a collection of statistical procedures that synthesize the "findings of studies that investigate the same research question using the same methods of measurement."[7(p153)] This technique results in calculating an average effect for the selected outcome across the studies, which need to have similar study designs and participants. The selected outcome or *effect size* may need to be standardized for a proper comparison. The process of standardization will depend on the type of variable, with the most common being standardized mean difference, odds ratio, risk ratio, and correlation coefficient. Also, a weight is given to each study based on sample size and precision.[20] Next, the level of similarity is subjectively assessed and calculated by a *test for heterogeneity*. If the studies are found to be homogeneous, a *fixed effects analysis* is conducted. If the level of heterogeneity is not too high, a *random effects analysis* is completed, which is a more conservative estimate, making it less likely to conclude that the intervention is effective when it is not. If studies are too heterogeneous, a meta-analysis cannot be conducted. The results of these analyses are presented in a *forest plot* (see **Figure 5–3**), which presents the *point estimate* of the outcome for each study (usually represented by a square) along with its *confidence interval (CI)* as a horizontal length of line and indication of the relative number of participants in the study by the size of the square. A vertical line called the *line of no effect* is added for a quick visual comparison. The calculated average effect size is represented by a diamond.[4]

Step 5d: Integrative Synthesis

Integrating both quantitative and qualitative studies into one synthesis can provide conclusions that highlight the strengths of both types of studies. Quantitative studies demonstrate evidence of effectiveness or size of relationships between variables, whereas qualitative studies reveal perspectives on appropriateness or acceptance, why/how interventions work, and contextual issues. Two mixed methods synthesis processes have been formalized and described. A *realist synthesis* works well with

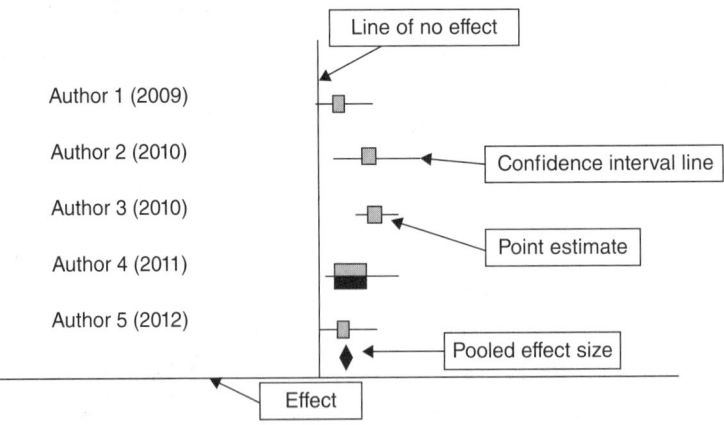

Figure 5–3 Example of a forest plot.

complex interventions by identifying when and how interventions work.[21] *Bayesian meta-analysis* is "a method of synthesis where a summary of qualitative data is used to develop a probability distribution (prior distribution), which can be tested later using a more conventional synthesis of quantitative data."[7(p157)] A *probability distribution* "shows how the total probability (which equals 1) is distributed among the different possible values of a variable."[22(p473)] In addition, this analysis recognizes the value of subjective judgment within evidence-based practice and considers the views of prospective users of the review.

Step 6: Analyze and Write

The final step is to analyze the overall meaning of the evidence synthesis by summarizing the strength of the evidence and its generalizability, determining its limitations, providing recommendations for action, and writing the review in appropriate formats for the selected audience.

Step 6a: Analyze the Strength of the Evidence

The strength of the evidence can be described by scrutinizing the results of the synthesis from various perspectives. First, assess the generalizability of the synthesis and the level of representativeness for various populations and settings. Next, evaluate the weight given to studies in the synthesis, whether done explicitly or not, to ensure that those studies given the most weight were the right studies to do so. Then, examine the influence of outliers on effect size or of unusual contexts or settings on synthesis. Finally, consider views of stakeholders and any competing explanations.[7]

Step 6b: Assess Limitations

In determining limitations, author(s) should consider the potential gaps in the literature sample and measure publication bias if needed, and should acknowledge risk of bias in the included studies. No matter how extensive the literature search, the sample could be missing relevant studies. Reporting bias, discussed in Step 4, is a collection of biases that has been well documented, showing "that it is more likely that significant positive findings will be published (publication bias), in a timely manner (time lag bias), in English (language bias), in multiple places (duplicate publication bias), cited more often (citation bias), and in journals that are widely indexed (location bias)."[23(p144)] Publication bias can be evaluated by a funnel plot.[16] The bias within the included study depends on the internal and external validity. In the analysis, detail the overall biases found in the literature, answering: How reliable are the studies? Do the outcomes in the studies vary due to quality? Are results influenced by one or two studies, without which the overall conclusions would change?[4]

Step 6c: List Recommendations for Action

Two types of recommendations are typically provided by systematic review authors: implications of the review's findings and recommendations for further research. Many journals request authors to include suggestions for practitioners; however, the *Cochrane Handbook* warns against listing these inferences, because the Cochrane Collaboration considers it to be outside of a systematic review's scope to provide these implications. The *Handbook* states that "the highest level of explicitness would involve a formal economic analysis with sensitivity analysis involving different assumptions about value and preferences."[6(p380)] If needed, recommended actions should be placed in the context of specific values, preferences, and settings explicitly found in the evidence. A list of potential future research should also be thoughtfully written. Some questions to consider are: Is a conceptual map or theoretical framework available for this topic? Is there a lack of representation of any population groups? Are all appropriate outcomes reported?[7]

Step 6d: Write the Report

In writing the formal review protocol or final report, use the PRISMA checklist to provide report elements and sequence, although some of the

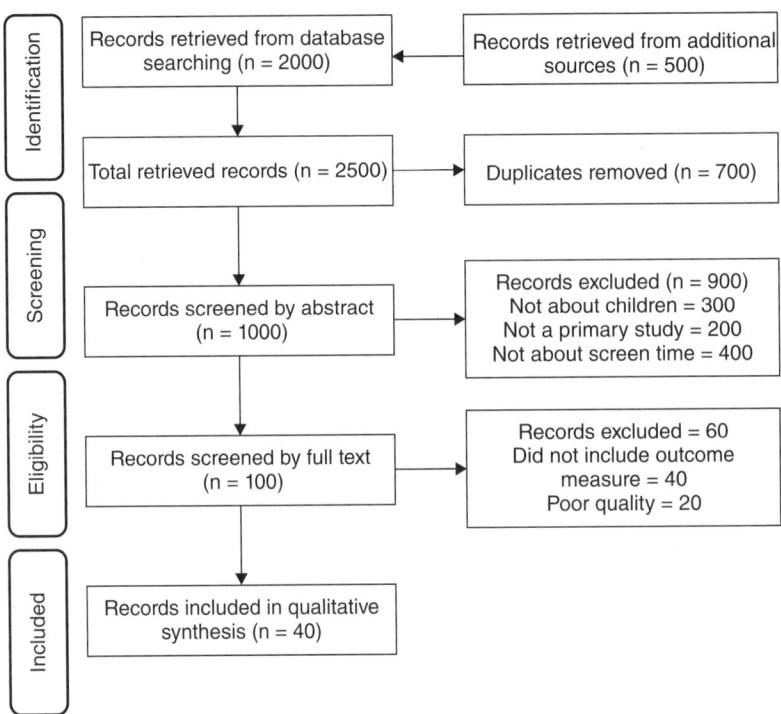

Figure 5–4 Example of a PRISMA flowchart.

Modified from Liberati A, Altman DG, Tetzlaff J, et al. The PRISMA statement for reporting systematic reviews and meta-analyses of studies that evaluate healthcare interventions: Explanation and elaboration. *BMJ*. 2009;339:b2700.

elements are not appropriate for all systematic reviews.[24] PRISMA also advises review author(s) to depict the flow of articles through the review process in a flowchart (see **Figure 5–4**). Most journals place limits on the number of words, tables, and figures that can be included, so author(s) must carefully select information to be reported, while not being overly selective in a manner that hides important outcomes and influences conclusions. In disseminating the review it may be necessary to write in other formats for various audiences including patients, policymakers, media, research funders, practitioners, or the public in general.

SUMMARY

Systematic reviews will continue to be the method of choice when a synthesis of the literature is required. By summarizing and appraising primary studies, authors provide practitioners, policymakers, patients, and researchers with evidence-based answers. Authors should follow standards to minimize bias and deliver an effective synthesis. Findings should be distributed to appropriate stakeholders.

REFERENCES

1. Grant MJ, Booth A. A typology of reviews: An analysis of 14 review types and associated methodologies. *Health Inform Libr J*. 2009;26(2):91–108.
2. Feldstein DA. Clinician's guide to systematic reviews and meta-analyses. *WMJ*. 2005;104(3):25–29.
3. Montori VM, Saha S, Clarke M. A call for systematic reviews. *J Gen Intern Med*. 2004;19(12):1240–1241.
4. Gough D, Oliver S, Thomas J. *An Introduction to Systematic Reviews*. London: Sage; 2012.
5. The Cochrane Collaboration. Home page. Available at: http://www.cochrane.org. Accessed February 26, 2014.
6. Higgins J, Green S, Cochrane Collaboration. Cochrane handbook for systematic reviews of interventions.

Available at: http://handbook.cochrane.org. Accessed September 16, 2014.
7. Booth A, Papaioannou D, Sutton A. *Systematic Approaches to a Successful Literature Review*. Thousand Oaks, CA: Sage; 2012.
8. Better Value Healthcare. Critical appraisal skills programme systematic review checklist. Available at: http://media.wix.com/ugd/dded87_ebad01cd-736c4b868abe4b10e7c2ef23.pdf. Accessed September 16, 2014.
9. Shea BJ, Grimshaw JM, Wells GA, et al. Development of AMSTAR: A measurement tool to assess the methodological quality of systematic reviews. *BMC Med Res Methodol*. 2007;7:10.
10. Booth A. "Brimful of STARLITE": Toward standards for reporting literature searches. *J Med Libr Assoc*. 2006;94(4):421–429.
11. Knobloch K, Yoon U, Vogt PM. Preferred reporting items for systematic reviews and meta-analyses (PRISMA) statement and publication bias. *J Cranio-Maxillofacial Surg*. 2011;39(2):91–92.
12. Eden J, Institute of Medicine, Committee on Standards for Systematic Reviews of Comparative Effectiveness Research. *Finding What Works in Health Care Standards for Systematic Reviews*. Washington, DC: National Academies Press; 2011.
13. Sampson M, McGowan J, Lefebvre C, Moher D, Grimshaw J. PRESS: Peer review of electronic search strategies. Available at: http://www.cadth.ca/index.php/en/publication/781. Accessed August 25, 2014.
14. Edwards P, Clarke M, DiGuiseppi C, Pratap S, Roberts I, Wentz R. Identification of randomized controlled trials in systematic reviews: Accuracy and reliability of screening records. *Stat Med*. 2002;21(11):1635–1640.
15. Heller RF, Verma A, Gemmell I, Harrison R, Hart J, Edwards R. Critical appraisal for public health: A new checklist. *Public Health*. 2008;122(1):92–98.
16. Dickersin K. Publication bias: Recognizing the problem, understanding its origins and scope, and preventing harm. In: Rothstein H, Sutton AJ, Borenstein M, eds. *Publication Bias in Meta-analysis: Prevention, Assessment and Adjustments*. Hoboken, NJ: Wiley; 2005:11–33. Available at: http://www.loc.gov/catdir/toc/ecip0516/2005021394.html.
17. Chadegani AA, Salehi H, Yunus MM, et al. A comparison between two main academic literature collections: Web of Science and Scopus databases. *Asian Soc Sci*. 2013;9(5):18–26.
18. Cochrane Center. Training manual for handsearches. Updated 2002. Available at: http://us.cochrane.org/sites/us.cochrane.org/files/uploads/pdf/Handsearcher%20Training%20Manual.pdf. Accessed January 12, 2014.
19. Briss PA, Harris KW, Zaza S. *The Guide to Community Preventive Services: What Works to Promote Health?* New York: Oxford University; 2005.
20. Leandro G. *Meta-analysis in Medical Research: The Handbook for the Understanding and Practice of Meta-analysis*. Malden, MA.: BMJ Books; 2005.
21. Rycroft-Malone J, McCormack B, Hutchinson AM, et al. Realist synthesis: Illustrating the method for implementation research. *Implement Sci*. 2012;7(33):7–33.
22. Bruce N, Pope D, Stanistreet D. *Quantitative Methods for Health Research: A Practical Interactive Guide to Epidemiology and Statistics*. Hoboken, New Jersey: John Wiley & Sons, 2008:471–525. DOI: 10.1002/9780470725337.
23. Foster M. Introduction to systematic reviews for healthcare design. *Health Env Res Design J*. 2013;7(1):143–154.
24. Liberati A, Altman DG, Tetzlaff J, et al. The PRISMA statement for reporting systematic reviews and meta-analyses of studies that evaluate healthcare interventions: Explanation and elaboration. *BMJ*. 2009;339:b2700.

THE RESEARCH PROCESS: DESIGN

SECTION II

CHAPTER 6

Methodology

Christopher E. Bork, PhD
Robert W. Jarski, PhD, PA-C
J. Glenn Forister, MS, PA-C

CHAPTER OVERVIEW

This chapter covers research design and methodology that become the methods section of a research project. Choosing the right design adds validity, reliability, and strength to the results and conclusions. The best of projects can be derailed by errors in experimental design and weakened by a poor choice of research design. Challenges to validity and reliability that may emerge at the peer-review stage must be considered when developing the methods for an investigation.

Learning Objectives

- Define research methodology.
- List the elements of methodology.
- Draw the schematic for selected research designs.
- List, define, and discuss the type of analysis for each research design.
- List and discuss the types of studies.
- Define, identify, and discuss the terms bias, error, reliability, validity, threats to validity, and types of data.

INTRODUCTION

Once the topic and specific research questions, or hypotheses, have been identified and the literature review has been completed, the investigator must choose a methodology suitable for achieving the project's objective. This objective is stated as a hypothesis, a purpose statement, or a clear and specific research question. Additionally, the primary objective should be evaluated by this criterion: Is it important to medicine, the profession, or society? That is, will the study make a significant contribution to the field's body of knowledge? Some journals refer to this as the "so what?" question. In many cases, authors are required to respond in writing to this question when submitting a manuscript for publication. Answering this question helps the investigator condense the meaning and value of the

Table 6-1 Selected Research Designs

Name	Design	Statistical Test
One-shot case study	X O	None
One group pretest–posttest	O X O	Dependent or paired t-test
		Wilcoxson matched pairs, signed ranks
Static group comparison	X O	Independent t-test
	O	Chi-squared
		Mann-Whitney U
Posttest-only control group	R X O	Independent t-test or ANOVA
	R O	Mann-Whitney U
		Kruskal-Wallis ANOVA
Nonequivalent control group	O X O	ANCOVA or ANOVA
	O O	
Pretest–posttest control group	R O X O	ANCOVA or ANOVA
	R O O	
Solomon four group	R O X O	ANCOVA or ANOVA
	R O O	
	R X O	
	R O	
Counterbalanced	X_1 O X_2 O X_3 O	ANOVA
	X_2 O X_3 O X_1 O	
	X_3 O X_1 O X_2 O	
Time series	O O O O X O O O O	ANOVA, trend analysis

X = experimental treatment or intervention; O = observation, measurement, or evaluation; R = randomization of a large number of subjects; ANOVA = analysis of variance; ANCOVA = analysis of covariance.

study. This question should be a guiding principle for most research endeavors.

The research methods should be driven by the research objectives. When choosing a methodology, two mistakes may distract novice investigators. The first mistake often made is selecting a familiar methodology without first defining the research objectives. The second most common mistake is planning to use already available data. Although convenient, this backward approach may produce trivial information that is unlikely to contribute to the field. The methodology should generate data that achieve worthwhile objectives.

THE METHODS SECTION

The methods section describes how the research study was conducted. It should be sufficiently clear and detailed so that others can duplicate the study. The methods section includes descriptions of the following:

- Subjects
- Instrumentation used (including questionnaires, when applicable)
- Procedures performed
- Analytic procedures used for evaluating and summarizing the data

Data analysis must be suited to the particulars of the study: the number of subject groups (e.g., two: an intervention and a control group), the number of subjects within each group, and the procedures used for data collection (e.g., single or repeated measures). Many healthcare researchers value a quantitative analytic approach using statistical methods. Although this is often the case, some questions in health care must be answered using a qualitative approach.

A Methods Scheme

Each study plan poses its own challenges. A system such as the one presented in **Table 6-1** is a useful tool for identifying some study options. First, the researcher must decide whether the approach will be analytic or descriptive by answering the question: Is there a comparison between groups in this study?

UNDERSTANDING RESEARCH DESIGN

Controlling Bias

When designing research, the investigator must limit or control factors and biases that could potentially contaminate a study. As mentioned in previous chapters, all research starts with an idea or a problem. The research hypothesis is the investigator's expectation for the outcome or the solution to the problem. The objective of a research study is to prove or disprove the investigator's hunch.

When selecting a research design, the investigator must consider the expectation (i.e., the research hypothesis) and create a means of controlling biases that may result from this expectation. In other words, an informed, objective observer must be able to conclude that the researcher's bias (or prior expectations) did not influence the results of the study. The investigator must design the research to eliminate bias, thus allowing the results of the study to truly represent the effect of the independent variable.

Other reasons for understanding research design include recognizing and minimizing the effect of threats to validity, both internal and external. In this chapter, the concepts of error and reliability, forms of validity, and a method of identifying and diagramming typical research designs will be discussed.

Error

All research involves measurement, and all measurements involve error. The common formula for a given measurement is

$$\text{Observed measurement} = \text{True measurement} + \text{Error}$$

As the concept of "error" decreases, the observed measurement begins to approximate the true measurement. In everyday life, errors in measurement are common; for example, anyone who has ever tried to cut a shelf to put inside a closet may be painfully aware of the formula for an observed measurement. If the observed measurement includes too great of an error, then the shelf will be either too large or too small and will not fit in the closet. Therefore, the error term can be either positive (too large) or negative (too small).

Types of Error

Error can be categorized into two forms, random and systematic. Random error consists of those errors that occur strictly because of chance; these errors are often thought of as "noise in the system." Small sample sizes tend to be more vulnerable to random error. For example, if five measurements are taken versus one measurement, the average of the five measurements is less likely to be incorrect or have a large error term. The carpenter's proverb of "measure twice, cut once" affirms the role of random errors.

Systematic error can be thought of as a series of consistent biases affecting a measurement. Typical researcher errors may be related to poor technique, such as sloppiness, or to inappropriate protocols or research designs, inappropriate measures, or incorrect statistical applications. For example, if a researcher is using heart rate (beats per minute) as an indicator and calculates heart rate using 10-second readings in some cases and 15-second readings in others, then the error risk increases. The measuring technique introduces errors of inconsistency.

Similarly, if a researcher uses a survey to assess a clinical outcome, error may be introduced by several factors including differences in verbal fluency among subjects or even the conditions under which the survey is completed. For instance, consider the differences in response to a telephone survey about practitioner satisfaction by an individual who has just experienced a 2-hour traffic jam versus a responder who has just exercised and feels wonderful. Differences in their levels of stress may affect their responses.

By choosing appropriate measurements, using reliable techniques, and employing valid instruments to obtain measurements, a researcher can eliminate a substantial number of experimental errors in data collection. Reliability and validity are fundamental to obtaining appropriate and useful data.

Reliability

Reliability focuses on the consistency with which a measurement is taken. If a measurement lacks reliability, then the data obtained may be useless because of error. In other words, if substantial error exists in the measurements, then the researcher cannot know whether observed changes in the dependent variable are caused by manipulation of the independent variable or by poor measurement. Reliability is also of paramount importance to the professional in clinical practice. If a clinician does not gather reliable data, then there is no way of knowing whether apparent changes in the patient are the result of actual physiological changes or poor technique. In other words, the clinician will not know if progress is taking place as a result of treatment.

Forms of Reliability

There are three common forms of reliability: instrument reliability, intrarater reliability, and interrater reliability. Instrument reliability indicates the consistency of measurement by a particular instrument. For example, if a weighing scale has a worn spring, it may measure lighter weights accurately but heavier weights inaccurately. The method to improve instrument reliability is to consistently calibrate the instrument.

Intrarater reliability indicates the consistency with which an individual takes measurements. For example, does the healthcare provider measure blood pressure in the same way each and every time? If not, there is a strong possibility that the measurements will differ because of technique rather than differences in the patient. One method of improving intrarater reliability is to consistently follow an established protocol and to routinely check for consistency.

Interrater reliability indicates the consistency in measurements among individuals taking the measurements. If more than one individual is taking a measurement, there must be adequate assurances that any changes are caused by changes in the true measurement, rather than fluctuations in human error. The concept of interrater reliability is often ignored and has important ramifications for clinical research. Inattention to interrater reliability may obscure differences in the research outcome. If individuals collecting data do not perform the related tasks in the same way, the researchers will not be able to ascertain whether differences are caused by differences in the patient or differences in the way the measurement was performed (i.e., an error). In other words, if data are not gathered in a consistent or reliable manner, their accuracy is questionable and, therefore, the data may be useless.

The "two P rule" (protocol and practice) applies when two or more individuals are taking measurements. Measurements should be taken using a standard protocol that has been practiced. Data collectors should also compare their measurements periodically; they may even wish to determine their consistency by performing one of the tests that assess interrater reliability, such as the kappa-statistic test. When reviewing any article that involves measurements, the reader should look for an assessment or other assurance that the data were gathered reliably.

Validity

Another concept that must be considered regarding data and measurement in an investigation is validity. Validity indicates the usefulness or appropriateness of the data being gathered. In a practical sense, reliability and validity are related concepts. Reliability focuses on consistency of measurement, whereas validity focuses on the appropriateness of a given measurement. A simple illustration is a game of darts. Reliability can be viewed as the consistency of the pattern or spread of the darts. Validity can be thought of as ensuring that the darts are aimed at a dartboard. There are two principal types of validity: measurement or test validity, and design or experimental validity.

Measurement or Test Validity

Measurement or test validity answers the question: Does the test or measure actually do what it is intended to do? For this to occur, a given measurement should have a defined purpose and should relate to a given phenomenon (e.g., a clinician routinely takes a temperature because this vital sign can be an indication of an inflammatory process). For the purposes of this chapter, we will focus on some common forms of test validity.

The first form is face validity, which addresses the question: Does the particular measurement or method appear to be appropriate? This form of validity often relies on the opinion of experts. Most authorities consider face validity the weakest form of test and measurement validity. Another form is construct validity, which assesses the degree to which the measurement is based on theory. In the example of measuring body temperature, the construct that an inflammation involves heat provides modest construct validity. On the other hand, content validity asks whether the test is broad enough to address the scope of the content. For example, if students' knowledge of anatomy were being tested but they were only tested on the anatomy of the upper extremity, then that particular test would lack content validity. Finally, criterion validity is an indication of how well the test performs and whether it is useful when judged against a standard. There are generally two subcategories of criterion validity: predictive validity and concurrent validity. Predictive validity assesses whether and how well a test predicts a specific phenomenon or outcome. For example, how well does a positive straight leg raise accurately predict a lumbar disc protrusion? Concurrent validity asks whether the test performs as well as an accepted test. Generally, this category is used to validate a short or noninvasive version of a test. For example, concurrent validity would be used to establish the validity of a urine test, as opposed to a serum glucose test, to monitor diabetes mellitus.

Design or Experimental Validity

There are two forms of design or experimental validity: internal and external. Internal validity is concerned with limiting or controlling factors and events other than the independent variable, which may cause changes in the outcome, or dependent variable. These factors or events are known as threats to internal validity. External validity, on the other hand, is concerned with factors that may affect the generalizability of the conclusions drawn from the study. These factors are referred to as threats to external validity. The next section examines these two concepts.

THREATS TO INTERNAL VALIDITY

As mentioned, threats and concerns related to internal validity are unintended factors and conditions that can affect the results. For example, if an investigator is assessing the effects of two dietary regimens and does not take into account the subjects' levels of activity, then the internal validity of the study is threatened.

There are two broad categories of threats to internal validity: temporal or time-based effects, and measurement effects. Temporal or time-based effects consist of history, maturation, or attrition. History refers to effects on the dependent variable that are a result of the passage of time. For example, suppose an investigator is interested in a new topical ointment for the common cold sore caused by the herpes simplex virus. The researcher treats one group of patients with a new drug or topical ointment for 7 days and obtains excellent results. However, cold sores from the herpes simplex virus are thought to be self-limiting anyway, with symptoms generally resolving in 7 days. Therefore, the passage of time has obscured the effect or noneffect of the topical ointment.

The next temporal effect or threat to internal validity is maturation, which can be thought of as threats that happen by changes as a result of development. Suppose an individual suggests that a particular type of rehabilitative therapy improves the development of infants' motor skills. In this example, the individual contends that the therapy helps infants walk sooner. The effects of that therapy and potential changes in the infants' motor skills may not be the result of the type of therapy involved, but rather of the developmental process. Thus, the experiment may be flawed by threats to internal validity, specifically maturation.

The third temporal effect or threat to internal validity results from attrition. When subjects leave a study prematurely, the results may be distorted. Consider the consequences of a study involving a new drug for migraine headache sufferers. In this hypothetical study, one group of subjects receives the new drug, and their results are compared with another group of subjects who receive a placebo. The subjects will be seen every 3 weeks for a period of 6 months. Suppose subjects taking the new drug no longer experience migraine headaches, so they no longer come to their appointments. The only participants left in the study are those for whom the drug did not work. Therefore, when comparing the placebo to the experimental drug after 6 months, there is apparently no difference between the groups because the majority of participants who continue to have migraine headaches remained in the study. The subjects who were helped by the drug dropped out of the study, thereby affecting and possibly even distorting the results.

Measurement effects are those threats to internal validity that result from an investigator trying to measure a phenomenon. The first threat is testing, especially when the test is repeated several times.

Sometimes the actual act of performing a test on a patient affects the results of the study. Consider a hypothetical investigation in which the researcher is interested in the effect of a particular type of setting on function in individuals who have suffered a cerebral vascular accident. One of the measurements may be a functional test (e.g., how well the individual is able to dress without help from others). In this example, the investigator decides to administer a pretest to determine the baseline time needed for an individual to self-dress. In this case, having the patient get dressed may help the patient discover new and better strategies for getting dressed, thus contaminating the results. As a second example, consider an investigator who wishes to compare two forms of drug therapy on patients with cardiac problems. In this hypothetical study, the investigator chooses to use a step test (i.e., have the subjects step up and down repeatedly) and record the number of times subjects can continue until the heart rate reaches a predetermined maximum percentage. In this study, the patient's performance may be affected by the motor learning that takes place. In other words, the patient's coordination may improve just by virtue of a pretest using the step test.

The next threat to internal validity is instrumentation. The type of instrumentation used may affect the results. Consider a study in which the investigator is interested in whether children with handwriting problems press their pencils harder on the paper. To measure the point pressure of the writing implement, the children are asked to use a pencil-type instrument containing a force transducer and a wire that leads to a recording device. The fact that the instrument represents an unnatural pencil may affect the results. Thus, the instrument itself is a threat to internal validity.

Another threat to internal validity is sampling. Sampling effects include the selection of subjects for a study according to some bias, whether recognized or not. If selected by virtue of a bias, the subjects are not representative of the population. For example, if subjects were surveyed in a study via a mail questionnaire that was sent only to residents in an affluent suburb, then the conclusions drawn from the results may be affected by the sample that was surveyed.

The final measurement effect that represents a threat to internal validity is statistical regression to the mean. Simply stated, this is the tendency for a group of outliers to move toward the mean (the average), not necessarily because of any difference in the subjects' characteristics, but because of the laws of probability. A classic example of statistical regression to the mean can be illustrated by what happened when students with developmental and learning challenges were mainstreamed into a classroom with so-called "normal" students. After a period of time, they were tested and their scores on a developmental and learning inventory improved. The researchers then hypothesized that, if scores improved by putting challenged students in a "normal" class, then perhaps putting "normal" students in a class with gifted students would bring the "normal" students' aptitudes up. However, when the students in the class were retested, the exceptional students appeared to do worse on the test. Did the exposure to "normal" students somehow contaminate these learners? The answer is no. What was happening was simply statistical regression to the mean. In both cases, the group that was being tested (the developmentally challenged and the gifted students) came from the ends of the distribution of test scores, that is, the highest and lowest scores. On the retest, their scores tended to migrate toward the mean or toward that typical score within a population. Therefore, investigations may be affected by statistical regression to the mean by utilizing subjects who may be considered outliers.

THREATS TO EXTERNAL VALIDITY

As previously mentioned, threats to external validity include factors and conditions that affect the ability to generalize the results of a study. Threats to external validity can be placed into two categories: threats related to the populations used and those related to the environment in which the study takes place (i.e., environmental threats).

Population-Related Threats to External Validity

The first population-related threat to external validity concerns the subjects' accessibility to the study. When one performs a study, one usually studies a portion of a given population—a sample. If the sample used in an experiment or investigation is substantially different from the population, then the ability to generalize the results to the population may be compromised. This threat may be of particular interest in clinical studies. In the majority of clinical studies, the subject generally has access to medical care and the ability to continue with treatment. Therefore, these subjects may not represent the entire population, which may include individuals who have compromised access to medical care.

The second threat to external validity in the population category is known as subject–treatment interaction. This threat can be described as the confounding effects of the subjects' attributes on the dependent variable. Because of genetic makeup, lifestyle, or other confounding variables, certain subjects react differently (i.e., either more positively or more negatively) to any given treatment. For example, some people are blessed with a metabolism that allows them to eat whatever they wish without gaining any weight. On the other hand, other people who follow the same diet may gain weight.

Environmental or Experiment-Related Threats to External Validity

One environmental or experiment-related threat to external validity is the description of the variables. If the variables used in a study are not described precisely and with sufficient detail, then it may be difficult for subsequent investigators to replicate the study or obtain the same results. For example, consider a new antihypertensive drug study where the control subjects receive "conventional therapy," but this is not specified in detail. A clinician may not be able to determine whether the new drug is preferable to current therapy if not enough detail is available to ascertain how similar the new drug therapy is to the control therapy. A second environmental threat takes place when there are multiple treatments involving test order. In some cases, when two treatments or two drugs are administered, one may potentiate the effects or affect the actions of the other. Failure to recognize the effect of treatment order or multiple treatments may hinder the practitioner's ability to apply the results of the study.

Named after a classic experiment by Elton Mayo, the Hawthorne effect is a threat to external validity. Mayo was looking at worker productivity at the Hawthorne Works plant located outside of Chicago. Mayo was interested in the effect of lighting on worker productivity. He explained to the workers that they would be in an experiment on productivity. Mayo then proceeded to increase the ambient lighting in the factory. As anticipated, productivity improved. In the next phase of his study, Mayo then dimmed the ambient lighting. Worker productivity increased again. Finally, Mayo raised the ambient lighting to the previous high-intensity level, and yet again productivity increased. Mayo concluded that the ambient lighting was unrelated to the workers' performance—rather, the fact that the workers knew they were being studied affected productivity. The Hawthorne effect is an effect on results caused by the subjects' knowing that they are participating in an experiment. Typically, subjects in clinical experiments have better compliance with treatment regimens than patients who are not participating in an experiment.

The Rosenthal effect refers to results caused by the involvement of the investigator in a study. The personal attributes, charisma, and abilities of the researcher can affect the results. For example, if an investigator is a charismatic practitioner, then patients may improve partially because of their belief in the clinician treating them. Other practitioners who attempt to obtain similar results are likely to be unsuccessful.

In every research study, the investigator must consider and try to control factors, conditions, and the effects of circumstances that threaten both internal and external validity. Similarly, professionals critically reading the literature must be aware of these threats to validity in order to determine the credibility of the conclusions and the applicability of the work in their practice. In many cases, the choice of research design affects the investigation's susceptibility to threats to validity.

TYPES OF STUDIES

Descriptive Studies

Descriptive studies generate data that are either numerical or non-numerical. Non-numerical information may be presented as verbal commentaries about subjects' clinical characteristics and behaviors, histologic slides, radiologic images, and so on. For these data, descriptive methods from the sub-discipline of qualitative research are appropriate. For ethical and legal reasons, subjects' personal information must always be de-identified when qualitative findings are presented.

Similarly, numerical data on individual subjects are almost never presented in a research report. Numerical information is usually presented as statistical summaries such as averages and measures of variability. The mean, median, and mode are all measures of central tendency. The measure of variability most often used in medical literature is standard deviation. Occasionally, a range or standard error (SE, also called standard error of the mean, SEM) is used. When confidential information is not disclosed, numerical reports may be supported by exemplar, anecdotal, or model information that conveys valuable research or teaching lessons.

Analytic Studies

Analytic studies test for the following:

- Differences between groups (e.g., a group of patients receiving a drug compared to those receiving a placebo)

- Relationships among variables (e.g., the correlation between cholesterol levels and coronary artery occlusion)
- Both differences and relationships

A "true experiment" is a prospective design in which the researcher controls as many subject, treatment, and environmental variables as possible.

A cross-sectional study is a database of "snapshots" of subjects at one period. For example, childhood bone maturation may be studied by describing bone densities in a group of children ages 1, 3, 6, and 9 years old. A longitudinal approach would follow a group of 25 one-year-old children over the next 8 years. If the researcher could control all or most variables over time, then a longitudinal study could also be experimental. However, it would be difficult to determine whether intervening variables had corrupted the design. Therefore, long-term experiments involving human subjects are rare.

When there is substantial risk to human subjects, it is not always possible to conduct a true experiment ethically. The risk may be caused by inducing the disease or condition being studied or by testing an experimental intervention or treatment. As an alternative, it may be possible to study a disease (e.g., cervical cancer) by identifying those who already have it and those who do not and then comparing the two groups for factors that might have been responsible for the disease (e.g., human papillomavirus exposure). This type of study is known as a case-control study design.

Another experimental approach is to identify people who have or do not have a particular risk factor (e.g., human papillomavirus exposure) and then examine the two groups over time to identify those who develop the disease or condition. This type of study is known as a cohort study design. Whether a cohort or case-control study design is used, a control or reference group is necessary. For example, if a newscast reports all subjects in a group of heroin addicts have used marijuana, can we conclude that marijuana use leads to heroin addiction? If the heroin addicts were found to have consumed whole milk, can we conclude that whole milk leads to heroin addiction? A control or reference group composed of people who do not use heroin is likely to show many have used marijuana or have consumed whole milk.

Prospective Versus Retrospective Designs

Data collection for prospective studies is planned in advance. Prospective designs include true experiments and concurrent cohort studies. The concurrent cohort design involves subjects who do not have the disease in question but have a suspected risk factor and are tested at a later time to determine whether the disease developed in them. In many cases, the prospective approach is the only way to obtain information about a new or recently discovered phenomenon, such as a previously unrecognized disorder or a newly developed technique.

True experiments attempt to gain strict control over the conditions of the study, including subject selection, instrument calibration, and the experimental environment. Compared to retrospective designs, prospective designs are credited with having better control of variables and a greater possibility of having valid and reliable standardized measurement methods. Disadvantages include cost (which may limit subject numbers) and the difficulty of extrapolating the results of strictly controlled methods to the clinical setting, where a similar level of control is not possible.

Retrospective studies examine data that already exist, including chart reviews and case-control studies. A retrospective approach may be the only ethical way to study the mechanisms of certain interventions. For example, thalidomide was widely prescribed outside the United States for nausea and vomiting during pregnancy, but later it was found to cause developmental defects. Looking back at the unexpected adverse events associated with a previously approved therapy is an example of a retrospective approach. In hindsight, the harms discovered provide valuable information that cannot be ethically studied in a prospective manner.

Because the researcher may not know exactly how and under what circumstances the data were collected, it may be difficult to verify that retrospective data were collected properly. Collecting data retrospectively is usually inexpensive, and data are readily available in large quantities. A large N value (the total number of participants in a study) may be used to compensate for variability. Therefore, the value and usefulness of a study should not be based solely on whether the data were collected prospectively or retrospectively. The particular method of data collection should be evaluated on its own merit.

Uses of Statistics

Many skilled clinicians are skeptical or even fearful of statistics. They contend that "anything can be proved or disproved," and that readers are easily fooled. This is not true for those who have knowledge about research methods and the basic statistical principles presented in this chapter. Statistical information is common in medical literature. A few easy-to-learn concepts enable clinicians to become informed consumers of medical information. This ability is invaluable for interpreting study results in journal articles, conference presentations, and drug advertisements. Because we rely on scientific information throughout our professional careers to understand new information, a healthcare provider should be familiar with clinical research methods and basic statistical terminology.

Statistics are used primarily in three ways in medical literature. First, statistics are used to describe and summarize group information. Second, they allow us to infer or generalize sample results to the larger population, which is essential because it is impossible or impractical to measure each and every individual. Third, statistics test for significant relationships or differences between groups of subjects.

Types of Data

A datum (singular of data) is a unit of information about a subject. An example would be the total cholesterol value of 178 mg/dL on a subject participating in a lipid study. Data may be non-numerical (nominal or ordinal, also referred to as nonparametric because of the statistical tests that can be legitimately performed on these types of data) or numerical (interval or ratio, also called parametric).

Nominal data are characteristic names that have no numerical value; examples include male or female, black or white, osteoarthritis or rheumatoid arthritis, smoker or nonsmoker. Ordinal data have characteristics that are comparative and can be ordered by rank; examples are shorter or taller, less painful or more painful, darker or lighter, or an increased size of a palpable mass. Interval data have numerical values between units but no actual zero point; examples include degrees centigrade and blood glucose (i.e., a patient could not have a body temperature or blood glucose value of zero). Ratio data have numerical values between units, and a zero value is possible; examples include milligrams of alcohol per deciliter, basophils per cubic millimeter, and number of pack-years smoking history (number of packs smoked per day multiplied by the number of years smoked).

Like clinical data, numerical research data are preferred to non-numerical data. For instance, in a study on smokers, knowing the number of pack-years (numerical data) provides better information than knowing only that a patient smokes (non-numerical). The more powerful parametric statistical tests can be applied to numerical data.

Although it is not always possible to quantify data, data can be valuable in the descriptive, qualitative form. For example, a narrative about a radiograph of a hairline fracture with a detailed description of its important characteristics, landmarks, and possible origin may be more informative than just a report of a "hairline fracture: present or not present" on 100 films.

When it is not possible to use numerical data, nonparametric statistical tests (such as the Spearman's correlation or chi-squared) must be used. The application of parametric tests (e.g., Pearson's correlation or the t-test) to nonparametric data is a mistake because a falsely low p value (probability value) is likely to be fabricated (i.e., referred to as an alpha or type I error). A falsely high *p* value is likely to result when nonparametric tests are used for analyzing numerical (parametric) data. In this case, it is unlikely that a false hypothesis will be accepted, but consequentially a true one may be overlooked (i.e., a beta or type II error). This may occur especially when the calculated *p* value is close to the desired alpha level.

These classifications of numerical data are commonly used in most scientific articles. However, qualitative research methods also serve invaluable roles in some medical studies and are used as extensively in clinical research as in clinical problem solving.

Experimental Designs

An investigator must decide whether a qualitative or quantitative approach will more effectively address the research objective. A second decision is whether the study will involve retrospective data (e.g., clinical records) or prospective data (i.e., information that will be newly generated as part of the project). The implications of these decisions have been discussed earlier in this chapter.

If the investigator decides to use an experiment to answer the research question, then choosing the appropriate experimental design is imperative. In a project proposal, the investigator describes the methods to be used for analyzing the study's data. Many proposal guidelines suggest creating mock data that are likely to resemble the study's actual data. This process also helps the investigator plan for both computer needs and possibly consultation with a statistician or methodologist.

The selected research designs presented in Table 6-1 are likely to accommodate the needs of most investigators. Although experimental and epidemiological studies share some methodological similarities, epidemiologists have developed specialized techniques for the needs of their discipline. Some investigators may need to use advanced epidemiological techniques for their studies. In these cases, consulting an epidemiology textbook or an epidemiologist is appropriate. The statistical principles presented here apply to most experimental and epidemiological studies, whether prospective or retrospective. Familiarity with these principles should enable the clinician to converse knowledgeably with most clinical research methodologists and consultants.

Pre-Experimental, Experimental, and Quasi-Experimental Designs for Research

The purpose of this section is to provide the reader with a simple way to recognize common research designs and the associated threats to validity inherent in those designs. Most of the work conducted in this area can be attributed to Campbell and Stanley, who wrote the classic text *Experimental and Quasi-Experimental Designs for Research*.[1] They developed a shorthand method for diagramming research designs similar to the way English grammar has been classically taught—by diagramming sentences, students learn to understand proper grammar and sentence construction. Similarly, individuals can more easily recognize a research design by diagramming it.

Campbell and Stanley and others have used certain conventions. For the purposes of this section, the following symbols are used:

- An R represents randomization and indicates a particular group was randomly selected or assigned.
- An M indicates the groups were matched.
- An X (with or without a subscript) indicates a treatment.
- An X_0 indicates no treatment or, in some cases, the control condition.
- An O indicates a measurement. If multiple measurements are taken, then subscripts, such as O_1, O_2, O_3, and so forth, may be used.
- A dashed line indicates nonequivalency and denotes the groups may be substantially different.

PRE-EXPERIMENTAL DESIGNS

The pre-experimental designs are the weakest of the research designs and are subject to many threats to internal and external validity. They are characterized by the lack of a control group, sensitivity to temporal threats to internal validity, and poor generalizability.

One-Shot Case Study

The first pre-experimental design, the one-shot case study, is diagrammed as follows:

$$XO$$

In this design, a treatment is given and a measurement is made. This particular design is typical of survey research. A group of respondents is identified based on one or more pre-existing criteria and are administered a questionnaire that is then measured. Another example of the one-shot case study is the typical high school or college classroom. The instructor assumes the students have a certain level of baseline knowledge when they enter the class, but this baseline is not measured. The treatment consists of the exposure in the class, and the measurement is the students' performance in the class. If the students do well, then the instructor may conclude it is because the students learned a great deal from the class. However, the instructor cannot justifiably arrive at that conclusion because the students' prior level of knowledge in the subject is unknown. This demonstrates how the one-shot case study is a weak design because of its vulnerability to threats to both internal and external validity.

Even with its limitations, the one-shot case study is useful for certain types of research, such as descriptive studies in which the investigator wishes to describe what currently exists. For example, most surveys can be characterized as one-shot case studies. Often the data they yield are very useful to clinicians and, therefore, are published in the medical literature. For example, Levine was interested in the clinical practice of lung transplantation and wanted to ascertain if there were wide differences among transplantation programs.[2] To describe the state of clinical practice, he surveyed 65 active lung transplantation programs. By requesting information on key areas of practice, such as lung preservation and posttransplantation care, he was able to conclude that there was substantial consensus as well as a few areas of variance among transplantation centers. The results could not be generalized to centers that did not respond. In addition, these studies do not have a long "shelf life" because a survey is most often a snapshot of a phenomenon at a specific time. However, the information could be considered valuable because lung transplantation centers may be able to determine if the practices at their center are consistent with those at other centers.

One Group Pretest–Posttest

Slightly more robust is the one group pretest–posttest design. In this particular design, subjects receive a pretest, the treatment, and a posttest or retest:

$$OXO$$

This design is characteristic of clinical practice in which a patient (or a group of patients) is evaluated and diagnosed, a treatment is administered, and the patient (or a group) is then subsequently re-evaluated.

For example, a group of high school students is provided with education about alcohol abuse. The pretest and posttest may be a questionnaire on alcohol use. This design is particularly vulnerable to the temporal threats to internal validity, and therefore the investigator theoretically cannot conclude the outcome was the result of treatment because the illness may have been self-limiting or the subject may simply have outgrown the problem as a result of development. In the case of high school students, changes in alcohol use may be related to the time of year and lack of parties where alcohol is served rather than to alcohol abuse education.

Without the ability to compare the study group to a reference or control group, the effects of temporal threats to internal validity cannot be evaluated. Similarly, the results cannot be generalized because it is not known whether the patient (or group) is representative.

In a study on the effects of a 5-day immersion leadership development experience on current and aspiring nursing leaders, Tourangeau et al. assessed and compared self-appraisals by participants and assessments by colleagues before and 3 months after the experience.[3] Although they concluded "a concentrated leadership experience is effective in strengthening leadership behaviors," critical readers may point out several issues that challenge their conclusions. Because participants' colleagues assessed leadership behaviors before the experience and knew they would be completing another assessment later, they may have become more sensitive to observing leadership behaviors. In other words, some of the observed differences may be due to changes in the raters rather than in the participants. The study could have addressed the concern about differences in the raters by having them also rate individuals who did not undergo the leadership program. Ideally, the raters would have been blind to the subjects' participation, or in other words, they would not know whether a person they were rating had or had not participated in the leadership development program. If changes in leadership were observed for individuals who had not participated in the program, then at least some of the observed change could possibly be attributed to the changes in the raters. This concern about the raters is further supported by the fact that the participants' self-report on leadership behaviors was not significantly different after the program. Finally, because the subjects were volunteers, those who felt they would benefit from the program may have self-selected to participate. Hence the subjects may not have been representative of aspiring nurse leaders.

Static Group Comparison

The third pre-experimental research design is entitled the static group comparison. In this design, a group that has received a treatment, or been exposed to a condition, is compared to a group that did not receive the treatment or was not exposed to the condition:

$$X O$$
$$\text{-------}$$
$$O$$

The dashed line indicates that these groups are not equivalent. This design, which attempts some form of control with the group that was not treated or exposed, is better than the previous designs. However, because the groups were not randomly assigned, it cannot be concluded that they are equivalent.

This design is commonly used in environmental or occupational epidemiological studies. For example, one may be interested in a group of people who are living in an area that might be contaminated with a carcinogenic agent. The investigator may hypothesize that living in this area may result in a greater incidence of certain types of cancers. People who live in the contaminated area are compared with similar people who live in an uncontaminated area. If there is a greater and statistically significant difference in the number of people with cancer in the contaminated area, then the researcher could conclude the suspected carcinogen might be related. Please note that one cannot conclude causality from this type of design. Correlation and causation are different concepts. Correlation helps to identify a relationship between variables and the direction of that relationship.

The usefulness of the static group comparison is that it allows the study of variables that generally cannot be manipulated by the investigator. Legally and ethically, an investigator cannot require people to live in an area that is suspected to cause a disease or disability. On the other hand, if individuals choose to live in that area, then one can measure and analyze the effects and compare them to a similar group of individuals who live in a different "control" area.

An example of a static group comparison from the medical literature is a study by Lynch et al.

that compared residency choices by medical students who did or did not participate in an optional rural health awareness program.[4] One group of medical students participated in an enrichment initiative entitled the Rural Health Scholars Program (RHSP), which included both didactic and experiential learning focusing on practice in underserved and rural areas. The proportion of participants that chose residencies in primary care, family medicine, community hospitals, and known underserved areas were compared to their classmates who did not participate in the RHSP. Although the results demonstrated that significantly more students who participated in the RHSP chose residencies in family medicine and community hospitals, the authors could not conclude that the RHSP was the "cause." Because the groups were nonequivalent, the possibility that medical students self-selected participation in the RHSP because of a possible interest in a rural primary care setting could not be ruled out.

In summary, one of the major problems with a static group comparison occurs because the groups are nonequivalent. Therefore, there is always the possibility that some factor other than the treatment is causing the results.

EXPERIMENTAL DESIGNS

The next series of research designs are the true experimental designs. These studies are characterized by randomization of the subjects and a control group. Randomization does not mean the groups are identical. Randomization works on the law of probability, which suggests that when a group is selected or subjects are assigned randomly, the traits, characteristics, and conditions that may affect the outcome (confounding variables) are distributed roughly equally among the groups, thus canceling out their effect.

Pretest, Posttest, Control Group Design

The first experimental design includes a pretest, posttest, and control group. In this design, subjects are randomly assigned to a group, pretested, given a treatment or not given a treatment, and then tested after exposure to the treatment or no treatment:

$$R \ O_1 \ X_0 \ O_2$$
$$R \ O_1 \ X_1 \ O_2$$

In this diagram, two groups are compared on a single variable with two conditions (X_0 and X_1), but more than two groups or conditions can be analyzed using this design. In addition, it is possible to examine more than one variable.

The pretest, posttest, control group design effectively rules out most threats to internal and external validity. Because it is the most rigorous design, the pretest, posttest, control group design is commonly accepted as the "gold standard" and is typically used in randomized clinical trials. It should be noted that in clinical trials and other research involving human subjects, it is unethical and often illegal to withhold treatment. Thus the control group may be the group that receives the conventional treatment while the experimental group receives the new treatment. In other words, the conventional treatment is sometimes used as a control or the baseline.

In a study to examine whether fortified cereals actually increased subjects' blood levels of selected B vitamins, Tucker et al. compared two groups of older adults—one who ate a fortified cereal and one who ate a cereal that was not fortified.[5] Their approach was to measure blood levels of homocysteine (an amino acid), folic acid, vitamin B_6, and vitamin B_{12} in subjects on two occasions to obtain baselines. According to the authors, "High homocysteine and low vitamin B concentrations have been linked to the risk of vascular disease, stroke and dementia."[5(p805)] After obtaining baseline measures, the subjects were randomly assigned to a group that ate either a cup of fortified cereal daily or a cup of cereal that was not fortified. At 12 and 14 weeks the blood levels of homocysteine, folic acid, B_6, and B_{12} were measured[†].

Neither the subjects nor the investigators performing the tests knew whether a subject was consuming fortified cereal or not. When the group membership is unknown to the subject and the investigator (until the tests are concluded), the study is called a double-blind study. Both the subject and the investigator are "blind" to the treatment. Comparisons between the two groups revealed significant differences between them. Homocysteine levels were lower, whereas folic acid, B_6, and B_{12} levels were higher in the group that ate the fortified cereal. Because of the rigorous design of the study, the authors concluded that eating a fortified cereal benefits older adults.[6] Because major threats to internal and external validity were controlled, the observed differences were due to the treatment. Therefore, the results may be generalized to similar groups of individuals; that is, eating a cereal fortified with B vitamins benefits older adults.

Posttest-Only Control Group Design

The second experimental design is termed the posttest-only control group design. The subjects are randomized, given a treatment, and then the results are measured and compared:

$$R\ X_0\ O$$
$$R\ X_1\ O$$

Typically, this type of design is used when a pretest is inappropriate or unavailable for other reasons. For example, an orthopedic group may be interested in the outcomes of a total hip replacement when using one particular appliance versus a second appliance. In this case, a pretest is inappropriate because patients who require total hip replacements generally lack substantial range of motion at the hip joint, often because of pain. In this example, the outcomes such as time to ambulation, pain, and range of motion may be appropriate to measure after the surgery. Because it is impossible to know the baseline or the pretest condition of the individuals, there might be some threats to internal validity based on pre-existing conditions. However, randomization minimizes these effects.

Gallo and Staskin investigated the effect of external cues on patient compliance in performing pelvic-floor exercises.[5] Because compliance is measured after a patient is educated about a treatment program, a pretest was not appropriate. In this study, 86 women with stress urinary incontinence were given a program on pelvic-floor exercises and then were randomly assigned to a group that either received an additional audio cassette or did not. They were subsequently evaluated for compliance to the pelvic-floor exercise program, and the results were compared. The women who received the audio cassette, labeled an external cue by the authors, demonstrated significantly better compliance than the group who received only instruction.[5] In this case, the robust experimental design, a posttest-only control group design, controlled major threats to internal and external validity, allowing the authors to conclude that external cues improve compliance for women with stress urinary incontinence.

Solomon Four-Group Design

The next experimental design is the Solomon four-group design. In this design, groups with and without pretests are exposed to one of two treatments and are subsequently tested after treatment:

$$R\ O_1\ X_0\ O_2$$
$$R\ O_1\ X_1\ O_2$$
$$R\ X_0\ O_2$$
$$R\ X_1\ O_2$$

The Solomon four-group design is actually a combination of the previous two designs: the pretest, posttest, control group design and the posttest-only control group design. This particular design is useful because it allows an investigator to assess whether an effect occurs because of the pretest. On the other hand, this design requires twice as many subjects.

Danley et al. investigated the effect of a multimedia learning experience designed to prepare dental students and dentists to recognize and respond to domestic violence.[7] The investigators were interested in ensuring that observed changes in the subjects between the pretest and the posttest were not due to the fact that the subjects completed the pretest. When the subjects who completed the pretest, the multimedia learning experience, and the posttest were compared to subjects who completed the multimedia learning experience and the posttest, but no pretest, investigators found no significant differences between the groups. On the other hand, the two groups who completed the multimedia learning experience were more knowledgeable than the subjects in the control group.[6]

QUASI-EXPERIMENTAL DESIGNS

The final group of research designs is termed quasi-experimental designs. Although they are more rigorous than the pre-experimental designs, they are not as rigorous or as robust as the true experimental designs. Typically, they lack one or more of the characteristics that would make them true experimental designs. Generally, randomization or multiple measurements are lacking, thereby making testing effects a potential problem.

Nonequivalent Control Group Design

The nonequivalent control group design is similar to the pretest, posttest, control group design, but because the groups are not randomized they must be considered nonequivalent:

$$O_1 \ X_0 \ O_2$$

$$O_1 \ X_1 \ O_2$$

An example of the use of this design is a hypothetical comparison of patient satisfaction with care from two clinics: one clinic hired a clinician 6 months previously (X_1) and one clinic had no clinician (X_0). Many ways in which the patients differ might affect the outcome, such as age, years seen by the provider, and so forth. Because the groups are nonequivalent, the results obtained from studies using this particular design must be viewed with caution; pre-existing conditions in the subjects may account for the changes after treatment.

Kristjansson et al. studied the effectiveness of a short-duration learning experience for teenagers that focused on preventing skin cancer.[8] Because the presentation was given in a classroom, they compared the classes that received the presentation to classes that did not. In this example, randomly assigning students would have made the study very complex and unmanageable. Although their results suggested the short-duration learning experience was successful, the fact that the groups were nonequivalent suggests that they should be viewed with caution. For instance, it is not known if one or more classes were composed of students who were more concerned about their health or more motivated to accept the content presented.

Separate Sample Pretest, Posttest Design

The separate sample pretest, posttest design is used when the investigators suspect that the pretest will significantly bias the posttest results:

$$O \ X$$

$$------$$

$$X \ O$$

Although measuring a change from pretest to posttest is appropriate when using a physical test such as blood level or heart rate, a pretest of a mental, psychological, or performance variable often affects the posttest. For example, a pretest for manual dexterity may result in some motor learning that could affect subsequent performance. If the investigator were interested in evaluating the effect of a new treatment, the observed changes could be due to motor learning from the pretest. The separate sample pretest, posttest design addresses concerns about the pretest biasing the outcome.

Markert et al. used a separate pretest, posttest design to assess the knowledge acquired by professionals who attended continuing medical education (CME) programs.[9] The investigators noted in this article that pretesting and posttesting attendees was an inappropriate approach for assessing knowledge. They felt that a pretest would bias performance on a posttest. Given the observation that most medical professionals are bright individuals who are committed to learning, it seems logical that they would remember items from a pretest. Instead, Markert et al. randomly assigned attendees to either a pretest group, which they considered a "control" group, or a posttest-only group, which they considered the "treatment" group. Upon comparing the groups, the treatment group demonstrated significantly more knowledge in selected topic areas.[9]

Time Series Design

A third quasi-experimental design is the time series design. In these designs, groups are compared to each other and there are multiple tests:

$$O_1 \; X_0 \; O_2 \; O_3 \; O_4$$

$$O_1 \; X_1 \; O_2 \; O_3 \; O_4$$

Because there are multiple measurements, one cannot conclude that changes or differences are not a result of sensitization or learning. In other words, the threat to validity of repeated testing is of concern, as well as the threat that groups may be nonequivalent.

In a study that compared nursing and medical interventions for skin care, Pokorny et al. examined differences in patients who developed pressure sores and those who did not.[10] Data were gathered on the day of admission, the day of surgery, and the following 4 days. Because the patients were admitted for cardiac surgery, it was anticipated a subject would average 6 days in the hospital. The investigators in this study looked for differences in the daily nursing and medical interventions between patients who developed pressure sores and those who did not. For this study, the dependent variable (what was measured) consisted of the documented interventions, specifically differences. The authors concluded that multiple assessments of skin condition by nurses were important in preventing pressure sores.[10] Because patients were not randomly assigned to groups that received standard or optimized skin assessment, differences in patients may have affected the results.

SUMMARY

The designs presented are by no means exhaustive of the pre-experimental, experimental, and quasi-experimental designs found in the literature. By recognizing the common designs, one can quickly focus on threats to validity. When designing a study, knowledge of common research designs may help avoid pitfalls. Although one can have a robust research design, failure to obtain reliable measurements using a valid instrument may render the conclusions of the study inaccurate or erroneous. Finally, reading research critically or performing research is a learning experience that generally requires a great deal of practice.

When evaluating the methods section of published research reports, this information should help clinicians to knowledgeably critique the methods used and evaluate the study's results before applying them to practice. For all clinicians, this information should help in interpreting new medical information presented in literature, professional conferences, and through other sources. Well-informed clinicians may be able to interpret and apply clinical information in new or better ways.

By definition, original research studies are unique. Applying the principles presented in this chapter should help beginning investigators select an effective research method for a planned research study and, when necessary, communicate effectively with methodological consultants.

REFERENCES

1. Campbell DT, Stanley JC, Gage NL. *Experimental and Quasi-Experimental Designs for Research*. Chicago Ill.: R. McNally, 1966.
2. Levine SM. A survey of clinical practice of lung transplantation in North America. *Chest*. 2004;125:1–16.
3. Tourangeau AE, Lemonde M, Luba M, et al. Evaluation of a leadership development intervention. *Nurse Leaders (Toronto)*. 2003;16(3):91–104.
4. Lynch DC, Pathman DE, Teplin SE, Bernstein JD. Interim evaluation of the rural health scholars program. *Teach Learn Med*. 2001;13:36–42.
5. Tucker KL, Olson B, Bakun P, Dallal GE, Selhub J, Rosenberg IH. Breakfast cereal fortified with folic acid, vitamin B-6 and vitamin B-12 increases vitamin concentrations and reduces homocysteine concentrations: A randomized trial. *Am J Clin Nutr*. 2004;79:805–811.
6. Gallo ML, Staskin DR. Cues to action: Pelvic floor muscle exercise compliance in women with stress urinary incontinence. *Neurourol Urodyn*. 1997;16:167–177.

7. Danley D, Gansky SA, Chow D, Gerbert B. Preparing dental students to recognize and respond to domestic violence. *J Am Dent Assoc.* 2004;135;67–73.
8. Kristjansson K, Helgason R, Mansson-Brahme E, Widlund-Ivarson B, Ullen H. You and your skin: A short-duration presentation of skin cancer prevention for teenagers. *Health Educ Res.* 2003;18:88–97.
9. Markert RJ, O'Neill SC, Bhatia SC. Using a quasi-experimental research design to assess knowledge in continuing medical education programs. *J Cont Educ Health Prof.* 2003;23:157–162*.
10. Pokorny ME, Koldjeski D, Swanson M. Skin care intervention for patients having cardiac surgery. *Am J Crit Care.* 2003;12:535–544.

* Readers interested in a full discussion of reliability measurement are advised to consult Bartko JJ & Carpenter WT. On the method and theory of reliability. *The Journal of Nervous and Mental Disease.* 1975;163:307–317.

† The astute reader will undoubtedly observe that the example used is a slight variation from the classical pretest, posttest, control group design because the investigators used two baseline measurements and two posttest measurements, so the design was:

$$R\ O_1\ O_2\ X_{\text{not fortified}}\ O_3\ O_4$$
$$R\ O_1\ O_2\ X_{\text{fortified}}\ O_3\ O_4$$

Ordinarily one might also be concerned about pretest–posttest sensitization with multiple tests, but in this study the dependent variable was blood levels of homocysteine, B_6, B_{12}, and folic acid, which should not be affected by repeated testing.

CHAPTER 7

Survey Research

J. Dennis Blessing, PhD, PA

CHAPTER OVERVIEW

Surveys are one of the most commonly used methods to gather information and data in the world. Surveys are used to gather information as important as the U.S. Census or who we plan to vote for in the next election or as mundane as the type of dishwashing soap we use or our favorite movie. Surveys can reveal trends, attitudes, opinions, lifestyles, needs, expectations, knowledge/information, behaviors, demographics—the list of uses is infinite. Surveys can be used in almost every aspect of our lives, and health care is no exception. A large amount of data from any number of people on a wide variety of subjects and issues can be gathered using surveys. Several formats are used to deliver and conduct surveys; they can be long or short, simple or complex. Surveys can use words, symbols, written responses, and simple or complex choices, and can collect quantitative or qualitative data. Despite its somewhat eclectic nature, survey research must still conform to the exacting requirements of design and methodology to have true value, meaning, and impact.

This chapter presents the basic concepts of survey research, including design, item construction, data analysis, and conducting the research. Emphasis is placed on designing items and developing concepts that are valid to survey research in health care. A short discussion of sample size is presented. The use of surveys in research and practice environments will be included.

Learning Objectives

- Discuss and evaluate the purpose of surveys.
- List the advantages and disadvantages of surveys.
- List the various types of surveys.
- Define verbal frequency scales and develop a verbal frequency scale.
- Develop survey items.
- Construct a survey.
- Discuss and identify survey analysis procedures.

WHAT SURVEYS CAN AND CANNOT DO

Surveys are used to gather many types of information: information on demographics, opinions, preferences, expectations, knowledge, and outcomes. They can be conducted by mail (including email), in person, via telephone, and through the Internet. Survey samples can be very specific for selected individuals, less specific for groups of individuals, or more general for large populations. Sample subjects can be defined by almost any characteristic. Samples can be randomized or assigned, stratified or open, well defined or ill defined, or a sample of convenience. As shown in **Table 7-1**, surveys have several advantages for data collection; they can be a relatively easy, inexpensive, fast, and consistent research tool.

As shown in **Table 7-2**, surveys also can pose some disadvantages. One major disadvantage is difficulty in establishing causality.[1] Causality involves manipulating a variable and determining

Table 7–1 Some General Advantages of Surveys

Advantage	Reason
Costs	Relatively low cost, but depends on survey and methodology
Sample size	Can vary from small to extremely large; can be targeted
Issues	Can gather information on single or multiple issues or topics
Format	Can vary: mail, Internet, interview, telephone
Impact	Can yield very influential results

Table 7–2 Some General Disadvantages of Surveys

Disadvantage	Reason
Respondent self-report	There is no way to ensure individuals will respond to surveys or choose to participate.
Respondent interpretation	There is a risk that respondents will interpret survey items in a manner different from investigator intent.
Respondent bias	There is a risk that people who choose to respond may be different from the population being studied.
Extrapolation to nonresponders	Can the response of a few be extrapolated to the population? Can the data be generalized?
Item bias	Is there bias in the way an item is worded or interpreted?

the effect on another variable. This is very difficult to do with a one-time survey. However, well-designed surveys can be effectively used as preintervention and postintervention assessment tools in experimental and quasi-experimental designs.

Other challenges associated with surveys revolve around reliability of respondent self-reporting, respondent interpretation of survey items, extrapolation of results to a population, nonrespondent influence, and respondent bias. Although these challenges to survey research cannot be completely avoided, good design and item construction should help to limit the impact and influence such issues have on outcomes.

TYPES OF SURVEYS

As shown in **Table 7–3**, surveys are delivered in different formats. The choice of delivery format (distribution) is part of the methodology and research design. Each format has advantages and disadvantages. The research purpose(s), study population, and sample size are factors that must be considered in the decision on the survey delivery. Surveys can be conducted by mail, telephone, Internet, and interview.

Most of this chapter will concentrate on Web-based surveys and those delivered by mail. The construction of the survey itself is very similar for both formats. Many Web-based surveys and paper surveys are delivered by email. Internet surveys have become the standard format for surveys. Telephone and interview surveys are briefly discussed.

PLANNING IS KEY

Performing a survey investigation or study is more than thinking up some questions, putting them on paper or on the Web, and sending them out. The meticulous planning required is just as important for surveys as for any other type of research effort. One of the first steps is to define what is to be achieved in the study. Not much can be accomplished beyond a literature review until the study goals are conceptualized and what is to be achieved and learned are defined. The survey must have specific goals or objectives, or aims that can be

Table 7–3 Comparison of Survey Methods

Characteristic	Mail	Telephone	Interview	Internet
Cost	Moderate, depends on sample size	Low to moderate, depends on local versus long distance costs	Relatively high	Variable, but becoming the least expensive
Cost examples	Printing, postage, paper, envelopes	Telephone costs, personnel training, and expense to conduct interview	Personnel training and expense to conduct interview	Professional help with Web design
Response rate	Potentially low	Dependent on willingness of subjects to participate	Relatively high; only willing subjects are interviewed	Variable, but instant; respondents must have Internet access
Investigator time	Relatively limited	Requires training of interviewers and/or time to conduct interviews	Requires training of interviewers and/or time to conduct interviews	Relatively limited
Respondent time	Completed as convenient	Telephone time	Interview time	Completed as convenient
Study time	Relatively long; must allow for mail and response times	Relatively short, but subject contact time may be long	Relatively short, but subject contact time may be long	Relatively short, dependent on subject time to respond
Anonymity	Survey form can be completely anonymous	Phone number is known	Person-to-person interaction	Web address can be identified
Sample size	Can be very large	Usually small to medium	Limited, usually small	Can be very large
Respondent bias	Respondent item interpretation	Interviewer voice influence	Interviewer influence is high	Must be computer literate
Investigator bias	Generally very limited except for item construction	Voice influence; interpretation of survey items	Influence by voice, facial expression, body movement; interpretation of survey items	Generally very limited except for item construction
Other	Requires mailing lists	Multiple interviewers conducting survey	Multiple interviewers conducting survey	Computer access required

researched. Once the goals, objectives, or aims of the investigation are defined, everything that follows will reflect the research effort. This planning generates the research questions, hypotheses, or null hypotheses.

RESPONSE RATES

Response rates are a threat to any survey. Generally, response rates tend to be low, particularly when used without a well-defined target population or sample.

Here are some helpful guidelines for surveys of health professionals, students, and educators.

- An introductory statement (cover letter if using regular mail) should accompany the survey. A personal salutation should be used if the subject is known to the investigator. Otherwise Mr., Ms., Mrs., or a professional title such as Dr. should be used.
- The survey instrument must be well designed in its content (items) and visually appealing.
- A respondent should be able to complete the survey in a short period of time. The longer it takes to complete the survey, the less likely that it will be completed.
- Some sort of inducement or gift may be included. However, this adds to the study expense, and there is no guarantee the response rate will be increased.[1]
- A follow-up request may spur some respondents. An email reminder may suffice.

With regard to the form and format of an email survey, these additional suggestions may be helpful.

- Begin with interesting questions.
- Use graphics and various question-writing techniques to ease the task of reading and answering the questions.
- Use capital or dark letters for readability.
- Limit the length of the survey.
- Send notices and reminders at carefully spaced times.
  - Notice by email that a survey is coming
  - Email with the survey attached
  - A reminder
  - A second reminder (optional)
- If an identifier is used, explain that it is for recordkeeping only and that the respondent's confidentiality is protected.

Much literature on survey research is available. A literature or Web search or book on survey research will help to develop and guide the survey research skills of the investigator.

SURVEY INTRODUCTION

The introductory information is presented at the beginning of the survey. The survey introduction to a subject is accomplished in two ways. The introduction, of course, depends on which survey format is used. For paper or Internet surveys, the introductory information is the first thing the subject should see. If a survey is sent by email with an attachment or a Web URL, the introductory information can be in the body of the email. For telephone or face-to-face delivery, the introductory information is read or provided in some physical way such as an agreement to participate. (For telephone surveys, the subject should voice his or her agreement to participate.) Regardless of the manner of introduction, certain basic points must be included. A well-worded, informative introduction (in mail body, cover letter, voice agreement, or face-to-face agreement) helps to increase the response rate. If the subject understands the purpose and need for their input or information, they are more likely to respond.[1]

The key points for an effective introduction are summarized in **Tables 7-4** and **7-5**. A well-defined and informative introduction may induce subjects to participate by appealing to their sense of responsibility and the importance of their information or input. The introduction statement should be concise, well written, informative, and easy to understand, as exemplified in **Exhibit 7-1**. The level of wording, grammar, and writing style should fit the subjects to be surveyed. Unless you are dealing with highly educated professional people, the introduction statement (like newspapers) should target an audience with middle school reading ability.

Proofreading and editing are essential. It is a good idea to have individuals who are not part of the investigation read and interpret the introduction, or an investigator may choose individuals who may be representative of the subject sample to review the introduction and provide feedback. For either choice, include the introductory statement in any prestudy evaluations or pretests of the survey instrument and pilot studies.

Table 7–4 Key Points for the Introductory Statement or Cover Letter

Key Point	Example
Who you are	Describe yourself and/or organization and/or business in the opening paragraph
Background for study	In our practice, we have been using an appointment system …
Purpose of the study	We want to learn …
What will be done with the data	The information you provide will help us to …
Why they were chosen	We are asking you to take part because …
Assurance of confidentiality	You do not have to identify yourself in any way. All information will be reported in aggregate. All responses will be coded for study purposes.
What respondents need to do	Please take a few minutes to complete the survey. Please follow the instructions for each question.
Who respondents can contact if they have questions	If you have any questions or concerns, please contact …
Approvals for the survey, if applicable	This study has been approved by the Institutional Review Board of …
Return deadlines	If possible, please complete and submit the survey by …
Statement of importance	The information you provide will be helpful in determining …
Acknowledge support	This study is supported by a grant from … This study is being conducted for ABC, Inc.
Statement of appreciation	We greatly appreciate your help in this matter and for taking the time to …
Closing	Sincerely, Your name, degree, titles
Signature	Co-investigators, degree, title

FOLLOW-UP

Follow-up notices or reminders to complete and return surveys may help to increase responses. A follow-up email, letter, or postcard can be used. Be aware of reminders for surveys that deal with sensitive or very private information. For example, an investigator is studying the rate of sexually transmitted diseases (STDs) in corporate executives who travel frequently. Any reminder must be private and protected from outside eyes. Good wording for such a reminder is "This is to remind you to take a few minutes to complete and return the survey we recently sent you." In the follow-up, add or use language that will encourage a response, such as, "Your opinion is very valuable to us, and we want to include your input in our study." The wording of reminders should be general and neutral to encourage survey completion and return. Do not threaten or even appear to be negative. For example, do not say, "If you do not complete and return the survey, no one will care what you think or know about STDs."

A follow-up or reminder should have enough information for the recipient to identify the survey. Alternately, the survey (or link to the survey) can be re-sent with the survey reminder note. How many reminders to send and when to send them should be part of the decision making that is done in the methodology planning for the research

Table 7–5 Construction of a Hard Copy Cover Letter

Construction Point	Explanation
Limit to one page.	The longer the letter is, the less likely it is to be read completely.
Use common block format with a readable font (e.g., Times New Roman, font size 12).	Script, serif, calligraphy, and the like are hard to read.
White, beige, or light gray paper, black print	Easy to read; visually pleasing.
Common language.	Readability and ease of understanding are key.

project. Although there are no hard-and-fast rules for follow-ups, 10 to 14 days is usually reasonable. Subsequent reminders can be sent at 4 weeks. More than two reminders is probably a waste of time.

Exhibit 7-1 Example of an Introductory Statement from the Author's Research

Dear < Participant >,

I invite you to participate in a survey on the importance of ranking health professions programs. You may access this survey by clicking on the URL below. You were selected to participate in this investigation by random selection from your professional organization's membership list. You do not have to identify yourself in any manner. Results will be reported in aggregate form. This is the first investigation on the opinion of health professionals on the ranking of educational programs. Your input will guide us in recommendations to the public and organizations. This investigation was approved as exempt by the IRB of State University. Please contact me at the address below if you have any questions.

Thank you,
J. D. Blessing

Exhibit 7-2 Example of a Reminder via Email or Mail

REMINDER

A few weeks ago you received a "Learning Assessment Survey" from me. It was distributed through your program via email. If you have not completed the survey, please take a few minutes to do so and hit the submit button. If you need the survey site, please contact me. The information you provide through this survey will be helpful to me in my study of how students learn and, hopefully, to education in the future.

Thank you for your time.

Dennis Blessing, State University
(123) 555-9776

Follow-up reminders can be done in several ways. One way is to send a reminder to everyone who was sent a survey. The other way is more economical if surveys have identification codes. If the survey is coded, the investigator can identify who has returned a survey and send follow-up reminders only to those subjects who have not responded. An explanation must be done for any codes that appear on a survey or a reminder. Subjects should be informed about what the number is and how it is used. Remember, if some type of code is used the respondents are not anonymous, but their information is kept confidential. **Exhibit 7-2** is an example of a reminder message used by the author.

TYPES OF SURVEYS

Web-Based Surveys

Web-based surveys have become the most common delivery method used to gather data on healthcare professionals. Typically, the survey is distributed using an email that contains a Web address (URL) for the survey. This format has become the norm. Two key advantages to

Table 7–6 Aspects of Web-Based Surveys

Aspect	Comment
Cost	Low; usual cost is a fee required by the Web company
Personnel	Investigators only; requires no training of interviewers or field workers
Sample size	Can be very large; can be general or a specific population set; can be geographically wide or distant from investigator; requires an email address and subjects must have a computer
Response rates	Potentially low; a response rate greater than 30 percent is rare[1]
Data	Potential for quantity, but quality is limited by respondent interpretation of survey items; only survey item data can be collected
Bias	Relies on respondent interpretation of survey items; nonrespondent bias is high
Subjects	Not under pressure to respond; less intrusive than person-to-person contact

Web-based surveys are (1) the sample size can be large and dispersed, and (2) a large amount of data can be collected. Another advantage of Web-based surveys is that results can be downloaded to a database, eliminating data entry and its associated errors, time, and costs. Major limitations of Web-based surveys are the potential for a low response rate and respondent misinterpretation of items. In addition, the target sample or population must have a computer. **Table 7–6** lists some of the positives and negatives of Web-based surveys.

An obvious advantage of Web-based surveys is that they can incorporate attractive photographs and illustrations in color that are difficult and costly to reproduce in print. A Web-based survey can be longer without increasing the costs of delivery. In fact, the cost of administering a Web-based survey is the hosting fee, which is not dependent on the amount of activity at the site. A number of commercial companies design surveys and help with data collection. Typically, these sites are user-friendly and economical if the investigator does not have the time, skill, or tools to develop their own surveys. Intuitively, it would seem that Web-based surveys are more cost-efficient, but some analyses bring this into question.[2] The Internet, Web knowledge, and computer skills of the investigator may affect overall costs.

Internet surveys are associated with certain advantages:

- Data are immediately available when the respondent submits the survey.
- Results can be loaded directly into a database for analysis.
- High-quality graphics and great detail can be used.
- Respondents can be "skipped" to appropriate items based on responses.
- Statistical analysis is facilitated because data are in a format for analysis.

Of course, one significant disadvantage of Internet surveys is that respondents must have a computer. The United States Census reports that 76.5% of US households have a computer with 71.7% with Internet access.[3] One limiting factor is that computer users tend to be adults younger than age 55. The rate for computer use by adults over 55 years drops to 61.7%.[3] Therefore, a consideration in using the Internet in survey research is the demographics of the study population. Sampling may also be a problem because access to Internet addresses or some form of notification is required to facilitate subjects to log on to an Internet survey. Email may be one way to contact subjects and provide an URL to a survey, or subjects may have to be contacted by direct mail. Whether or not response rates are higher with Internet surveys is open to question, and evaluations of Internet survey responses are mixed.[2]

Telephone Surveys

Political parties and pollsters seem to love telephone surveys, particularly near election time. Interviewing by telephone can provide very timely information. **Table 7-7** presents some key aspects of telephone interviewing as a survey format.

One obvious limitation of telephone surveys is that subjects must have a telephone. Telephone interviews allow for some personal contact between the respondent and the interviewer while maintaining a moderate level of anonymity. This may be very valuable when dealing with sensitive or personal information. Speaking directly with a subject allows the interviewer (or investigator) to interpret survey items, to move through the survey based on responses, and to clarify responses. Cost may be a major factor in telephone surveys because interviewers often must be trained and paid. Telephone costs increase if long distance is needed or if a large number of subjects must be contacted. The "annoyance factor" must be considered. Individuals may not want to be called or to have their routines interrupted by the phone ringing. The length of time a respondent is willing to be on the phone will influence their responses. The longer the subject is on the phone, the more likely they are to hang up.[1]

An investigator must also consider the type of responses that will be allowed in a telephone interview. Are subjects asked to respond to specific choices or are they allowed to respond in an unrestricted manner? Quantifying open-ended responses may present some analysis difficulties. Response recording must also be considered, particularly with open-ended questions. Remember, if a telephone interview is recorded, the respondent must be informed and agree.

Personal Interview Surveys

Person-to-person, face-to-face interviewing has a number of advantages and disadvantages

Table 7-7 Aspects of Telephone Surveys

Aspect	Comment
Cost	Actual telephone costs, such as long distance.
	Training costs of interviewers.
	Interviewer time costs.
Personnel	May require multiple interviewers.
	Interviewers can telephone from one location.
	Skilled interviewers get better and more complete responses.
Sample size	Subjects must have a telephone.
	Size determined by investigator and funding.
	Can be large.
	Can be geographically dispersed.
Response rates	Vary, due to willingness of subjects.
	Timing of call may influence willingness of respondent to participate.
Data	Potential for moderate amount and quality of data based on number of subjects willing to participate.
Bias	Interviewer's manner, voice inflections, and interpretation of survey items may influence subject responses.
Time	Study can be conducted over a short period of time.
	Responses are immediately available.

(**Table 7-8**). Interviews must occur where people are (e.g., office, mall, hospital room, home, clinic, school, etc.). Special sites can be utilized, but something must entice the subject/respondent to travel to a special site. If a special site is used for the survey, specific scheduled appointments for the interview may work best. Person-to-person interviewing requires contact between the subject and the investigator or interviewer.

Unlike a telephone respondent, who can be influenced by the interviewer's voice, a personal interview respondent can be influenced by the physical being and bearing of the interviewer and

Table 7–8 Aspects of Personal Interview Surveys

Aspect	Comment
Cost	High; takes time and people
Personnel	Requires training
Sample size	Tends to be relatively small because of the time needed to conduct interviews
Response rates	Can be high once respondents agree to be interviewed; face-to-face encounters may improve or facilitate response and allow for clarification of responses
Data	Varied, time may limit amount
Bias	Interviewer bias, interviewer influence on subject
Time	Training and interviews take time

the site of the interview. In addition, the interviewer's voice inflections, facial and body movements, personality, and animation may influence responses. For these reasons, interviewer training must be more exact and extensive. Supervision of interviewers may be required. Risk of interviewer bias is high. The time needed to train interviewers and the required time for interviews are factors to consider in personal interviews.

Interviews can be used to collect qualitative and quantitative data. They can allow for greater exploration of subject responses and can add detail that may help interpret or understand responses. Certainly, if a product is being investigated, subjects can see and handle the product. The types of allowed responses must be considered in a personal interview process. How responses are handled is something that should be planned for as part of the methodology. A decision on how responses will be handled cannot be made after data collection.

✳ SURVEY ITEM CONSTRUCTION

Survey items must provide data that answer the research questions, hypotheses, or null hypotheses. Before any survey is constructed, much less applied, the purposes of the study must be defined. Generally, the best format for defining and guiding survey research is to use research question(s) or hypotheses as outlined in **Table 7–9**. This does not exclude use of null hypotheses.

Table 7–9 Definitions

Type	Definition	Example
Null hypothesis[4]	A negatively worded statement about the relationship among or between variables. It does not necessarily mean or refer to zero or no difference, but provides a hypothesis that is "rejected" or "accepted."	There is no difference in 5-year myocardial infarct rates between angina patients treated with a calcium channel blocker (CCB) and those treated with a beta-blocker.
Hypothesis[4]	A statement about the relationship among or between variables. This statement may be a conjecture or prediction of a relationship or outcome.	Patients with angina who are treated with a CCB will have a lower number of myocardial infarctions after 5 years than patients treated with beta-blockers.
Research question	Similar to a hypothesis, but is constructed as a question.	Will angina patients treated with a CCB have fewer myocardial infarctions after 5 years than patients treated with a beta-blocker?

Without a well-developed and defined research question, hypothesis, or null hypothesis, a well-designed survey cannot be developed. As a survey item is constructed, the investigator must ask, "How does the information or data gathered by this item help me answer my research question, hypothesis, or null hypothesis?" If the survey item does not provide part of the answer to the research question, it is not needed.

DEMOGRAPHIC DATA

Surveys almost always collect some type of demographic data. In many instances, the demographic data provide the basis for comparison groups. Demographics can be used to define and identify your study sample. Some common types of demographic data are age, gender, occupation, and education. For healthcare professionals, some types of demographic data are practice location, practice specialty, length of time in practice, number of patients seen, and procedures performed. Demographic data are the information that describes or characterizes the subject, sample, or population in some way. Demographics often strengthen the extrapolation of a sample result to a population by demonstrating how similar the sample is to the population. Most demographic data comprise nominal data. In the past, demographic information was usually collected at the beginning of the survey, but there is no reason it cannot be collected at the end. In an interview setting, it may be best to get to the heart of the survey first and save the routine demographics for the end.

Demographic survey items should be straightforward questions about the information sought. Here are some examples:

- What is your gender?
- How old are you?
- What degree did you receive from your program?
- What is your practice specialty?
- How long have you been in practice?

When constructing these survey items, a direct response is probably better than using a range as a choice. An example is age. You may want to group respondents by age, but it is better to have each respondent give their exact age and then group the responses if that method fits the project needs. **Box 7-1** gives an example.

Box 7-1 Example: Age Demographic Questions

What is your age in years? _____

Versus

What is your age group in years?
A. 21–25
B. 26–30
C. 31–35
D. 36–40
E. > 40

When collecting sensitive or private information, however, it may be better to group responses. One example is the salary demographic. Respondents may be more willing to provide salary data in a range rather than their exact salary. This provides some degree of privacy. Data in ranges may also be useful when respondents cannot recall information precisely, as shown in the example in **Box 7-2**.

Box 7-2 Example: Salary Question

What is your annual salary? _____

Versus

What is your annual salary?
A. < $25,000
B. $25,000–49,999
C. $50,000–74,999
D. > $75,000

The following are some points to remember when gathering demographic data:

- Be specific with the statements or questions. Specify the unit of measure. For

example, if time-related information is sought, specify whether the time interval is in weeks, days, months, or years.
- When using ranges, make sure they do not overlap; this could lead to confusion. Using salary as an example, how can a respondent accurately answer the question shown in **Box 7-3**, when the options overlap?

Box 7-3 Example: Unclear Salary Question

What is your annual salary?

A. $50,000 or less
B. $50,000–60,000
C. $60,000–70,000
D. $70,000–80,000
E. $80,000 or more

- Avoid asking for the same data in more than one statement or question.
- Use short, to-the-point, but understandable statements or questions.
- Ask only for information that is relevant to the study. The construct of a survey item should make it clear to the respondent why a piece of data is needed for the investigation. Do not be overly invasive unless the data are essential to the project.

THE SURVEY INSTRUMENT

The heart of the survey consists of items that provide the data for the investigation. The construct of these items influences respondent rates, willingness to answer, and quality of the data for analysis. Survey items that provide unequivocal data help ensure reliability and validity. *Survey items must be short, clear, exact, understandable, and answerable.* Items must be designed to provide the data needed to answer the research questions, hypotheses, or null hypotheses. An investigator must decide on a format for the survey items and questions; however, it is not unusual for surveys to include a variety of item formats.

First Things First

Developing survey items is a process that goes from very general to very specific. One way to start is to sit down and write down every possible question even remotely related to the investigation. This brainstorming approach helps develop a list of considerations for the survey. This list does not have to be neat, orderly, grammatically correct, or even very specific; it is the beginning of the critical thinking for the development and building of the survey. A brainstorming list is often very expansive and far longer than the final product. Team members and colleagues can provide valuable assistance at this stage. Seek consultation on ideas and specific points, if needed. Good research surveys are rarely the result of one person's efforts.

Once general thoughts have been recorded, the investigator can begin to edit, define, delete, combine, categorize, and develop the specific survey items. Refining the survey and its items is often a long process, always aimed toward improving the survey. Although there is always room for improvement, at some point development has to stop and the survey must be finalized before it is administered. One question that may help decide when a survey is ready is: Does each survey item provide some aspect of the answer to the research question?

Item Format

The format of survey items is dependent on the information sought. There are two basic forms of survey items: structured and unstructured (or open-ended).[1] Some examples of open-ended questions are listed in **Box 7-4**.

Box 7-4 Example: Open-Ended Questions

1. What do you think are the benchmarks for a quality medical practice?
2. What do you do to stay up-to-date for your practice?
3. What is the best way to deal with noncompliant patients?

Table 7–10 Examples of Survey Item Formats[1,5,6]

Item Format	Example
List responses	A checklist of responses or multiple choices.
Semantic differential scale	A scale defined by its extremes, with a range between the extremes.
Comparison scale	Choice between two or more items.
Visual analogue scale	Indicates the intensity of a subjective experience along a continuum.
Picture scale	Series of pictures/drawings indicate a response; may be useful for children or people who cannot read.
Forced ranking	All items in a list are ranked.
Ranking versus rating	With rank items, each ranking value is used once; rating values may be repeated for different items.

These types of questions may remind healthcare professionals (and students) of the essay questions that everyone hated (or hates) in school. Open-ended questions certainly have value, but they may be difficult to quantify or interpret. Structured survey items, in contrast, allow the investigator to control responses to a large degree as well as define the responses as values that are more statistically useful to the study. The formats of structured survey items vary; examples are presented in **Table 7–10**.

The choice of format depends on the data sought. When constructing the survey items and the possible responses to those survey items, it is important to state whether more than one option can be selected. This prevents misunderstanding by the respondents. **Box 7-5** provides an example

---

Box 7-5 Example: Wording Format

What activity do you prefer for earning CEUs?

(Check all that apply.)

A. _____ Formal lectures
B. _____ Hands-on exercises
C. _____ On-the-job experiences or consultations
D. _____ Patient/case studies
E. _____ Seminars/expert panels

Versus

What activity do you most prefer for earning CEUs?

(Check only one.)

A. _____ Formal lectures
B. _____ Hands-on exercises
C. _____ On-the-job experiences or consultations
D. _____ Patient/case studies
E. _____ Seminars/expert panels

---

using activities related to earning continuing education units (CEUs).

Generally, ranking is a more robust method for obtaining meaningful results.

Specific wording can be used in the item stem, as shown in **Box 7-6**. (The items in Box 7-5 also could be worded in this manner.)

Box 7-6 Example: Alternate Wording

Check all the activities you prefer for earning CEUs.

Versus

Check the one activity you most prefer for earning CEUs.

In developing survey items, an investigator must try to eliminate subject interpretation errors as much as possible. Ultimately, no investigator can guess how respondents will interpret what is written or asked. It may be clear to the investigator but not to the subjects. A pilot test helps reduce interpretation errors.

Rankings

The ranking of responses is valuable in many cases. An example using the previous material may resemble the example presented in **Box 7-7**.

In this case, the investigator ensures that the ranking numbers (1–5) are defined and specifies whether or not all items should be ranked. This example could state "Rank in order of preference those items you use to earn CEUs: 1 = most preferred, 5 = least preferred. Do not rank items you do not use." This may be a long statement, but it clarifies both what data are sought and what the respondent is to do. In some instances, it may be desirable to rate some items with the same value. Two examples of the rating approach are given in **Box 7-8** and **Box 7-9**.

Box 7-7 Example: Ranking

Rank each activity in the order of your preferences for earning CEUs.

(1 = most preferred, 5 = least preferred)

Rank all items.
A. _____ Formal lectures
B. _____ Hands-on exercises
C. _____ On-the-job experiences or consultations
D. _____ Patient/case studies
E. _____ Seminars/expert panels

Box 7-8 Example: Rating

Rate the value to you of each of the following CEU delivery formats.

(Rate all)

1 = Preferred, 2 = Acceptable, 3 = Not preferred
_____ A. Lecture
_____ B. Workshop
_____ C. Video
_____ D. Computer program
_____ E. Monographs

Box 7-9 Example: Alternate Rate Format

Rate the value of each of the following CEU delivery formats.

Rate all items 1–5, with 1 being the most valuable and 5 being the least valuable.
_____ Lecture
_____ Workshop
_____ Video
_____ Computer program
_____ Monographs

In some instances a two-level question may be a better construct, where respondents indicate "preferred" items, then rank their preferred choices.

Ranking or rating systems should be defined clearly. Using the number 1 is a common format for the most preferred or highest value, but sometimes a reverse rating (e.g., 5 as the most preferred to 1 as the least preferred) may be useful or desired. The instructions to the respondents must be very clear. The item format must be completely consistent. If more than one item format is used, group similar format items together. This not only is space-efficient, but also will help in survey presentation and will be less likely to confuse respondents.

The Likert and Verbal Frequency Scales

Verbal frequency scales are very common tools in survey research. One of the most common types of verbal frequency scales is the Likert Scale (pronounced Lickert). This is an ordinal scale used to gather information about respondents' opinions or positions on the subject under investigation. The true Likert Scale uses the values shown in **Box 7-10**.

The descriptors can be reversed where descriptor 1 is *strongly disagree* and 5 is *strongly agree*. Remember, the number does not matter because this is ordinal data, not continuous data; however, these types of scales are often treated as interval

Box 7-10   The Likert Scale

1. Strongly agree
2. Agree
3. Neutral
4. Disagree
5. Strongly disagree

data in large samples with normal distributions. Analysis by parametric tests may be misleading. A statistician should be consulted with regard to handling ordinal data as continuous data.

Investigators sometimes use a scale similar to this one, but with different descriptors or an increase in the number of descriptors. In these cases, the scale should be termed a "Likert-like scale" or, more accurately, a "verbal frequency scale."[1] An example of a verbal frequency scale with regard to angiotensin-converting enzyme (ACE) inhibitors used for treatment of high blood pressure is given in **Box 7-11**.

Box 7-11   Example: Verbal Frequency Scale

How often are ACE inhibitors given as the first drug in hypertension therapy?

A. Always
B. Often
C. Occasionally
D. Infrequently
E. Never

Regardless of the descriptors used, verbal frequency scales are very powerful and popular research tools.[1] **Table 7-11** lists keys for using verbal frequency scales.

Items in a verbal frequency scale ask the respondent to state his or her level of agreement with that item. However, a verbal frequency scale may indicate some responses other than agreement. Likert and other scales are generally used with a series of related survey items. Instructions for respondents should lead with a direction statement such

Table 7-11 The Likert and Verbal Frequency Scales: Keys for Their Successful Use

Be clear in the instructions.
Use direct statements.
Avoid redundancy.
Address one element in each item.
Group survey items in sets of 5–10.
Make sure word responses are appropriate for the item statement or question and scale responses are logical.
Allow for neutral responses if possible.
Use terms that are easily understood.
Be consistent in format as much as possible.
Avoid overlap of grouped responses, and make sure response options are logical for the questions asked.
Have a survey pilot tested or reviewed by expert.
Always proofread everything that is distributed to subjects.
Make it short and simple; the shorter the survey, the more likely it will be completed.
Number the pages: 1 of 4, 2 of 4, etc.
Allow respondents to comment at the end of the survey.

as, "Indicate your level of agreement or disagreement to the following statements." **Box 7-12** is an example from the author's research.[7]

In addition, the instructions should ask respondents to respond to all survey items. Unanswered items lead to questions of validity, extrapolation, and analysis. Before the survey is administered, investigators should make a plan to handle nonresponses in the analysis.

When constructing survey items, ensure that the statement can be answered by the scale used. Avoid redundancy. Each item should address only one idea or concept. An example of a conflicting statement is shown in **Box 7-13**.

The statement in Box 7-13 contains two separate components. A respondent may agree that ranking benefits society but disagree that ranking should be part of accreditation. Item clarity is key to accurate responses and sound interpretation of results.

Box 7-12 Verbal Frequency Scale

For each of the following items concerning the ranking of programs, indicate your degree of agreement or disagreement using the Likert scale:

1. Strongly Agree 2. Agree 3. Neutral 4. Disagree 5. Strongly Disagree

	SA	A	N	D	SD
1. Physician assistant programs should be ranked.	1	2	3	4	5
2. Ranking programs will benefit society.	1	2	3	4	5
3. Ranking programs will help ensure the quality of PA education.	1	2	3	4	5
4. Only the top 25 ranked programs should be published.	1	2	3	4	5
5. The rankings of all programs should be published.	1	2	3	4	5
6. Program rank should be a component for accreditation.	1	2	3	4	5
7. Ranking creates ill will or loss of collegiality among programs.	1	2	3	4	5
8. Ranking creates unnecessary competition among programs.	1	2	3	4	5

Box 7-13 Example: Conflicting Statement

Ranking health professions programs will benefit society and should be part of accreditation decisions.

When using verbal frequency scales, be sure that the choices reflect the responses that will provide the information needed by the investigation. Some examples of descriptors used in verbal frequency scales are given in **Box 7-14**.

For some surveys, choices of "Not Applicable," "Unsure," "No Answer," "Unknown," and the like may be needed. In some instances more or less than five responses may be needed. Regardless, there must be consistency in the options presented. Items and their responses must provide adequate choices along a continuum for the subjects' responses. Consistency allows for appropriate analysis, which leads to more accurate conclusions.

Another key to developing survey items is that each item should have an equal number of positive and negative responses with a neutral response, if possible. This is not always necessary. For example, not offering the opportunity for a neutral response forces the subject to make a choice. This is called a *forced response*. One risk of the forced response approach is that respondents who are neutral may not answer. Therefore, decisions must be made as to whether the risk of a respondent not answering the question is acceptable or whether a neutral or noncommittal response is acceptable. Another option is to have a choice such as "does not apply" or "no experience" or "no knowledge."

Box 7-14 Descriptors for Verbal Frequency Scale

Very Satisfied	Satisfied	Neutral	Dissatisfied	Very Dissatisfied
Very Good	Good	Neutral	Poor	Very Poor
Highly Positive	Positive	Neutral	Negative	Highly Negative
Excellent	Good	Fair	Poor	Very Poor
Very Important	Important	Somewhat Important		Not Important

PUTTING THE SURVEY TOGETHER

Once the research question has been developed, the appropriate literature search completed, the methodology designed, and the survey items developed, the survey has to be constructed. Some type of introduction must be first. Few people will respond to a survey that begins with just the survey items. This is true for Web-based surveys, paper surveys, telephone surveys, and face-to-face interviews. For Web-based and paper surveys, a plain, easily read, black print on white background introduction is probably best. If a colored background is desired, light beige or gray may be acceptable. The survey should be organized so that like items are grouped, particularly if some type of scale is used. Demographic questions, in the past, have been presented first, but recent trends have moved toward placing them at the end of the survey. It is the investigator's decision.

Assess the visual quality of the survey. Does it appear organized with well-defined borders, sections, and the like? Ensure the method of submission is clear. The submit button for an Internet survey must be very apparent and visible. A decision must be made about whether respondents already logged in to Web-based surveys can log out and return to the survey later. Proofread everything, and then have someone else proofread the survey. It is difficult to proofread one's own work, particularly if the work has been repeatedly reviewed by its developer.

PILOT TESTING THE SURVEY

A pilot test is an excellent way to help ensure the survey is understandable and the survey items gather the data desired, but a large group of subjects is not needed. Ask pilot test subjects to evaluate the survey, that is, give feedback on their feelings, interpretations, and suggestions for improvement. The pilot-test group or a separate group can participate in a focus group for review, feedback, and critical comment. Do not take critical review personally. The critical review is an important step toward making the survey as perfect as possible.

Some of the things to ask pilot study or focus group participants are:

- Are there too many survey items?
- Is the time needed to complete the survey too long?
- Are the survey items clear, concise, and easy to understand?
- Are item responses appropriate for the survey item?
- Are the directions for completion clear and understandable?
- Does the survey provide the data and information sought?
- Are there biased responses or leading items?
- Is the survey format visually acceptable or pleasing?
- Are there suggestions for improvement?

Remember that even before a pilot study, appropriate institutional approval is required. Institutional review board (IRB) or research ethics committee approval must be obtained in writing and maintained in study files. If approval by the IRB, research ethics committee, or another body is required, do not conduct the survey until approval is granted in writing. To do so, even if approval is forthcoming, would be unethical. Once all of these small steps are completed, start the study.

When results begin to accumulate, work on the investigation regularly. The most efficacious way to proceed is to set aside a specific period each day for working on the project. Keep good records, protect confidentiality, do the follow-ups, and set a deadline after which no further data will be accepted. Data cannot continually be added indefinitely. At some point, data analyses must start. Once analyses are completed, the conclusions can be drawn. *Remember:* If the methodology is sound, the analyses are appropriate, confounding variables are controlled, and study biases are minimized, the results are the results. As a researcher, the search is for "truth," not "hoped for" outcomes. Ultimately, the most that the majority of research efforts contribute is just one very small piece in the universe of knowledge.

HOW MANY SUBJECTS?

How many people (subjects) should be surveyed? This is a simple question, but a tough one to answer. If the population of interest is small, survey the entire population. One good example of a fairly easy population to sample is a specific healthcare profession's educational programs. Another example might be all of the occupational therapists who work only in nursing homes in communities with a population of less than 5000. In these cases, the sample and the population are the same. In some instances, a convenience sample may be used. As the name implies, the sample subjects are convenient for the investigator to survey. One example is faculty members who survey students in their program or classes. These subjects are convenient; however, a convenience sample may *not* be representative of a population. In this example, students in a healthcare profession program may be demographically different from students in another or similar program. A convenience sample presents problems with extrapolation to the larger population. Convenience samples are of very limited benefit.

An investigator wants the sample to represent the population to be studied. However, consideration of costs and logistics in setting the sample size must be part of the methodology. In other words, an investigator has to be able to afford the costs of the study and to handle the survey distribution and analysis. Remember, a larger number of respondents does not necessarily increase accuracy of the results; a good response rate from a smaller sample may be better; however, the sample must represent the population. Small sample groups are more likely to be different from the population than large or multiple sample groups.[1] The survey instrument must be valid and reliable.

Confidence Level and Interval

Every investigator has to accept the fact that there is always a chance of error. There are some ways to try to control some inherent errors. First, set a confidence level and a confidence interval. (See **Box 7-15**.)

The confidence level is usually set at 95% or 99%. This means that one can state with 95%

> **Box 7-15 Confidence Level and Interval**
>
> Confidence level: A desired percentage of scores that falls within a certain range of confidence limits. It is calculated by subtracting the alpha level from 1 and multiplying the result by 100.[7]
>
> Confidence interval: A range of values of a sample statistic that is likely to contain a population parameter. The wider the interval, the higher the confidence level.[7]

or 99% confidence that the results are within the margin of error. The confidence interval is the margin of error, usually expressed as a range (e.g., 3–5). The size of the population must be known. With these pieces of information, the sample size can be calculated. Many statistical texts and websites have tools for determining sample size. Some statistical computer programs will do the job. If there is difficulty in determining sample size, consult a statistician.

WHAT STATISTICS TO USE?

Again, it may be wise to consult a statistician to determine the best statistical tests to use for analysis of the results. Statistical tests can be bewildering, and most of us need help from an expert. However, make the analysis decisions part of the initial planning for the methodology, not after the data are collected. Consult a statistician early in the planning. Demographic data can be presented as percentages and, if necessary, can be compared to known population data. This is a good way to demonstrate the sample is similar to the population of interest.

Another key to successful survey strategies is to understand what the statistical tests mean and what they demonstrate. Use statistical tests that fit the data and meet the study needs. The questions about evaluating ordinal data with continuous data analysis is one of contention within the healthcare research community.

SUMMARY

Surveys can provide a wealth of useful information. Survey research requires the same attention to detail as any other part of any research project. The same process is used in survey research as with any other type of research. Survey and survey item construction are the keys to success.

REFERENCES

1. Alreck PL, Settle RB. *The Survey Research Handbook*. 2nd ed. Boston, MA: Irwin McGraw-Hill; 1995.
2. Sharp K. White papers: Public sector use of Internet surveys and panels. Available at: http://www.decisionanalyst.com/Downloads/PublicSectorUseofInternetSurveys.pdf. Accessed September 8, 2014.
3. US Census Bureau. Computer and Internet Use in the United States, May 2013. Available at: http://www.census.gov/prod/2013pubs/p2-569.pdf. Accessed September 8, 2014.
4. Fricker RD Jr, Schonlau M. Advantages and disadvantages of Internet research surveys: Evidence from the literature. *Field Methods*. 2002;14(4):347–367.
5. Cui WW. Reducing error in mail surveys. *Practical Assess Res Eval*. 2003;8(18). Available at: http://pareonline.net/getvn.asp?v=8&n=18&cmd=View+Article. Accessed September 8, 2014.
6. Blessing JD, Hooker RS, Jones PE, Rahr RR. An investigation of potential criteria for ranking physician assistant programs. *Persp Phys Asst Educ*. 2001;12(3):160–166.
7. Vogt WP. *Dictionary of Statistics and Methodology*. 2nd ed. Thousand Oaks, CA: Sage; 1999.

CHAPTER 8

Qualitative Research

Elsa M. González, PhD
J. Glenn Forister, MS, PA-C

CHAPTER OVERVIEW

The complexity of the healthcare environment often demands a different methodology than the quantitative approach. The purpose of this chapter is to provide an introduction and overview of qualitative research as it relates to health care. The terminology in qualitative research differs from that of quantitative research, so a comparison of terms is provided. This chapter also discusses how to design and implement an essential qualitative investigation in health care, as well as some appropriate ways to assess the quality of a qualitative study.

Learning Objectives

- Define qualitative research.
- Discuss the differences between qualitative research and quantitative research.
- Describe when a qualitative design is the preferred methodology for a project.
- List and discuss the techniques used in qualitative research.
- Design a research project combining qualitative and quantitative methods.

INTRODUCTION

Qualitative research answers different kinds of questions than does quantitative research. Quantitative studies answer questions that begin with the words "how much" or "how many."[1] In contrast, qualitative studies answer questions that begin with the words "what," "how," or "why." The two approaches are often complementary in healthcare studies. When both types of investigation are employed concurrently, the study is termed a *mixed-methodological* study.[2]

Historically, many healthcare researchers have criticized and avoided qualitative methods. Those investigators believed that all research should be objective and that subjectivity should be eliminated to ensure reliable findings.[3] However, healthcare researchers are becoming more familiar with qualitative methodologies; their potential to enhance understanding of the phenomenon that patients, physicians, nurses, and others face; and the expansion of the knowledge obtained quantitatively.[3]

In many cases, healthcare professionals are interested in objective proof that a treatment works. Quantitative studies are the preferred way to measure such outcomes. However, healthcare professionals treat human beings, unique individuals who are suffering and feeling in different ways. Qualitative studies shift the investigation away from the lab and into settings where the care is rendered. Truth is revealed in human experiences rather than in blood tests or imaging. Interviews and observations are used to collect data. The patient interview and observation are familiar ways to gather data about medical conditions; however, interviews and observations can reveal much more than the patient's health history. Healthcare professionals may choose a qualitative research approach to study such topics as:

- The human experiences of illness
- The human experiences of care
- Interactions among clinicians, patients, and families
- Lifestyle interventions
- Quality of life
- Cross-cultural perspectives
- The caregivers' experience

Qualitative investigations can produce meaningful results that humanize and alter healthcare practice. The purpose of this chapter is to provide an introduction to essential qualitative research as it relates to health care.

A multitude of terms fall under the umbrella of *qualitative research* including approaches such as case studies, naturalistic inquiry, phenomenology, ethnography, grounded theory, life history, content analysis, and narrative analysis.[1,4] The authors acknowledge this chapter is introductory and risks oversimplifying complex topics related to various qualitative methodologies. However, it is possible to introduce many of the key aspects of qualitative research by discussing an essential qualitative study.[1] After completing this chapter, the reader should recognize the applied qualitative process in healthcare research and be able to discuss how to understand and critically evaluate a qualitative study. Those individuals interested in becoming qualitative researchers will need to seek additional training and resources beyond this introductory text. At the end of this chapter, a list of references and additional readings are provided for that purpose.

PHILOSOPHICAL PERSPECTIVE

In contrast to the rationalistic or positivist paradigm of quantitative research, qualitative research falls within intepretivism, also called constructivist paradigm. The paradigm operates on the assumptions of subjective reality and multiple truths, rather than an objective reality and a single truth.[5] Furthermore, the paradigm values the lived experiences of individuals.[5] For this reason, interpretive study designs are sometimes more suitable than rationalistic and traditional designs to understand the human being and his/her experiences. Although many approaches to qualitative research exist, naturalistic approaches focusing on the clinical environment are well suited for healthcare research. The primary purpose of such studies is to understand and interpret reality as defined by individuals through their experiences in natural settings.[1]

COMPARING QUANTITATIVE AND QUALITATIVE RESEARCH IN THE HEALTHCARE FIELD

Qualitative research can feel foreign to individuals accustomed to the traditional quantitative perspective, particularly in the healthcare field. Although the two approaches are often complementary, it is important to understand some key differences between qualitative and quantitative studies in this field. To some extent, the researcher's role, reasoning, sampling, data collection, analysis, reporting, and study validation measures differ between quantitative and qualitative studies. **Table 8-1** outlines some of the key characteristics of these two

Table 8–1 Key Differences Between Quantitative and Qualitative Studies in Health Care[5]

Element	Quantitative	Qualitative
Researcher's involvement	Detached	Participatory
Researcher's stance	Objectivity	Subjective confirmability
Setting	Controlled	Naturalistic
Sampling	Random population-based	Case-based/purposeful
Methodology	Positivist method	Naturalistic inquiry
Data	Numbers	Words
Analysis and reasoning	Hypothesis testing Deductive	Hypothesis generation/working hypothesis Inductive
Reporting	Statistics	Themes/categories
Study validation	Internal and external validity	Trustworthiness

Table 8–2 A Comparison of Quantitative and Qualitative Studies Terminology Regarding Validation and Rigor[5]

Traditional Terminology	Qualitative Terminology	Purpose
External validity (generalizability)	Transferability	Establishes a relationship between the study's results and the world outside of the study
Internal validity	Credibility	Ensures the study's processes are performed in an appropriate and rigorous manner
Reliability	Dependability	Signifies the level of confidence in the study's data collection methods
Objective reproducibility	Confirmability	Assesses the ability of researchers to accomplish a similar study and replicate the results

methodologies in the healthcare field. Furthermore, the terminology used by qualitative researchers often differs from the terminology used by quantitative researchers. **Table 8–2** includes a comparison between terms regarding rigor and validity in both traditions.

Researcher's Role

One of the key beliefs of positivism is that the researcher is objective and distant. Interpretivism, however, does not require adherence to the belief in objectivity.[5] The qualitative researcher gains access to the participants' natural environment and is the main research instrument used to collect data. Subjectivity is seen as valuable and inevitable; however, the qualitative researcher also understands that bias may influence study outcomes. Acknowledging that it is difficult to eliminate bias, qualitative researchers present their biases "up front" in a positionality statement that is included with the study results.[1]

This positionality statement allows subjectivity to be revealed and gives the reader the opportunity to consider the researcher's stance in relation to the research findings.[5] The positionality statement typically includes the researcher's assumptions, values, and reasons for choosing the research topic. The researcher reflects on potential biases and makes them transparent to the reader. Quantitative investigations rarely contain such explicit descriptions of the researcher's views. In contrast to the quantitative researcher who relies on the assumption of objectivity, the qualitative researcher relies on confirmability and transferability,[6] a topic discussed later in this chapter.

Settings

Many quantitative investigations occur in laboratory settings where potentially extraneous influences on the study's outcome can be controlled. Traditional researchers working outside of the lab also attempt to control the participants' environment. In contrast, qualitative investigations often take place in natural social settings without imposing controls. Healthcare settings are a source of rich qualitative data. An investigation may occur in a single setting or multiple settings. For example, an investigator may interview several patients in a single dialysis center or conduct focus group interviews in multiple centers. Researchers can observe different treatment settings and explore how patients experience health care in those settings.

Sampling

In quantitative studies, researchers seek to provide answers for a population by using a statistical representative random sample, a process called generalization.[7] Although these researchers obtain their samples in different ways, the most common approach is through random population sampling. Random sampling is performed to minimize the chance of forming a participant group that differs from the population from which the sample is drawn.

In contrast, most qualitative researchers employ nonrandom purposeful sampling to select sources of rich data. Qualitative researchers may study the story of a single individual or the experiences of a large group of individuals. When sampling, qualitative researchers consider the comparisons and distinctions needed to answer their research questions.[8] The individuals sampled may have shared and differing characteristics with each other. Therefore, the researcher may wish to limit the study to a homogenous group, or may purposefully sample individuals who are heterogeneous to provide for maximum variation and representation.[9] In contrast to quantitative researchers, who often determine the size of their samples based on statistical measures, qualitative investigators initially estimate how many participants are needed to reach thematic saturation.[5] Thematic saturation occurs when the information obtained is redundant and no new information is forthcoming.[10]

Methodology

Traditional/positivist research designs include pre-experimental, experimental, and quasi-experimental designs. Quantitative investigations test for group differences, variable relationships, and causal explanations. In contrast, qualitative methodologies are primarily exploratory and descriptive.[5] Many of these methodologies are designed to find meaning and evaluate social settings.[4] Some of the more common qualitative research approaches include naturalistic inquiry, grounded theory, ethnography, phenomenology, and action-oriented research.[2] Naturalistic studies focus on the realities associated with real contexts.[6] Grounded theory generates theoretical explanations for social phenomena.[2] Ethnography explores the activities and relations within cultural groups.[2] Phenomenology looks to understand a particular phenomenon in a particular context of a group, community, or society. Action-oriented research seeks solutions to local practical problems.[2] Most importantly, qualitative investigators use the methodology that fits the research purpose and research questions.

Data Types

Quantitative researchers measure things. The different types (scales) of quantitative data include nominal, ordinal, interval, and ratio. In contrast, qualitative researchers collect data from a variety of sources using different methods such as interviewing, observation, and document analysis.[6] Words, images, non-verbal communication, documents, and artifacts; not numbers, are the data.

Analysis and Reasoning

Traditional research involves hypothesis testing. The researcher forms a hypothesis prior to collecting data; this timing is called *a priori* or before the fact. In contrast, as qualitative studies evolve, working hypotheses are generated and are not based on a priori hypothesis testing. Qualitative researchers use inductive, not deductive, reasoning. In traditional investigations, the analyses are based on descriptive and inferential statistics; however, the qualitative approach to analysis is interpretive. The ultimate purpose of qualitative data analysis is to answer the research questions through methods such as content analysis, narrative analysis, and discursive analysis, among others.[1]

Reporting

Traditional results are reported using various numeric values such as the mean, standard deviation, and p value. Quantitative results are often presented in tables and graphs. In contrast, qualitative results are presented as themes, not statistical results. The final thematic structure emerges through induction and is supported by units of meaning.[1] Many qualitative reports are organized by the research questions and are supported by direct quotes from the study's participants, which constitute the data or units of meaning.

APPLYING QUALITATIVE RESEARCH IN HEALTH CARE

Now that the differences between quantitative and qualitative research have been presented, the remainder of the chapter will review the essential steps of qualitative research. One approach of qualitative research that healthcare researchers use is the case study. The case study design is well suited to reporting qualitative research findings and generating working hypotheses.[5] Case studies in health care may resonate with the reader in a way that is concrete, contextual, and participatory.[1] Case studies are defined by the unit of analysis and any bounding conditions or criteria.[11] The unit of analysis can be an event, a person, a group, a program, an institution, or a process.[11] Bounding conditions can be geographic, temporal, or concrete.[11] For example, a case could be defined by a group of patients who are bounded by a shared medical diagnosis and specific treatment location.

Figure 8-1 illustrates the flow of a basic qualitative study. The research purpose allows the investigator to define the research questions. The research questions then drive the methodology and methods of the study. In Figure 8-1, a purposeful sample is obtained and different data collection methods are used. Data collected during the study are then systematically managed and analyzed. This process includes breaking the large volume of data into small units of meaning and then reassembling the units into emergent categories and themes.

The figure includes the option to use a computer or index cards to carry out this process. These options are a matter of personal choice; many times choices depend on the volume of data. In each case, the ultimate goal is to generate a report that contains rich data organized thematically to capture the essence of the case studied. The report should address the research questions and contain excerpts of data that support the researchers' results, conclusions, and recommendations.

Suggested Steps for an Essential Qualitative Study

1. Identify the research problem.
2. Define the purpose of the study and design the research questions.
3. Ensure the study design is consistent with the research purpose and research questions.
4. Complete a literature review on the topic and identify the theoretical framework.
5. Refine the research purpose and questions.
6. Reflect on potential personal biases, values, and assumptions.
7. Consider how participant sampling will occur.
8. Give a rationale for participant selection and define the criteria.
9. Obtain institutional review board (IRB) approval for the study.

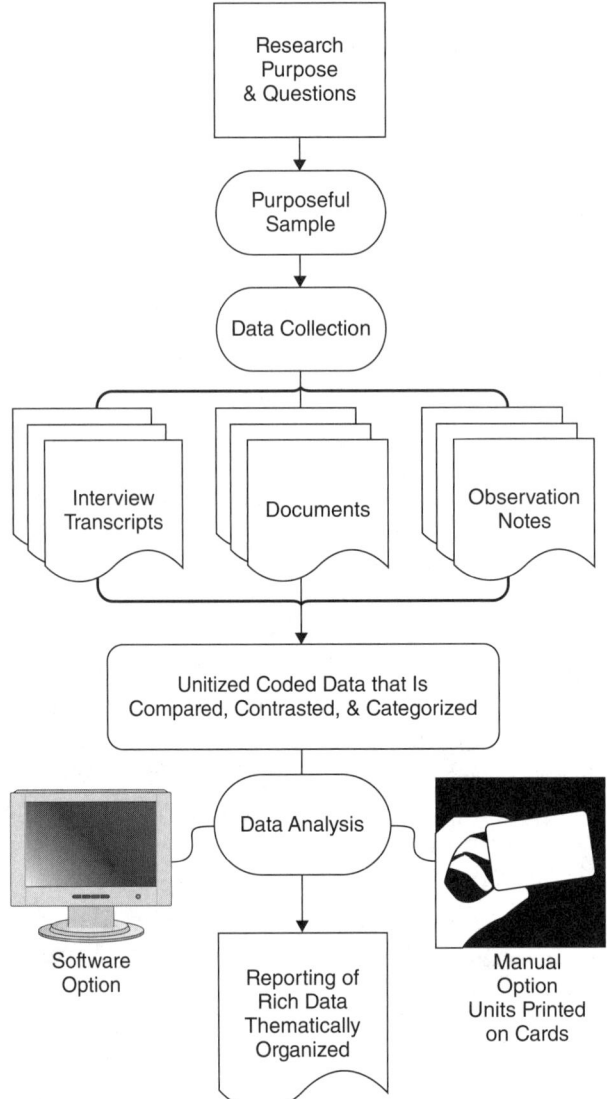

Figure 8–1 Flow of an essential qualitative study.

10. Gain access to participants.
11. Choose data collection methods (observation, interviews, and/or document analysis).
12. Obtain informed consent from the study participants.
13. Collect a comprehensive data set (transcripts, field notes, and documents).
14. Assess the adequacy and depth of the data collected considering the research questions.
15. Divide data into smallest units of meaning (unitize).
16. Analyze data and assemble information into categories and themes using constant comparative analysis, content analysis, and inductive reasoning.
17. Evaluate the theoretical framework/value of the results (novel theory, supports known theory, refutes known theory).

18. Define the clinical utility of the study in relation to similar patients or contexts and research questions
19. Conduct the study in a systematic, auditable manner.
20. Report results, conclusions, and recommendations.

Qualitative Design and Implementation

The design plan must be flexible and adapt to field conditions; the design in qualitative research is called "emergent design."[6] Despite this flexibility, some preplanning is required. The initial plan includes gaining access, participant sampling, data collection, data management, data analysis, and trustworthiness techniques to be used.[6,8,12]

Access

Investigators need to consider how they will access study sites by negotiating effectively with institutional gatekeepers.[5] Some researchers may ask questions that are sensitive and intrusive. Gatekeepers may refuse access when the investigation covers delicate issues. Even when access is allowed, researchers cannot assume that it will continue. Access should be considered an ongoing process that requires continued negotiation.

Participant Selection

Qualitative researchers use a multitude of sampling strategies, most of which are nonrandom and purposeful. **Table 8-3** contains a list of the more commonly used nonrandom sampling approaches with brief descriptions.

Data Collection

In qualitative inquiry, the investigator attempts to collect rich data not readily captured by other types of research instruments. To gather such data, researchers should use a variety of sources, different methods, and multiple senses.[6] Interviewing is the most common data collection method used by qualitative researchers, but it can be successfully combined with observation and document analysis.[6] Health professionals frequently use interviewing

Table 8-3 Purposeful Sampling Strategies for Qualitative Research

Sampling Strategy	Description
Maximum variation	A wide range of individuals are selected to capture multiple perspectives.
Homogenous	Similar individuals are selected based on specific shared characteristics and criteria of the study.
Critical case	Individuals are selected based on their perceived value in addressing the research problem.
Theory-based	Participants are selected for their ability to support the generation of a theory.
Snowball	Individuals participating in the study help the researcher find and recruit additional participants.
Extreme case	Participant(s) are selected due to an outlying characteristic that makes them different from others.
Typical case	Participant(s) are selected because they are representative of what is usual.
Stratified purposeful	A group of individuals is divided into subgroups to allow for comparison.
Convenience	Sample is selected based on accessibility.

Data from Onwuegbuzie AJ, Leech NL. A call for qualitative power analysis. *Qual Quant.* 2007;41:105–121.

to gather information when taking a patient history. This process is systematic, sensitive, and well-suited for research in the healthcare field. During the interview, researchers should listen carefully and avoid peppering the subject with questions. The interview is a conversation with a purpose that remains faithful to the research questions.[6] Investigators should avoid interruptions, leading questions, and conversational deviation. Data can be captured using audiotapes, digital recordings, handwritten notes, or a combination. Interview transcripts can be transcribed verbatim or with verbal fillers and extraneous pauses removed. Verbatim transcripts, however, allow researchers to assess the potential meaning of long pauses and verbal fillers. In addition, field notes can be incorporated into the transcript or left as a separate data source.

Data can also be obtained by observation. Qualitative researchers can collect observations as a participant or as a nonparticipant. Participant observation allows the researcher to experience the conditions of an insider. Such in-depth observation may yield insights unobtainable by other methods; however, the researcher risks "going native" and losing focus in the research problem unless they keep a critical distance.[4] Nonparticipant observation is direct but more detached than participant observation. The amount of information collected in both types of observation can be vast; therefore, qualitative researchers usually devise a plan or protocol to direct and focus the observations.[2]

Documents and artifacts are another source of data available to healthcare researchers. Documents are not just written items, but can include photographs, videotapes, or DVDs.[6] Artifacts are other physical items that convey information about the participants or setting.[11] For example, the artwork generated by pediatric oncology patients would be considered artifacts in qualitative research.

Data Management and Data Analysis

A large volume of data can be collected in a naturalistic study. The volume may be a challenge to manage. A codebook, or coding database, helps the researcher keep track of the voluminous data. Qualitative research software, such as NVivo, ATLAS.ti, and Dedoose, can help researchers manage and access the data. Still, some researchers prefer to manage the data on index cards that can be color coded and sorted manually when the volume of data allows it. Although the data management choice is a matter of preference, staying organized is the key to maintaining data integrity. Once the data are collected they must be put into a useful form for the purpose of analysis. The data must be unitized. A single unit of meaning is the smallest meaningful piece of content that can stand alone.[5] Each single unit of meaning must be coded. Coding is a way of tagging the units to associate them with the source and begin the categorization process. In the following example, a patient is interviewed and a transcript is generated. The coding process will be illustrated.

Interviewer: *I am interested in learning about people's experiences when they are hospitalized. You recently had a serious injury that caused you to be a patient in the hospital. Would you talk to me a little about what it felt like to be a patient?*

Jane: *I think that the biggest thing is that not many people have a sensitivity to a person who has back problems because that's what I had—a herniated disc—and I really don't think for days that they realized how much pain that was associated with injury. Um, they were making kind of light of the situation, asking me to move in positions of just getting out of normal clothes into a hospital robe and that didn't seem like a major task to them but, uh from my side it was excruciating to where I wanted them to cut the clothes off but they insisted on literally moving my body around to get the clothes off to get the robe on, which gave me the sense that they had no earthly idea of what kind of pain I was in.*

Interviewer: *So it sounds to me like you were really concerned that the staff did not understand the pain that you were in, how did that make you feel?*

Jane: *Starting from the emergency room, I think that they would not even sometimes give me time to complete a sentence, that they would ask me something and before I—they would kind of judge how much*

I could tell them, um and they would always either cut me off or say oh that's fine, that's all we need to know for now. And they would never keep me posted, like I was in the emergency room for hours and if you'd ask them if my doctor had been called or whatever—well we will get back with you in a minute—and it'd be another hour or two. Um so you were laying there not necessarily being kept updated on your condition or what work they were doing and the a that just left you in a state of fear because you did not know what was going on and maybe they were doing the right things. But if they had just come in and said "you know we've called your physician and he's on his way" or "we haven't got a call to him in yet" or "we are tracking him down" or something, it would have allowed me to know that, it would have eased my mind knowing that they were doing their job and because the way it looked it was like I was just in another world—that they were doing their thing and I just happened to be the thing that they were kinda focusing on but not really paying much attention to. They were doing their thing kind of like outside of my issue. And it even happened in the hospital room. And even the nurses and whatever. You really had to hand-tie nurses and literally put them on the spot sometimes and make them stop and listen to you and answer your questions completely or hear you out because they were constantly cutting you off or saying "well it's in your chart." Well this pill I've never taken before why am I taking it. "Well, because" < nurses >. And I just think a patient needs to know a little bit more than that. And deserves to know more than that, than being cut off and not being listened to.

Interviewer: *So it sounds to me like one of the biggest concerns that you experienced was that the communication you received was not helpful to you as a patient. Maybe we could explore that a little bit more and talk about what would have helped you more. You gave me a few examples, but what other kinds of things would have helped you as a patient to have understood what was happening to you?*

Jane: *I think when they were, I think that just extra time not feeling like you were being rushed to the point that where I think if they had just come in and done a little TLC or whatever and saying you must be in pain here, we are trying to do everything that we need to do. Tell me what happened, tell me where it hurts. Um, to the point of listening to my pain, not just seeing it. But listening to the pain; I think that would have helped me as a patient knowing that I was being cared for and that I just wasn't part of the shift; and that I was somebody that did need help. And I really felt that a lot of times, especially in the emergency room, that I was just a part of their paycheck. And that if the shift had changed, I don't know if I'd have known the difference. I don't think that one nurse—a new face would have come in and just taken right over and that made me feel like I was part of the shift; that I was not a person in pain that I was just a body that was in pain. And I don't think they had any perception of how scared people are in that situation and maybe need a little coddling and maybe need just a few minutes of their time to settle the anxiety down. You know before all the other stuff starts happening.*

Qualitative researchers often prefer that transcripts include the printed line numbers as shown in **Figure 8-2**. This procedure allows for data tracking. In addition, the researcher may prefer transcripts with wide margins to allow for annotations.

With these annotations, researchers document their first impression about the meaning of each unit. At some point, each of the units will be separated from the larger source document, either by computer software or manually on index cards. Figure 8-2 shows how a unit of data is transferred and coded by source and category.

Although the figure shows only a single coded unit, readers are encouraged to read the entire excerpt and practice unitization and coding.

As a reminder, the ultimate purpose of data analysis is to answer the research questions.[1] The process is comparative, iterative, and inductive.[1] A frequent approach to qualitative data analysis is content analysis. In content analysis, the unitized and coded data from transcripts, field notes, and other artifacts are categorized to form a thematic structure.[13] Data are analyzed using constant-comparative analysis, so categories and themes are defined.[5] The themes are combined or subdivided as necessary until the final structure is revealed. Ideally, this process should begin even during the data collection phase.[1] Tentative themes will likely change as the process evolves. Induction occurs when these individual pieces of meaning are joined together to represent general concepts, or themes. The final themes and categories will support the responses to the research questions.

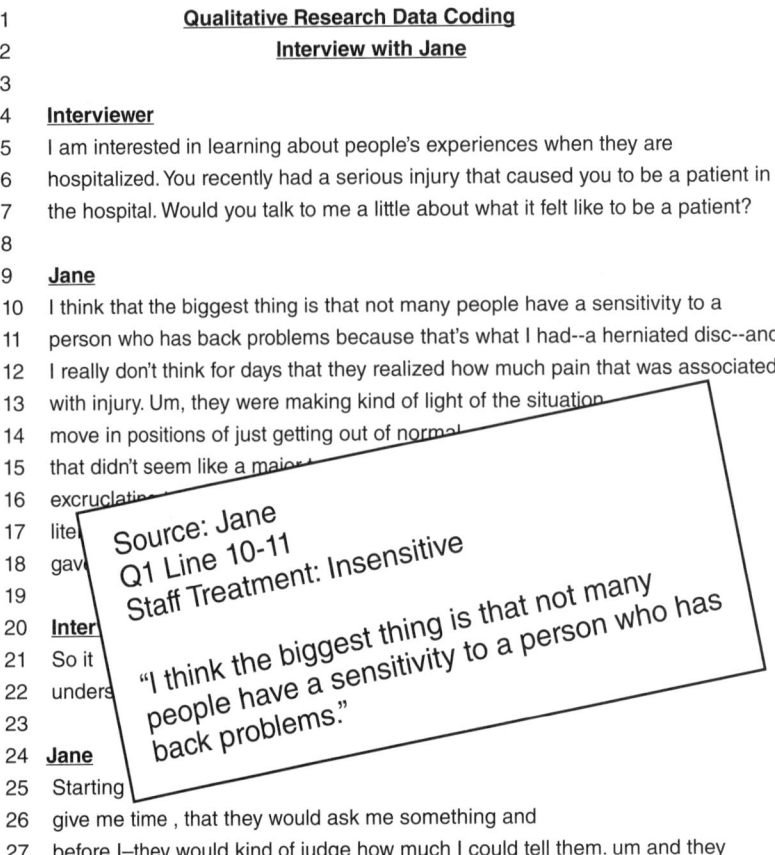

Figure 8–2 Unitization and coding example.

ASSESSING THE QUALITY OF A QUALITATIVE STUDY: ENSURING TRUSTWORTHINESS

Although the reader determines if a qualitative study is trustworthy, specific criteria have been established. Trustworthiness covers all areas that ultimately determine the study's integrity: its truth value, plausibility, rigorousness of design and method, and the credibility of both data and researcher.[5] The four trustworthiness criteria used in qualitative research are credibility, transferability, dependability, and confirmability.[5] Each of these criteria has a set of corresponding techniques.

Credibility

Analogous to internal validity, credibility can be achieved through prolonged engagement, persistent observation, and triangulation.[5] Additional techniques that help establish credibility include peer debriefing, negative case analysis, referential adequacy, member checking, and reflexive journaling.[6] These techniques demonstrate the researcher's commitment to scholarly standards and the rigorousness of the study.

Prolonged Engagement

Investigators must first establish credibility with the participants. Prolonged engagement allows researchers to learn about the social setting while establishing a trusting relationship with the participants.[6] Prolonged engagement facilitates candid and truthful responses during interviews. Furthermore, researchers can learn details about the organization not discoverable in a single visit. Immersion allows researchers to experience the participants' reality.[12] During prolonged engagement, however, investigators should avoid psychological fusion with the participants or the organization. This fusion is called "going native," and it might compromise the research perspective.[5,6]

Persistent Observation

Early research findings can be superficial and incomplete. Persistent observation can be defined as a process of going deeper. Participants may give politically correct or deceptive responses.[6] Investigators must be alert for long pauses, verbal fillers, and body language that may indicate more information is lurking under the surface. The researcher is the measurement instrument and must be able to discern what is atypical versus what is irrelevant.[5]

Triangulation

Even a single experience or opinion can be meaningful. Credibility is enhanced, however, when the single experience can be verified. Triangulation can be employed when selecting sources, methods, and theories.[5] Triangulation enhances credibility by supporting or refuting research findings in a way not achieved by a single source, method, or theory. Researchers can triangulate sources by purposefully selecting individuals likely to experience a given phenomenon from a different perspective. The triangulation of methods is exemplified by a research design that uses a variety of ways to collect data. Triangulation of theories is achieved when the data collected are checked against multiple theories.

Peer Debriefing

In peer debriefing, researchers consult a knowledgeable peer for advice and ideas.[4] By using this external check, researchers are demonstrating that they consider other perspectives and lenses to see data and the study. Peer debriefing allows researchers to deal with emotions, test working hypotheses, and take a momentary outside stance during the study.[6] Ethical dilemmas can be discussed and resolved. This technique keeps the study on course.

Negative Case Analysis

Some researchers begin with fixed ideas about the anticipated results of their study. Negative case analysis is used in analytical induction and theory building. Using this technique, researchers "purposefully seek cases that apparently do not fit the explanation as formulated."[1] This iterative process allows researchers to reformulate their hypotheses by accounting for aberrant data.[5] Credibility is enhanced when researchers look for additional explanations for findings that do not initially fit.

Referential Adequacy

A control group is often used in traditional studies for the purpose of comparison. In a qualitative study, referential adequacy refers to the use of a separate set of materials collected in the study environment to reinforce the research findings.[6] For example, a subset of the data collected can be archived for later comparison.[5] Video recordings, photos, and other materials can be collected for the same purpose.[6]

Member Checking

Distortions often occur in human communication. Member checking is a frequently used technique that helps to minimize such distortions. Member checking is also the most direct means of testing research interpretations.[5] The most basic form of member checking occurs when investigators ask for clarification during the interview. Investigators can also summarize their understanding at the end of the interview and ask if the data collected accurately reflect the participant's statements. Participants can also check the transcripts and the researcher's interpretations after data collection happens.

Reflexive Journal

The reflexive journal serves a dual purpose: (1) it is a diary that documents the evolving nature of the researchers' relationship to the study, and (2) it is a place to keep track of logistical information.[6] The qualitative research process involves making meaning that is enhanced when researchers track their thoughts and experiences in a reflexive journal.[13] Reflexivity involves critical self-reflection.[4] The journal entries document the internal dialogue of the researcher during the course of the study. In addition, the journal allows the researcher to continually examine biases, assumptions, and tentative hypotheses. Reflexive journaling is valuable and enhances the study's credibility.

Transferability

The concept of transferability is similar to external validity. Qualitative investigators do not make statements that generalize the results to others outside of the study. Although external generalizability is not a qualitative research goal, thick descriptions may direct readers to draw conclusions about the relevance of the collected data in relation to similar contexts, which allows for transferability and replicability.

Thick description is not simply a detailed description, but one that has interpretive value.[4] The study's results can provide concrete examples that others use as a platform for additional inquiry and understanding.[1] Thick description also includes a detailed explanation of how the study was conducted. The description should allow other investigators to replicate the study in a different setting. The following questions should be considered:

- How well does the author describe the lived experiences of the participants?
- How well does the author describe the participants and who they are?
- Does the author provide enough detail about the social, cultural, and physical context of the study?

Thick description answers these questions of relevancy without making claims about the application of findings outside the study's context. Human stories evoke human responses across contexts, thus making the research and sometimes the results transferable.

Dependability and Confirmability

Dependability, analogous to reliability, can be established by (1) using different methods, (2) splitting the data, and (3) conducting dependability audits.[5] A study that demonstrates internal consistency is dependable. Confirmability is similar to objective reproducibility and demonstrates an attempt to make the investigators' steps traceable. Dependability and confirmability rely on auditing procedures.

Audit Trail

Similar to a tax audit, the auditing process allows for an external review of documentation and decision making after the study is completed. All of the documents and materials generated during the study can be examined, including the data, field notes, codebooks, and other records. By following an audit trail, the external reviewer can determine if the research was conducted in a systematic and reliable manner.[4] The auditor verifies that the described research steps were actually followed.[5] Like tax records, research records should be retrievable and include dates. The auditor should be able to access raw data, communications, schedules, thematic summaries, and graphical representations of the interpretations.[6] Producing an audit trail enhances interpretation because researchers work with the data more than once.[4]

SUMMARY

It is likely that healthcare research will continue to evolve and include more qualitative research approaches alongside the traditional study designs. The essential qualitative study described in this chapter provides an introduction to the way qualitative researchers may approach different questions in health care. By adhering to the basic concepts and steps discussed in this chapter, healthcare professionals can embark on their own investigations of the human experiences of their patients and others. Those not interested in conducting their own qualitative study will at least be familiar with the ways in which a qualitative study can be assessed. Healthcare professionals are advised to seek out supplementary explanations for the terms and methods discussed in this chapter. Mentors who are familiar with this type of research can provide additional assistance for those wishing to conduct their own qualitative investigation. Suggested readings that may provide clarification of the topics introduced in this chapter can be found in the Resources list at the end of the chapter.

REFERENCES

1. Merriam SB. *Qualitative research: A guide to design and implementation.* 2nd ed. San Francisco, CA: Jossey-Bass; 2009:xvi.
2. Creswell JW, ed. *Educational Research: Planning, Conducting, and Evaluating Quantitative and Qualitative Research.* 4th ed. Boston, MA: Pearson Education; 2012.
3. Pope C, Mays N. *Qualitative Research in Health Care.* Oxford, UK: Blackwell; 2006.
4. Schwandt TA. *The Sage Dictionary of Qualitative Inquiry.* Thousand Oaks, CA: Sage; 2007.
5. Lincoln YS, Guba EG, eds. *Naturalistic Inquiry.* Newbury Park, CA: Sage; 1985.
6. Erlandson DA, Harris EL, Skipper BL, Allen SD, eds. *Doing Naturalistic Inquiry.* Newbury Park, CA: Sage; 1993.
7. Vogt WP, ed. *Dictionary of Statistics and Methodology: A Nontechnical Guide for the Social Sciences.* 3rd ed. Thousand Oaks, CA: Sage; 2005.
8. Flick U, ed. *Designing Qualitative Research.* Thousand Oaks, CA: Sage; 2007.
9. Onwuegbuzie AJ, Leech NL. A call for qualitative power analysis. *Qual Quant.* 2007;41:105–121.
10. Bourgeault IL, Dingwall R, DeVries RG, eds. *The Sage Handbook of Qualitative Methods in Health Research.* London: Sage; 2010.
11. Yin RK, ed. *Case Study Research.* 5th ed. Thousand Oaks, CA: Sage; 2014.
12. Marshall C, Rossman GB, eds. *Designing Qualitative Research.* Newbury Park, CA: Sage; 1989.
13. Lincoln YS, Guba EG, eds. *The Constructivist Credo.* Walnut Creek, CA: Left Coast Press; 2013.
14. Denzin NK, Lincoln YS, eds. *The Sage Handbook of Qualitative Research.* Thousand Oaks, CA: Sage; 2011.
15. Morse JM. *Qualitative Health Research: Creating a New Discipline.* Walnut Creek, CA: Left Coast Press; 2012.
16. Sobo EJ. *Culture and Meaning in Health Services Research: A Practical Field Guide.* Walnut Creek, CA: Left Coast Press; 2009.
17. Littlewood R, ed. *On Knowing and Not Knowing in the Anthropology of Medicine.* Walnut Creek, CA: Left Coast Press; 2007.
18. Richardson L. *After a Fall: A Sociomedical Sojourn.* Walnut Creek, CA: Left Coast Press; 2013.

Resources

- *The Sage Handbook of Qualitative Research*, 4th ed., Denzin & Lincoln, 2011.
- *Qualitative Health Research: Creating a New Discipline*, Morse, 2012.
- *Culture and Meaning in Health Service Research: A Practical Field Guide*, Sobo, 2009.
- *On Knowing and Not Knowing in the Anthropology of Medicine*, Littlewood, 2007.
- *After a Fall: A Sociomedical Sojourn*, Richardson, 2013.

CHAPTER 9

Community-Based Participatory Research

Scott D. Rhodes, PhD, MPH
Christina J. Sun, PhD, MS

Learning Objectives

- Define and describe community-based participatory research.
- List and discuss research paradigms.
- Describe common research methods used.
- Define, describe, and discuss four CBPR study designs.

INTRODUCTION

Community-Based Participatory Research Defined

Emerging evidence suggests that through a process of partnership that includes lay community members, organization representatives, and researchers, advances in health status and reductions in health disparities can occur as health promotion and disease prevention approaches, strategies, and efforts increase in authenticity. Lay community members and organization representatives participate in the research process to provide insight into the knowledge generated, guide the study and intervention design, ensure the accuracy of measurement, and support the interpretation of results. However, partnership is not easy; researchers must establish and maintain trusting, authentic co-learning partnerships with community members if partnerships are to function well and improvements in health are to occur within communities, especially within the most vulnerable communities.[6-8,12-14]

CHAPTER OVERVIEW

Despite the strides made to improve the overall health status in the United States, not all communities are benefiting equally from current medical and health advances. In fact, many of the complex health problems that persist in the United States have proven to be ill-suited for traditional "outside expert" approaches to health research, health improvement, and intervention development and implementation.[1-8] To decrease the growing gaps in health status among vulnerable communities such as minority (e.g., racial/ethnic communities and sexual minorities), economically disadvantaged, and other underserved communities, alternative approaches to medical and health research, health promotion, and disease prevention are being explored and promoted. Community-based participatory research (CBPR) is an approach to research designed to promote community and population health through the establishment and maintenance of community partnerships.[5-9] A partnership approach to research involves and benefits lay community members, representatives from community-based organizations (CBOs) and health departments, and medical and health researchers alike. Partnerships enhance both the quality of data collected and the validity of findings and their interpretation.[2-11]

In this chapter we define and describe the advantages and processes of CBPR. We also describe why CBPR is an appropriate approach to research. We then introduce four research methods and describe how a CBPR approach may be applied and incorporated. Finally, we offer a case example of the application of CBPR in a behavioral research study.

> **Box 9-1 CBPR**
>
> CBPR is a collaborative research approach that is designed to ensure and structure participation by communities affected by the issue being studied, by representatives of organizations, and by researchers in all aspects of the research process, from conception, study design and conduct, data analysis and interpretation, to the dissemination of findings.

CBPR (see **Box 9-1**) is an approach that ensures community participation in research. CBPR establishes structures for full and equal participation in research by community members (including those affected by the issue being studied), organization representatives, and researchers to understand and improve community and population health and well-being through multilevel action, including individual, group, community, policy, and social change.[7,8]

CBPR emphasizes co-learning and the reciprocal transfer of expertise, decision-making power, and the ownership of the processes and products of research. This approach involves a strong partnership in which all parties (e.g., lay community members, organization representatives, health department representatives, and researchers) participate and share control over *all* phases of the research process. These research phases typically include:

1. Identifying research questions
2. Assessing community strengths, assets, and challenges
3. Defining priorities
4. Developing research and data collection methodologies
5. Collecting and analyzing data
6. Interpreting findings
7. Disseminating findings
8. Applying the results to address community concerns through action or intervention

Although participation of the affected community in all research steps is critical to CBPR, another hallmark of CBPR is the translation of findings into action.[6-8] The accumulation of knowledge is important for the progression of science and understanding; however, the priority for most community members and organization representatives is the application of findings to improve the health status of community members, including friends, neighbors, families, consumers, patients, and clients. Furthermore, growing concern exists that the pendulum has swung too far towards "research for research's sake" without the application of new knowledge to affect change to improve the health outcomes of populations and community members.[3,10,12]

CBPR relies on community participation to ensure the research questions asked are important not only to the researcher for the generation and accumulation of knowledge, but also to lay community members themselves. CBPR also helps to ensure the methods used are reasonable and authentic to existing community structures and experiences and are as noninvasive as possible. Finally, the increased validity of findings from CBPR yield more effective actions and successful interventions to positively affect health and well-being because of the inherent insights that emerge from partnership. **Table 9-1** illustrates the advantages of using a CBPR approach, as summarized from the literature.

Research Paradigms

All research approaches, including the design of a study and the methods selected, reflect a specific research *paradigm*. Research paradigms are defined as a set of basic beliefs about the nature of reality that can be studied and understood.[15] These basic beliefs are accepted simply on faith; however well argued, no way exists to establish their ultimate truth. The *positivist* and *postpositivist* research paradigms, for example, hold that a single reality on how things really are and really work exists to be studied and understood. The *positivist* research paradigm posits that this single reality can be fully captured; this paradigm is reflected in *experimental* research designs and methods, which are used most often in the basic sciences. In contrast, the *postpositivist*

Table 9–1 Advantages of Community-Based Participatory Research (CBPR)

- Enhances data relevance, usefulness, and use
- Improves the quality and validity of the research by blending local knowledge and local theory based on the lived experiences of community members, expertise from organization representatives, and scientific perspectives
- Recognizes the limitations of the concept of value-free science and encourages reflexive and critical thinking among all partners
- Recognizes that knowledge is power, and thus knowledge gained can be used by all partners to direct resources and influence policies that will benefit the community
- Reduces the separation of the individual from her or his culture and context
- Aims to increase the health and well-being of the communities involved, both directly through examining and addressing identified needs and indirectly through increasing power, control, and skills (e.g., capacity building)
- Joins partners with diverse skills, knowledge, expertise, and perspectives to address health
- Strengthens the research, program, and problem-solving capacity of all partners
- Creates theory grounded in social experience, and creates better informed and more effective action guided by such theories
- Increases the possibility of overcoming the understandable distrust of research by communities
- Has the potential to bridge "cultural gaps"
- Involves communities that have been marginalized on the basis of, for example, race, ethnicity, class, gender, and/or sexual orientation in examining the impact of marginalization and attempting to reduce or eliminate it

frequently used in the social and behavioral health sciences. Both experimental and quasi-experimental methods require the goal of objective detachment between researchers and participants so that any influence in either direction on what is being studied can be eliminated or reduced.

CBPR is often aligned with a *constructivist* research paradigm, which holds that multiple realities exist to be studied and understood.[15] Each reality is an intangible construction rooted in people's experiences with everyday life, how they remember them, and how they make sense of them. Individual constructions of reality are assumed to be more or less "informed," rather than more or less "true," because they are always alterable. This means that as researchers and participants encounter and consider different perspectives, they will alter their own views. The result is a *consensus construction of reality*[15] that is mutually formed by variations in preceding constructions (including those of the researchers) and that can move both participants and researchers toward communicating about action, intervention, and change.[16] The methods of constructivist research require researchers and participants to be interactively linked so that the consensus construction of reality is literally created as the study proceeds. Researchers using a CBPR approach are cast, therefore, in the dual roles of participant and facilitator.

Principles and Values of CBPR

Successful use of CBPR relies on various partnership principles and values[17-19] that tend to include:

- Mutual respect and genuineness
- Establishing and utilizing formal and informal partnership networks and structures
- Committing to transparent processes and clear and open communication
- Roles, norms, and processes evolving from the input and agreement of all partners
- Agreeing on the values, goals, and objectives of research and practice
- Building upon each partner's strengths and assets

research paradigm holds that this single reality can only be *approximated*; human knowledge is based not on absolute "truths," but rather upon human supposition. Postpositivism often is reflected in *quasi-experimental* research designs and methods

- Offering continual feedback among members
- Balancing power and sharing resources
- Sharing credit for the accomplishments of the partnership
- Facing challenges together
- Developing and using relationships and networks outside of the partnership
- Incorporating existing environmental structures to address partnership focuses
- Taking responsibility for the partnership and its actions
- Disseminating conclusions and findings to research and clinical audiences, community members, and policymakers[6-8,17]

Often, the researcher feels that she or he must make decisions on behalf of the community. This is a natural inclination given the years spent in school, in training programs, and/or in the field. The researcher may be highly motivated to apply and use her or his resources for the benefit of the community. After all, the researcher is armed with intellectual resources: training and experience in the reduction of bias and the traditional approaches to increase validity with the hope of increasing generalizability; and perhaps financial resources or, at the minimum, increased access to financial and material resources to conduct research (e.g., grant funding and students), among other tools. Thus, the researcher may forget that community members and organization representatives have perspectives that are key for inclusion during the research process.

For community members the textbook of life is living. With this axiom in mind, researchers must recognize that lay community members have perspectives that can greatly enhance all phases of the research process. Community members have firsthand knowledge of the health issue of concern. They can contribute to identifying and understanding the most salient health needs of their community; giving context to epidemiological data; and building local theory about needs, challenges, and potential solutions that may not have occurred to or may not be easily understood by outsiders (e.g., researchers and other health professionals).

Each of these points can strengthen research and intervention design through the interpretation of data and the development, revision, and evaluation (and further revisions if warranted) of intervention strategies.

Although their training and experiences may or may not have been learned in formal educational or training programs, organization representatives who are on the "frontlines" also have an understanding of the community that is not readily available or apparent to the researcher. They know how systems (e.g., service provision) are organized and utilized and may have a wealth of experiences providing services to community members on the frontlines or at the "grassroots" level. However, their perspectives may lack detail, and they may miss insights that have not been well discovered or explored.

Many researchers might conclude that they themselves are on the frontlines in their capacity as health professionals (e.g., clinicians, counselors, health educators, pharmacists, providers of medical and mental health services, therapists, and other service providers); yet, they may truly know very little about the lived experiences of their patients or clients, especially the lives lived after patients or clients leave the office. To illustrate, having access to care and medications does not ensure that a patient will adhere to prescribed medication regimens for diabetes management. Patients and clients (and providers themselves) live in complex social contexts that cannot be easily understood or teased apart by outsiders. Thus, although organization representatives (e.g., individuals from community agencies like the health department, community clinics, agencies, etc.) may have useful knowledge, experiences, and theories, their insight alone is insufficient.

FOUR STUDY DESIGNS

CBPR can be infused into any research methodology; however, the following section highlights four research methods and briefly outlines how CBPR can be applied to each. These methods are action-oriented community diagnosis (AOCD), focus groups, photovoice, and in-depth interviews. Although this discussion is not meant to be exhaustive, it is meant to serve as a starting point for researchers who want to explore the use of CBPR within qualitative research.

Action-Oriented Community Diagnosis (AOCD)

The purpose of AOCD is to understand the health status, the collective dynamics, the functions of relationships within a community, and the interactions between community members and broader structures that can impede or promote the conditions and skills required to assist community members in making decisions and taking action for social change and health status improvement.[4] AOCD can be a critical first step in program planning, intervention development and implementation, and evaluation because it provides the foundation for:

- The establishment of baseline data from which objectives, intended outcomes, and measures of change can be derived
- The selection of intervention methods and delivery that are most appropriate based on the community's structure, including formal and informal power dynamics and community assets and strengths
- A collaborative relationship between professionals and communities, who can begin "closing the gap between what we do not know and what we ought to know"[4,20]

AOCD may serve as a process for *needs assessment* (**Box 9-2**) but actually goes beyond traditional interpretations of needs assessment. Although needs assessment is defined as a systematic examination and appraisal of the type, depth, and scope of needs for the purpose of setting priorities, AOCD also identifies and explores community assets on which intervention can be based. Philosophically true to CBPR, AOCD utilizes a *strengths-based approach* to research to identify both the needs and challenges faced by communities, and just as importantly, the assets and strengths within the community. To forego the identification of

---

Box 9-2 Needs Assessment

Needs assessment is the systematic examination and appraisal of the type, depth, and scope of needs for the purpose of setting priorities. It is the process of identifying and measuring gaps between what is and what ought to be.

---

community assets and strengths is to use a *deficits-based approach* that may miss key information vital to understanding the community's reality and lived experience and the strengths and resources on which successful intervention strategies can be based.

Like all research methods that adhere to a CBPR approach, AOCD begins with the establishment of a working collaborative relationship with community members. Representatives from the community, CBOs, and researchers come together to determine a research plan. Typically, existing community-specific data are reviewed. These data may include epidemiological data usually available from public health departments at the local or state level as well as other reports and resources available from local CBOs such as faith-based service providers and other agencies.

A *windshield tour* of the community can be an important initial step in the AOCD process. If the community consists of a geographical location, a researcher will explore the community guided by community members to gain an appreciation of the community's geography, size, physical characteristics, and important community venues (e.g., a corner store where people gather or a house of worship). This windshield tour is meant to be an introduction to a geographic community or a community of identity and its context through simple observation and community member guidance and commentary. If the community is less geographically defined—such as a community of elderly shut-ins, for example—a windshield tour may include the agencies and organizations that visit and offer support to these community members. A windshield tour for a virtual community might include exploring the chat rooms, mobile applications, listservs, bulletin boards, and newsgroups visited and used by the community and visiting sites that are advertised on pop-up and pop-under screens.

After the windshield tour and throughout AOCD, researchers document their experiences using *field notes*. Frequently kept in various study methodologies and often informal, field notes are documentation of details about the community that are interesting or noteworthy and when combined with other data might well prove to be important. Field notes may serve several purposes:

- Provide the opportunity to document first impressions about a community
- Assist the researcher to remember experiences encountered in the field
- Record names of individuals and places that may prove key in the execution of the AOCD process
- Document unusual characteristics within a community

Field notes also allow the researcher to track her or his own perspectives, impressions, feelings, and frustrations during the AOCD research process. Field notes can be simply reflective writings while the research "event," such as a windshield tour, is still fresh in the mind of the researcher. It is wise to keep field notes of all research efforts because field notes serve as a documentation source for decisions made that affect the research process and subsequent data interpretation.

Because researchers tend to be very different from the communities they study, researchers need to gain an *emic* or insider's perspective on how people live and the issues facing the community.[4,6,21-24] An insider's perspective is privileged knowledge that only members of a particular community have. Outsiders can guess and hypothesize, but those assumptions are not value free and may not be accurate or complete. Because no researcher can completely remove her- or himself from their research, an emic perspective provides the researcher insight into the perspectives of community members. For example, a homeless individual understands aspects of the lived experience of homelessness better than any outsider. Members from a disabled community can provide insights that may not be understood or correctly interpreted by an outsider.

Of course, some researchers may have started out as members of the communities they study and assume themselves to be insiders. However, the years of training in research methods and/or their content specialty and time outside of the community transform them into outsiders. In fact, outsiders who were once insiders may assume understanding that in fact is misunderstanding.[4,25]

Furthermore, one's social position in a community affects the "truth" of the experience of community life. For example, all African American gay men do not share a truth; in fact, among other influences, perception of truth is affected by the position within the community. Thus, AOCD allows for distinctions and differences to emerge that may be lost through other approaches such as quantitative approaches. However, these emerging distinctions and differences challenge researchers who must work with community members to merge varying—perhaps contradictory—data and perspectives and make useful sense of findings.

Although the emic perspective is important, a hallmark of ACOD, and in fact CBPR, is to move toward change through some type of action or intervention. Action may include, for example, a behavioral intervention to promote medication adherence or a policy change to increase access to medical or health care. Such movement also requires an understanding of *etic* or outsider perspectives. Outsiders are comprised of representatives from CBOs and other service providers such as those from the local public health department, and may include health professionals (e.g., clinicians, counselors, health educators, pharmacists, providers of medical and mental health services, therapists) and other researchers. Outsiders provide perspectives on the health and well-being of communities, their access to resources, and community strengths, as well as support for subsequent action or intervention. Like community members themselves, outsiders have a story to tell based on their experiences.

After reviewing and incorporating secondary or extant data and collecting, analyzing, and interpreting emic and etic data in partnership with community members and organization representatives, the researcher helps the community disseminate the findings. AOCD relies on a *community forum* to present the findings of a research process to *influential advocates* (e.g., local policymakers, service providers, healthcare providers identified by participants as potential collaborators and advocates for change). This forum highlights issues, may propose solutions, and allows the community to dialogue with influential advocates who are supporters, but who may also benefit from increased awareness and greater understanding of the situation. The forum is an opportunity to initiate dialogue and come together during a facilitated discussion to explore potential action or intervention.[17,26] Without the forum, AOCD merely explores root causes but does not move to improving the health status of the community. Dissemination of findings within the community and movement towards action are important steps in both AOCD and CBPR.

AOCD requires the involvement of both insiders and outsiders to ensure the collection of accurate (defined as reliable and valid) data and the most correct interpretation of these data. AOCD might include understanding both the emic and etic perspectives of uninsured families within a cultural and geographic community. This understanding may lead to action and, perhaps, policy changes that reduce barriers and/or increase access. For example, monolingual Spanish-speaking Latinos may have little access to public health department services if their local health department does not have translation capacity. A forum can educate providers on the ramifications of the deficiency and spark new ideas and innovative approaches to solving problems. AOCD allows for solutions to emerge based on the compilation of realities that come from various perspectives. No one group or sector is responsible for change; rather, direction and change come from a negotiated process that includes multiple groups or sectors. The exchange of perspectives and ideas allows insiders and outsiders to see community health from fresh perspectives and builds partnerships that are stronger and can move forward in directions that positively affect health.

Often emic and etic perspectives are explored and interpreted through the use of qualitative methods. A CBPR partnership may choose to conduct focus groups, photovoice, or qualitative interviews—methodologies that also are outlined within this chapter. More quantitative methods may be less useful during the early stages of AOCD because they may not allow for sufficient flexibility and exploration of perspectives. However, they may provide important data in less exploratory or developmental research. Moreover, researchers, and in fact community members and organization representatives, often assume that CBPR requires the use of qualitative approaches. However, CBPR is useful during all phases of quantitative and mixed methods studies as well, including intervention outcome evaluation studies.[6,8,25,27-31]

Focus Groups

As a qualitative methodology, focus groups provide the opportunity to investigate participant responses and reactions related to an issue or topic more fully. They also allow new areas of inquiry to emerge. The methodology can reveal key nuances and perspectives that clinician researchers may not be able to foresee.[4,32-34] Briefly, focus groups usually are composed of 6 to 10 participants who are guided through a set of general predetermined open-ended questions outlined in a *focus group moderator's guide*. The guide may be based on behavioral theory[35,36] or may allow for theory that explains a phenomenon to be developed based on the findings, much like a *grounded theory* approach to research.[17,24,37] Either way, the guide should be agreed upon by the partners. Not only should the research objectives be mutually agreed upon, but the selection of focus groups as a methodology and the line of inquiry outlined within the guide should reflect the most meaningful approach and language as agreed upon by the research partners.

After an introduction to the focus group process (and of course getting informed consent to participate) as well as outlining ground rules (e.g., speaking one at a time, respecting various opinions, and maintaining confidentiality), the participants, who sit in a circle, respond to open-ended questions. Group interaction is an explicit component of this methodology. Instead of the researcher asking each person to respond to a question in turn, participants are encouraged to talk to one another, asking questions, exchanging anecdotes, and commenting on one another's experiences and perspectives.[17,32,35,36,38] The moderator must be skilled and experienced in soliciting discussion from all participants in a group, reminding participants that there are no wrong answers, affirming all opinions, and probing for detail. Probing for detail, whether through examples, clarification, or further exploration, is key to successful qualitative data collection, especially when using focus groups. In most cases, qualitative research requires the researcher to allow the design to emerge more fully during the project's evolution;[39,40] thus, all potential questions cannot be predicted. The moderator's guide is meant to serve as an outline, but the moderator must facilitate the discussion beyond what is written within the guide. The moderator may need to probe into a perspective to develop and understand it more fully. However, the moderator must be skilled at keeping the discussion on track. If the discussion deviates from the purpose of the focus group, the moderator must be able to bring the discussion back to the purpose.

In addition to a moderator, successful focus groups most often involve at least one *note taker* who documents participant speaking order, body language, and facial expression that cannot be captured by audio recording. These details may provide important insight during the data analysis and interpretation phases. Because anonymity may be desired, names of participants may not be used; rather, participants may be assigned numbers that are added to the focus group transcript in order to track which focus group participant is responding. It may not be important to know the name of a participant; however, it may be important to attribute certain quotations to certain participants. Perhaps only one participant has a certain perspective about a topic that she or he continues to reiterate. When analyzing the transcripts, it may be important to recognize this and weigh the findings accordingly.

The note taker also documents nonverbal communication. If a participant is noticeably uncomfortable with a discussion topic or the focus group discussion but does not assert her or his unease or disagreement, such observations should be noted by the note taker. Overall, the note taker is documenting what is going on during the focus group session that may be missed by the audio/digital recorder and by the moderator who is leading the session.

When applying a CBPR approach to focus group research, the research question, moderator's guide, and recruitment methods must be developed and agreed upon by the research partners. Data analysis and interpretation should be completed in partnership to allow for community participation.[5]

Photovoice

Photovoice is a qualitative method of inquiry that:

- Enables participants to record and reflect on their personal and community strengths and concerns
- Promotes critical dialogue and knowledge about personal and community issues through group discussions and photographs
- Provides a forum for the presentation of the lived experience of participants through the images, language, and contexts defined by participants themselves[26,41-45]

As a method closely aligned with CBPR, photovoice improves the quality and validity of research by drawing on local knowledge, developing local theory, and progressing toward action. Perhaps one of the most participant-driven research methodologies, photovoice engages participants in the following procedure:

1. Attend a training session to receive a disposable camera, and determine the topic for their first photo assignment.

2. Record through photography each photo assignment.
3. Share and discuss their photographs from each photo assignment during photo discussion sessions.
4. Organize a forum to present their photographic and thematic data to *influential advocates*.
5. Create plans of action.[44]

Photo discussions typically begin with a review and discussion of themes that emerged from the analysis of previous sessions followed by a "show and tell" activity that allows each participant to share her or his photographs and explain how the photographs relate to the photo assignment. These discussions often follow a Paulo Freirian–based[46] model of root-cause questioning and discussion known by the acronym SHOWED (see **Box 9-3**).[45,47,48] However, because SHOWED has proven to be unwieldy at times,[48] other guides or triggers are used. For example, a simpler approach has been effectively conducted using: (1) What do you see? (2) How does this make you feel? (3) What do you think about this? and (4) What can we do?[45] A Spanish-language version of SHOWED also has been developed and used.[49]

At the conclusion of each photo discussion, the group develops a new photo assignment by asking, "Given what we have learned so far, what should we explore next?"

The photo discussion data are analyzed like other qualitative data, through exploring, formulating, and interpreting themes. The participants share these themes with local community leaders, service providers, and policymakers. These photographs serve as the medium through which issues are discussed to raise awareness among a core group of allies, mobilize these allies, and plan for change.

Photovoice transitions from knowledge, or raised consciousness around issues and assets, to direct community action. Although a relatively new methodology, photovoice has been found to be a flexible method both in terms of the issues it has been employed to explore and address and the geographic and culturally diverse groups it has been employed with. It has been applied in partnership with a number of communities including Latino youth in the rural southeast;[48] women in Yunnan Province, China;[50,51] homeless men and women in Michigan;[51,52] heterosexual immigrant Latino men;[42,45] youth peer educators in Cape Town, South Africa;[53] urban lay health advisors;[10] HIV-positive persons;[26,43,54] and public health department leaders and constituents.[55]

Individual In-Depth Interviews

Individual in-depth interviews are another common data collection methodology. These interviews are *unstructured*, *semistructured*, or *structured* depending on the research goals. Unstructured interviews are characterized by questions that emerge during the interview process. The research partners may have general topic areas or categories, but the questions are asked as they are formulated in the natural course of the discussion. There is no predetermined wording of questions. This style is more conversational and increases the salience and relevance of questions. A problem with unstructured interviews is that different information is collected from different individuals based on different questions. Unstructured interviews may be useful for initial explorations or case studies. However, unstructured interviews can result in less systematic and comprehensive data, causing challenges in data analysis.

Semistructured interviews by definition provide more structure for the interviewer. Topics and issues to be explored and discussed are specified in advance, often in outline form. Semistructured and

---

Box 9-3 SHOWED

SHOWED follows the following discussion outline:

What do you *see* here?
What is really *happening* here?
How does this relate to *our* lives?
Why does this concern, situation, or strength exist?
How can we become *empowered* through our new understanding?
What can we *do*?

structured interviews require an *interview guide* that leads the interview process. Leading a semistructured interview, the interviewer often decides the order and sequence of the questions during the course of the interview. The interviewer may probe for detail and develop questions and their wording during the interview process. Data collection using this approach is more systematic than an unstructured approach. Because semistructured interviews remain conversational and situational, gaps in data can be explored and closed. However, important and salient topics may be inadvertently omitted as interviews go in directions that jeopardize comparability among interviews and the data collected.

Structured interviews are often well defined prior to the interview. The sequence and exact wording of questions are determined in advance. All interviewees are asked the same basic questions in the same order and manner.

Interview questions may be *open-ended*, *closed-ended*, or a combination of question types. Open-ended questions tend to provide more exploratory, developmental, and contextual data. Data from open-ended questions tend to be more descriptive. For example, an open-ended question that was asked of healthcare providers who worked in an undocumented Latino community was: "If you could envision an answer to meeting the healthcare needs of the local Latino community, what would that vision be?" Answers were descriptive and complex, providing not only ideas about how to meet healthcare needs in the short- and long-term, but also further information about what healthcare needs existed in this community and root-cause explanations and insight into the sociopolitical context pertaining to health.

Closed-ended questions are characterized by response options that are *fixed*. Participants choose among a list of fixed responses. An example closed-ended question from a structured interview implemented among Latino men was: "Some men report having sex with other men for a variety of reasons; have you ever heard of a male friend having sex, including oral or anal sex, with another man?" The response options were: "yes," "no," and "refused to answer."

Closed-ended response options simplify data collection and analysis because many questions can be asked in a shorter period of time and responses can be easily aggregated and compared. The disadvantage, however, is that participants must fit their experiences and feelings into predetermined categories. This may distort the true experiences and feelings of the participants by limiting their response choices. Closed-ended questions and responses may also reduce participants' ability to express why and the context of the phenomenon of interest.

Conventionally, closed-ended interviews collect data on a topic by asking individuals questions to generate statistics on the group or groups within a community or population that those individuals represent. Closed-ended interviews do not tend to be formative or exploratory; rather, they ask questions about a variety of factors that influence, measure, or are affected by health. For example, population-based or community-wide, closed-ended interviews may document and follow health status. Or, closed-ended interviews may provide local data and a baseline for evaluation of intervention efforts. After a local CBPR research project has evolved and developed a research intervention to effect change (e.g., individual behavior change, community change, or policy change), interviews comparing baseline data to intervention implementation or postintervention follow-up may provide information on how well the intervention is working.

When applying a CBPR approach to research, the research question, measurement method (e.g., interview, questionnaire), and items or questions to be included must be agreed on by the partnership. Furthermore, the process for recruitment and administration must be decided by the partnership. Basic questions the CBPR partnership will want to answer as members prepare a study include:

- How will participants be recruited?
- What type of compensation will be provided?
- Who will administer the interview or questionnaire?
- Will interviewers be used or will the questionnaire be self-administered?

Researchers may think they know the best way to recruit interviewees and administer data collection procedures; however, community partners may provide great insight that may increase recruitment and response rates as well as honesty in responses.[56,57] In fact, what seems scientifically sound to the researcher (e.g., reducing bias and threats to validity) may inhibit responses.

Qualitative and Quantitative Data Analysis

Analyzing and interpreting any type of dataset, whether qualitative or quantitative, using a CBPR approach is challenging. Ensuring the participation of all partners in the process can be daunting. Researchers may have a variety of data analysis software to choose from that community partners may not have the time or energy to learn and apply. Thus, creative ways to examine data may be necessary. During qualitative data analysis, community partners may review and provide perceptions on potential themes through their detailed reading and rereading of the transcripts separately. The researcher may choose to analyze the data using a software program to code and retrieve non-numeric data (e.g., NVivo, ATLAS.ti, Ethnograph, NUD*IST, and Dedoose). Coming together, the research partners compare broad categories, resolve discrepancies, and begin the process of interpreting the findings through the development of themes. Themes based in qualitative data are most often directional. Themes can be described as potential assertions that can be tested later through subsequent research. Examples of themes developed using qualitative analysis include: (1) Manhood is affirmed through sex.[17] (2) Undocumented Latinos felt that they have no right to access public health care.[58] (3) Familiar brand-name medicines are preferred by immigrants.[59] Quotations are usually abstracted from the qualitative transcripts to illustrate the themes.

Quantitative data analysis poses similar challenges.[5] How can community members, who lack quantitative data analysis skills or software training, participate in this phase? Researchers should communicate and solicit feedback with the partnership throughout the process, keeping the partners up to date on statistical approaches, decisions, and rationales. Furthermore, researchers should not assume that partners do not want to be engaged in the analysis process.[5] After all, CBPR promotes knowledge gain and skill development on all sides. As mutual co-learners, the researcher is learning about the partners, and the partners are learning as well; this learning may include building data analysis skills.

Because it may be difficult to ensure participation of all community partners, getting a commitment from one, two, or three partnership members who are from the community may be key to the data analysis.[5] The entire CBPR partnership may not choose to participate in all phases of the research process, but establishing guidelines that ensure community member representation in each phase of the process is key.

In this section only a few research methods were described. However, it is important to note that a researcher need not give up traditional research methods, but may infuse a CBPR approach into any research method.

INITIATING CBPR

Beginning the exciting work of CBPR requires a clear understanding of partnership principles and values, as outlined earlier in this chapter. In the following sections we outline some pivotal tasks in the researcher's effort to engage in CBPR.

Network, Network, Network

A first task in the CBPR process requires the development of a network with other individuals with a similar health area of interest or concern. A relatively easy and helpful initial contact for a researcher may be a local public health department. Providers and educators within health departments around the country are likely to have connections with community agencies working with those affected by and committed to a variety of health concerns. A clinician, administrator, nutritionist, intern, health educator, and/or epidemiologist within the public health department might already be working with established local health coalitions or community groups. Dialoguing with these potential partners represents a good solid start in this process and is well worth the effort. A simple review of a public health department website or a telephone call to the health department may offer initial guidance and contacts, and an informational interview with a health department staff member will begin the networking process essential throughout CBPR. As a researcher, casting a wide net facilitates networking contacts to identify overlapping health concerns and resources, including talent that may support the research process synergistically. Networking also initiates the establishment of trust that is key to success in CBPR.

The researcher must understand the local communities and work in collaboration, not through confrontation, with local *stakeholders*. Stakeholders typically are individuals who are affected by the health issue and those who will be part of the research as well as affected by the research and subsequent change. Stakeholders may include community members experiencing the problem, service providers, and community leaders, among others.

In addition to contacting and networking with a local public health department, making connections with those healthcare providers in the community who are working with individuals and community members affected by overlapping health and research priorities may provide access to potential partners. The researcher benefits from thinking broadly about those individuals providing care (e.g., counselors, exercise physiologists, mental health providers, nutritionists, physical therapists, etc.). Furthermore, becoming familiar with other local CBOs, other types of community agencies, and service providers and making contact with representatives from a variety of organizations will yield helpful results. The researcher may find partnerships for CBPR within the local school system, clinical settings, clubs and service agencies, and/or retirement communities, just to name a few more possibilities.

Build Trust

After commonalities have been identified, the researcher will begin a process of *trust building*. Trust building is especially important because communities have felt exploited as "living laboratories" for universities and medical centers. Often communities are inundated by research projects that test hypotheses, but do not benefit the community itself through some type of action or intervention to improve and promote health and well-being. Communities may be apprehensive about committing to a partnership, and the researcher may have to overcome a history of research that was not initiated and conducted in a respectful manner.[60] A positive relationship is built by working hand-in-hand with community members. A researcher may choose to spend some up-front time volunteering with a CBO and serving on local health coalitions. This level of commitment serves several purposes. First, it advances a genuine and mutually respectful relationship with key community leaders whom the researcher may need and want to have on board as partners in the research. It may also open other doors for the researcher; the researcher may be unfamiliar with all the players and may use the opportunity to identify informal community leaders who may be committed to a health issue and may be interested in the research. Third, it allows the researcher the opportunity to understand community structure, decision-making processes, and levels of influences through their role as a participant observer. Finally, community service allows community members to interact with the researcher in a setting that is not focused on any one agenda. By selecting the right place to volunteer and thus "be seen," the researcher may build community trust by association. If a Latino-serving CBO is well respected by the local Latino community, for example, the researcher will gain more immediate community favor, and thus participation, by spending time there. Such volunteer work not only builds trust, but also begins to offer emic and etic community perspectives to the researcher.

Building trust includes building relationships. Relationships among lay community members, organization representatives, and researchers may involve informal "working" meetings that allow partners to get to know one another. Community events such as street fairs, church gatherings, and forums as well as parties and celebrations are ideal places for lay community members, organization representatives, and researchers to convene. These types of opportunities show commitment to the community and allow for lay community members, organization representatives, and researchers to know one another better. This improves trust and communication, which improve the research process.

Maintain Relationships

Key to trust building is *relationship maintenance*. Although it may be easy to feel one has built trust, one must remember partnerships cannot be taken for granted. When things are being done behind the scenes, gaps in the research process may exist; the researcher must be present within the community. For example, getting a research protocol approved by an institutional review board (IRB) or ethics committee may require a delay in the research process, but the researcher must touch base with partnership members to provide informal status reports. This is important because the researcher does not want to lose community interest, motivation, or momentum. Community members do not necessarily understand the confusing steps required by universities, research institutions, and funders. Time should be spent in dialogue explaining these steps and their rationales.

Negotiate Partnerships

Subsequent tasks in the CBPR process include bringing key community members and organization representatives together. This may be easy if an existing community health coalition exists. The coalition can determine whether a health issue is of interest or not. If a health issue is not a focus and yet data suggest that it contributes profoundly to morbidity and mortality of the community that the coalition serves or represents, the researcher has to walk a fine line between asserting what she or he perceives to be "important information" and staying true to the priorities of the community. Exploring community priorities and perspectives may yield important insight or even areas of overlap. It may require thinking creatively or "outside of the box." The researcher may provide data and increase awareness, affirming her or his agenda, or she or he may decide the community-prioritized agenda is important and an opportunity to build trust and relationships. Nothing can impede or destroy trust between a researcher and the community members and organization representatives more than going into a community to "fix" something without asking community members what they prioritize. After all, community members are not inanimate objects to be "fixed"; they are potential partners. CBPR requires the researcher to be flexible, and no place is this flexibility more evident than in adaptations related to community priorities. A researcher may be required to take on other priorities as identified by the community in the spirit of partnership.

However, the importance of linking community needs and priorities with researcher interests and skills cannot be ignored. Just as community priorities must be respected, researchers must be honest with communities about where their interests and skills overlap and complement. Researchers should not prioritize community priorities without regard to the epidemiologic data; in fact, community members and organization representatives may rely on researchers to provide that epidemiologic data and thereby provide a context for their perspectives. Thus, education and negotiation among community members, organization representatives, and researchers are warranted to establish priorities. Through iterative negotiation, these priorities are more informed. Without negotiation of priorities, it is unlikely that anyone will be effectively served or community health enhanced.

The researcher may begin with a community health coalition or may need to identify and build a network of community members and CBO representatives. Through this network, the foundation of a partnership may be established. Although growth may occur throughout, this network may evolve into a partnership through the hard work of those involved.

A CASE STUDY

HoMBReS: Hombres Manteniendo Bienestar y Relaciones Saludables

HoMBReS, an acronym for *Hombres Manteniendo Bienestar y Relaciones Saludables* (Men Maintaining Wellness and Healthy Relationships), was an intervention research project in rural North Carolina that was initiated through a partnership of lay community members, organization representatives, and university health professionals and researchers.[5-8,13,28,31,61-63] A community health coalition known as Chatham Communities in Action (CCIA) was formed in 1991 as part of the North Carolina Community-Based Public Health Initiative (CBPHI).[6,36,64,65] Because of the rapidly growing Latino community in North Carolina and their early success in diabetes prevention within the African American community, CCIA, with expanding Latino membership, chose to explore Latino health concerns within their local community. A subgroup of CCIA members met with university researchers to develop a plan to explore the healthcare priorities of the Latino community.

The CBPR partnership, which initially was composed of members of CCIA, convened first to determine how to further develop the CBPR partnership to expand Latino representation. Local Latino-serving CBOs and interested individuals who were not involved with CCIA were invited to participate in the process. This inclusion required time to build trust and clarify goals. These added members included representatives from a local adult Latino soccer league, a local Latino *tienda* (grocery store), and a farm worker advocacy group. The soccer league was a nine-county Latino soccer league of over 1600 adult men. The league president, along with various other interested league members, became involved in the CBPR partnership. The research partners continued to build trust among themselves as research partners through personal relationships, genuineness, respect, and "being there." CCIA representatives and the researcher spent many dinners meeting with league representatives. Although CCIA had a history of working with the university, these relationships could not be assumed or taken for granted. Building and maintaining trust and communication always plays a paramount role in CBPR.

The expanded CBPR partnership gained consensus on the research aims. This process involved answering two equally important questions. First, the research partners had to ask themselves: "What do we want to know?" Second, the partners had to ask themselves: "Why do we want to know it?" This distinction is important because a CBPR approach recognizes that knowledge for knowledge's sake (i.e., the accumulation of scientific knowledge) is important, but the immediate application of knowledge to affect the health and well-being of the participating community is equally important. The researchers had many curiosities and theories they wanted to explore, but the partners kept the focus on the practical use of knowledge gain.

In this study, members of the CBPR partnership chose to explore health concerns of Latino men primarily because the majority of Latinos who had recently arrived to the United States were male, especially in rural North Carolina. Partners had to come to agreement on the research and recruitment design and the roles and contributions of each of the partners. They decided to use focus groups to explore health priorities. Partners created, reviewed, revised, and approved the focus group moderator's guide. The league president recruited focus group participants, and two partnership members served as the focus group moderator and the note taker. The note taker was the university public health researcher, who was proficient in Spanish. A Latino-serving CBO hosted the focus groups. Seven focus groups were completed.[5,36]

The first stage of data analysis involved members of a subgroup from the CBPR partnership sorting the focus group transcripts into broad content categories. After the initial sorting process was complete, the analysis team came together to compare broad categories and begin the process of interpreting the findings into conceptual domains. After themes were created, the themes were presented to members of the CBPR partnership and other community members including soccer league members for *number checking* and interpretation. This was done by writing themes on flip charts and presenting these draft themes to the CBPR partners and representatives from the soccer league to review, discuss, and revise. Several iterations of this process were completed to ensure the validity of the interpretation of the data.

Findings were disseminated through community and national presentations, report writing, and manuscript development. Because action is a key component of CBPR, the findings also were used for funding proposals and intervention design. All partners had equal access to the findings. For example, organization representatives used preliminary findings for service grant and programmatic grant preparation, and community members used the findings to advocate for Latino men's health within the health department. It was through the initial focus groups that human immunodeficiency virus (HIV) and sexually transmitted disease (STD) infection were identified as priorities by members of the Latino soccer league, as well as the potential use of the social network of the league to develop, implement, and evaluate a social network lay health advisor intervention.[36]

The HoMBReS intervention study was funded by the Centers for Disease Control and Prevention (CDC). The goal of this CBPR study was to reduce the risk of HIV/STD infection among Latino men through the development, implementation, and evaluation of a lay health advisor intervention. Briefly, HoMBReS was a multiyear quasi-experimental research study with four interrelated objectives:

1. Develop and implement a lay health advisor intervention to reduce HIV/STD risk behaviors among members of the soccer league.
2. Evaluate the efficacy of the intervention by comparing soccer league members in the intervention to those in the delayed-intervention comparison group using self-reported sexual risk behaviors and utilization of HIV/STD counseling, testing, and treatment services.
3. Evaluate the changes experienced by the lay health advisors by being trained and serving as lay health advisors.
4. Assess the feasibility of engaging a soccer league in implementing a lay health advisor intervention designed to reduce HIV/STD transmission among Latino men.

The lay health advisors (based in the social networks of soccer teams), known as *Navegantes* (Navigators), were trained to provide HIV/STD prevention education, information, and service and resource referrals to their teammates. They served as: (1) sources of HIV/STD information and referral, (2) opinion leaders to change risky behavioral norms resulting from culturally infused male gender socialization, and (3) community activists to work with organizations such as the local public health department to better address the needs and priorities of Latino men in culturally congruent approaches.

This project was successful in the recruitment and training of a strong cadre of Navegantes because of the initial buy-in of the Latino soccer league. Without their history of interest, support, and involvement, the idea for HIV/STD primary prevention and the use of team members as lay health advisors would not necessarily have been considered or possible. Had it been considered, the risks would have been higher because buy-in would not have been garnered. Less knowledge about whether men would want to participate in a 16-hour, theory-based training and what that training should include would have left more opportunity for misjudgment on the part of the researcher. Instead, the partnership approach ensured fewer problems were incurred; when unavoidable roadblocks did occur, creative solutions that had a higher potential for success were explored because more perspectives and options were identified.[13,61,62,66]

The HoMBReS intervention was found to successfully increase condom use and HIV testing.

At postintervention assessment, the intervention was found to have increased condom use and HIV testing among teammates in the intervention compared to their peers in the comparison control group.[28] Further, the success of this initial study that was conducted in partnership with lay community members and organization representatives has led to further interventions. The CBPR partnership developed a multisession small-group intervention designed to increase condom use and HIV testing among heterosexually active Latino men entitled *HoMBReS-2*, which in pilot testing was found efficacious.[29]

The partnership is currently testing two different interventions for Latino gay and bisexual men, men who have sex with men (MSM), and transgender persons. One intervention is a lay health advisor intervention entitled *HOLA*. This intervention is based on the original HoMBReS intervention; however, rather than utilizing the social structure of the soccer league, it harnesses informal social networks of Latino gay and bisexual men, MSM, and transgender persons. Lay health advisors, also known as Navegantes, are trained to work with their friends to increase condom use and HIV testing.[27] The second intervention is entitled *HOLA en Grupos*, a small-group intervention for Latino MSM, also designed to increase condom use and HIV testing.[14]

Since the partners began their intervention research with immigrant Latino men, Latinas (e.g., girlfriends, wives, partners, sisters, and female cousins of male participants) stepped forward and asked representatives of the CBPR partnership for HIV prevention programming tailored to their needs and priorities. Based on extensive formative research, partners developed a culturally congruent intervention entitled *Mujeres Juntas Estableciendo Relaciones Saludables (MuJEReS)*, translated as Together Women Establishing Healthy Relationships. The intervention, which is designed to reduce the disproportionate HIV burden borne among Latinas in the United States, trains Latina lay health advisors, known as *Comadres* from the community, to work within their existing informal social networks. Latinas chose the term *Comadre* because of its common use to mean a trusted friend or neighbor who can be relied upon for advice and assistance. Besides the formal and informal health advising in which Comadres engage, partners determined that each Comadre also holds six 60- to 90-minute group sessions during intervention implementation with their social network members. These group sessions include (1) hosting a *fiesta* (party) to inaugurate the Comadre's role as a resource within her social network; (2) learning and practicing correct condom use skills; (3) brainstorming and discussing ways to overcome communication barriers with sex partners; (4) brainstorming and discussing ways to overcome communication barriers with providers; (5) demystifying the HIV testing process through describing available testing options, delineating the process (eligibility, etc.), and illustrating challenges that will be faced and how they can be surmounted; and (6) exploring what it is like to be an immigrant Latina through facilitated dialogue designed to build positive self-images and supportive relationships.[67]

SUMMARY

It has been asserted that ensuring the health of the public will require clinicians, health professionals, researchers, and others to join forces with lay community members and organizations of both community insiders and outsiders to generate new understandings of health status, explore health status predictors and measures, and uncover innovative ways to effect change in the health status within vulnerable communities.[2,68] Although this may seem logical, the process of partnership requires time to establish trusted relationships, create a research infrastructure, and develop a history of partnership. The investment of time to build these trusted relationships is essential for successful CBPR; this effort is well worth the expense in time, energy, and resources if true changes in health status are to occur.

Although no road map exists to conduct CBPR, it is important to note that often individuals, including health professionals, researchers, and community members, who are unfamiliar with CBPR confuse *community placed* with *community based*. Community-placed efforts simply imply that clinicians, health professionals, practitioners, and researchers leave the traditional institutions such as the university, hospital, or medical center and go into the community to do their work. However, community-based efforts are more than going outside the physical walls of these traditional institutions. CBPR requires partnering with communities and basing efforts in the reality and structures *preferred* by the community.

Health research through community partnership is a viable mechanism for health promotion and disease prevention[2,3,6,8,10,11,69,70] because CBPR improves the quality of research, increases community capacity, and advances positive health outcomes by:

- Bringing community members into a study as partners, not just as *subjects*
- Using the knowledge of the community to understand health problems, take appropriate action, and design meaningful interventions
- Connecting community members directly with how research is done and how it is used
- Providing immediate benefits from the results of the research to the community that participated in the study

CBPR can be infused into any research design. In this chapter, four methodologies were briefly presented and one case study was described. Researchers who are exploring the use of CBPR in their own research and practice should remember two important issues. First, key to using a CBPR approach is the inclusion of lay community members, CBO representatives, health department and other agency staff, and university personnel, including students and faculty researchers.[10] Together these partners must share control over all phases of the research process, including community assessment, issue definition, development of research methodology, data collection and analysis, interpretation of data, dissemination of findings, and application of the results to address community concerns. CBPR recognizes that lay community members themselves are the experts in understanding and interpreting their own lives.

Second, inherent in CBPR is a commitment towards action or intervention. This action may be loosely defined, including community organizing and mobilization, the development of new and authentic community member and agency partnerships with concrete tasks, and measurable plans for action with assigned responsibilities and defined timelines. The actions may be focused on immediate changes to improve health-related conditions, such as changes in a clinical practice protocol that increases adherence to an AIDS medication, policies that increase access to community mental health services, or even improved lighting on an outdoor neighborhood running/walking track to encourage utilization. Furthermore, actions may be focused on long-term changes in social determinants of health, such as improved racial equality in administrative and political representation through community mobilization and organization.

CBPR not only may be an effective tool to address the complex health problems facing vulnerable communities, but also is considered to be a just and democratic approach to research, as has been noted by community members. "Nothing about me, without me," implies that community members have a *right* to participate in all aspects of the research endeavor. Although CBPR is a challenging approach to research, it offers the researcher the opportunity to participate in a co-learning process of sharing resources, knowledge, skills, and attributes to increase the quality and validity of research. Increased quality and validity thus yields more effective interventions and improved health outcomes.

REFERENCES

1. Centers for Disease Control and Prevention, Agency for Toxic Substances and Disease Registry, Committee on Community Engagement. *Principles of Community Engagement*. Atlanta, GA: US Department of Health and Human Services; 1997.
2. Institute of Medicine. *Unequal Treatment: Confronting Racial and Ethnic Disparities in Health Care*. Washington, DC: National Academy Press; 2003.

3. Minkler M, Wallerstein N, eds. *Community-Based Participatory Research for Health.* San Francisco, CA: Jossey-Bass; 2003:3–26.
4. Eng E, Strazza K, Rhodes SD, et al. Insiders and outsiders assess who is "the community": Participant observation, key informant interview, focus group interview, and community forum. In: Israel BA, Eng E, Schulz AJ, Parker E, eds. *Methods for Conducting Community-Based Participatory Research for Health.* 2nd ed. San Francisco, CA: Jossey-Bass; 2013:133–160.
5. Cashman SB, Adeky S, Allen AJ, et al. The power and the promise: Working with communities to analyze data, interpret findings, and get to outcomes. *Am J Public Health.* 2008;98(8):1407–1417.
6. Rhodes SD. Demonstrated effectiveness and potential of CBPR for preventing HIV in Latino populations. In: Organista KC, ed. *HIV Prevention with Latinos: Theory, Research, and Practice.* New York: Oxford; 2012:83–102.
7. Rhodes SD, Duck S, Alonzo J, Daniel J, Aronson RE. Using community-based participatory research to prevent HIV disparities: Assumptions and opportunities identified by The Latino Partnership. *J Acq Immunodef Synd.* 2013;63(Suppl 1):S32–S35.
8. Rhodes SD, Malow RM, Jolly C. Community-based participatory research: A new and not-so-new approach to HIV/AIDS prevention, care, and treatment. *AIDS Educ Prev.* 2010;22(3):173–183.
9. Viswanathan M, Eng E, Ammerman A, et al. *Community-Based Participatory Research: Assessing the Evidence.* Rockville, MD: Agency for Healthcare Research and Quality; July 2004:99.
10. Israel BA, Schulz AJ, Parker EA, Becker AB. Review of community-based research: Assessing partnership approaches to improve public health. *Annu Rev Public Health.* 1998;19:173–202.
11. Wallerstein N, Duran B. The conceptual, historical, and practice roots of community-based participatory research and related participatory traditions. In: Minkler M, Wallerstein N, eds. *Community-Based Participatory Research for Health.* San Francisco, CA: Jossey-Bass; 2003:27–52.
12. Eng E, Blanchard L. Action-oriented community diagnosis: A health education tool. *Int J Community Health Educ.* 1991;11(2):93–110.
13. Eng E, Rhodes SD, Parker EA. Natural helper models to enhance a community's health and competence. In: DiClemente RJ, Crosby RA, Kegler MC, eds. *Emerging Theories in Health Promotion Practice and Research.* Vol. 2. San Francisco, CA: Jossey-Bass; 2009:303–330.
14. Rhodes SD, Mann L, Alonzo J, et al. CBPR to prevent HIV within ethnic, sexual, and gender minority communities: Successes with long-term sustainability. In: Rhodes SD, ed. *Innovations in HIV Prevention Research and Practice Through Community Engagement.* New York: Springer; 2014:135–160.
15. Lincoln YS, Guba EG. Paradigmatic controversies, contradictions, and emerging confluences. In: Denzin NK, Lincoln YS, eds. *The Handbook of Qualitative Research.* 2nd ed. Thousand Oaks, CA: Sage; 2000:163–188.
16. Habermas J. *The Theory of Communicative Action.* Cambridge, MA: Polity Press; 1984.
17. Rhodes SD, Hergenrather KC, Vissman AT, et al. Boys must be men, and men must have sex with women: A qualitative CBPR study to explore sexual risk among African American, Latino, and white gay men and MSM. *Am J Mens Health.* 2011;5(2):140–151.
18. Seifer SD. Building and sustaining community-institutional partnerships for prevention research: Findings from a national collaborative. *J Urban Health.* 2006;83(6):989–1003.
19. Seifer SD, Maurana CA. Developing and sustaining community–campus partnerships: Putting principles into practice. *Partners Perspect.* 2000;1(2):7–11.
20. Steuart GW. Planning and evaluation in health education. *Int J Health Educ.* 1969;2:65–76.
21. Cassel JC. The contribution of the social environment to host resistance: The fourth Wade Hampton Frost lecture. *Am J Epidemiol.* 1976;104:107–123.
22. Kauffman KS. The insider/outsider dilemma: Field experience of a white researcher "getting in" a poor black community. *Nurs Res.* 1994;43(3):179–183.
23. Steuart GW. Social and behavioral change strategies. In: Phillips HT, Gaylord SA, eds. *Aging and Public Health.* New York: Springer; 1985: 217–247.
24. Rhodes SD, Hergenrather KC, Aronson RE, et al. Latino men who have sex with men and HIV in the rural south-eastern USA: Findings from ethnographic in-depth interviews. *Cult Health Sex.* 2010;12(7):797–812.
25. Rhodes SD. Authentic engagement and community-based participatory research for public health and medicine. In: Rhodes SD, ed. *Innovations in HIV Prevention Research and Practice Through Community Engagement.* New York: Springer; 2014:1–10.
26. Rhodes SD, Hergenrather KC, Wilkin AM, Jolly C. Visions and voices: Indigent persons living with HIV in the southern United States use photovoice to create knowledge, develop partnerships, and take action. *Health Promot Pract.* 2008;9(2):159–169.
27. Rhodes SD, Daniel J, Alonzo J, et al. A systematic community-based participatory approach to refining an evidence-based community-level intervention: The HOLA intervention for Latino men

who have sex with men. *Health Promot Pract.* 2013;14(4):607–616.
28. Rhodes SD, Hergenrather KC, Bloom FR, Leichliter JS, Montano J. Outcomes from a community-based, participatory lay health adviser HIV/STD prevention intervention for recently arrived immigrant Latino men in rural North Carolina. *AIDS Educ Prev.* 2009;21(5 Suppl):103–108.
29. Rhodes SD, McCoy TP, Vissman AT, et al. A randomized controlled trial of a culturally congruent intervention to increase condom use and HIV testing among heterosexually active immigrant Latino men. *AIDS Behav.* 2011;15(8):1764–1775.
30. Rhodes SD, Vissman AT, Stowers J, et al. A CBPR partnership increases HIV testing among men who have sex with men (MSM): Outcome findings from a pilot test of the CyBER/testing Internet intervention. *Health Educ Behav.* 2011;38(3):311–320.
31. Rhodes SD, Daniel J, Alonzo J, et al. A snapshot of how Latino heterosexual men promote sexual health within their social networks: Process evaluation findings from an efficacious community-level intervention. *AIDS Educ Prev.* 2012;24(6):514–526.
32. Krueger RA, Casey MA. *Focus Groups: A Practical Guide to Applied Research.* Thousand Oaks, CA: Sage; 2000.
33. Morgan DL. *Focus Groups as Qualitative Research.* Newbury Park, CA: Sage; 1988.
34. Stewart DW, Shamdasani PN. *Focus Groups: Theory and Practice.* Vol. 20. Newbury Park, CA: Sage; 1990.
35. Rhodes SD, Hergenrather KC. Exploring hepatitis B vaccination acceptance among young men who have sex with men: Facilitators and barriers. *Prev Med.* 2002;35(2):128–134.
36. Rhodes SD, Eng E, Hergenrather KC, et al. Exploring Latino men's HIV risk using community-based participatory research. *Am J Health Behav.* 2007;31(2):146–158.
37. Glaser BG, Strauss AL. *The Discovery of Grounded Theory: Strategies for Qualitative Research.* Chicago, IL: Aldine; 1967.
38. Kitzinger J. The methodology of focus groups: The importance of interactions between research participants. *Sociol Health Illn.* 1994;16:103–121.
39. Sandelowski M, Davis DH, Harris BG. Artful design: Writing the proposal for research in the naturalist paradigm. *Res Nurs Health.* 1989;12(2):77–84.
40. Tashakkori A, Teddlie C. Introduction to mixed method and mixed model studies in the social and behavioral sciences. In: *Mixed Methodology: Combining Qualitative and Quantitative Approaches.* Thousand Oaks, CA: Sage; 1998:3–19.
41. Wang C, Burris MA. Photovoice: Concept, methodology, and use for participatory needs assessment. *Health Educ Behav.* 1997;24(3):369–387.
42. Rhodes SD, Hergenrather KC. Recently arrived immigrant Latino men identify community approaches to promote HIV prevention. *Am J Public Health.* 2007;97(6):984–985.
43. Hergenrather KC, Rhodes SD, Clark G. Windows to work: Exploring employment-seeking behaviors of persons with HIV/AIDS through photovoice. *AIDS Educ Prev.* 2006;18(3):243–258.
44. Hergenrather KC, Rhodes SD, Cowan CA, Bardhoshi G, Pula S. Photovoice as community-based participatory research: A qualitative review. *Am J Health Behav.* 2009;33(6):686–698.
45. Rhodes SD, Hergenrather KC, Griffith D, et al. Sexual and alcohol use behaviours of Latino men in the south-eastern USA. *Culture Health Sex.* 2009;11(1):17–34.
46. Freire P. *Pedagogy of the Oppressed.* New York: Herder and Herder; 1970.
47. Shaffer R. *Beyond the Dispensary.* Nairobi, Kenya: Amref; 1983.
48. Streng JM, Rhodes SD, Ayala GX, Eng E, Arceo R, Phipps S. Realidad Latina: Latino adolescents, their school, and a university use photovoice to examine and address the influence of immigration. *J Interprof Care.* 2004;18(4):403–415.
49. Baquero B, Goldman S, Muqueeth S, et al. Mi Cuerpo, Nuestra Responsabilidad: Using photovoice to describe the assets and barriers to reproductive health among Latinos in North Carolina. *J Health Dispar Res Pract.* 2014;7(1):65–83.
50. Wang C, Burris MA, Ping XY. Chinese village women as visual anthropologists: A participatory approach to reaching policymakers. *Soc Sci Med.* 1996;42(10):1391–1400.
51. Wang CC, Yi WK, Tao ZW, Carovano K. Photovoice as a participatory health promotion strategy. *Health Promot Int.* 1998;13(1):75–86.
52. Killion CM, Wang CC. Linking African American mothers across life stage and station through photovoice. *J Health Care Poor Underserved.* 2000;11(3):310–325.
53. Moss T. Youth put their world on view. *Child First.* 1999;3(27):3–35.
54. Rhodes SD. Visions and voices: HIV in the 21st century. Indigent persons living with HIV/AIDS in the southern USA use photovoice to communicate meaning. *J Epidemiol Community Health.* 2006;60(10):886.
55. Wang C. Picture this: A snapshot of health in Contra Costa [unpublished report]. 1988.
56. Angell KL, Kreshka MA, McCoy R, et al. Psychosocial intervention for rural women with breast cancer: The Sierra-Stanford partnership. *J Gen Intern Med.* 2003;18(7):499–507.

57. Lauderdale DS, Kuohung V, Chang SL, Chin MH. Identifying older Chinese immigrants at high risk for osteoporosis. *J Gen Intern Med.* 2003;18(7):508–515.
58. Rhodes SD, Hergenrather KC, Wilkin AM, Alegria-Ortega J, Montaño J. Preventing HIV infection among young immigrant Latino men: Results from focus groups using community-based participatory research. *J Natl Med Assoc.* 2006;98(4):564–573.
59. Vissman AT, Bloom FR, Leichliter JS, et al. Exploring the use of nonmedical sources of prescription drugs among immigrant Latinos in the rural southeastern USA. *J Rural Health.* 2011;27(2):159–167.
60. Rhodes SD, Yee LJ, Hergenrather KC. Hepatitis A vaccination among young African American men who have sex with men in the deep south: Psychosocial predictors. *J Natl Med Assoc.* 2003;95(4 Suppl):31S–36S.
61. Painter TM, Organista KC, Rhodes SD, Sañudo FM. Interventions to prevent HIV and other sexually transmitted diseases among Latino migrants. In: Organista KC, ed. *HIV Prevention with Latinos: Theory, Research, and Practice.* New York: Oxford; 2012:351–381.
62. Rhodes SD. Tuberculosis, sexually transmitted diseases, HIV, and other infections among farmworkers in the eastern United States. In: Arcury TA, Quandt SA, eds. *Latino Farmworkers in the Eastern United States: Health, Safety and Justice.* New York: Springer; 2009:131–152.
63. Rhodes SD, Hergenrather KC, Montano J, et al. Using community-based participatory research to develop an intervention to reduce HIV and STD infections among Latino men. *AIDS Educ Prev.* 2006;18(5):375–389.
64. Margolis LH, Stevens R, Laraia B, et al. Educating students for community-based partnerships. *J Community Pract.* 2000;7(4):21–34.
65. Parker EA, Eng E, Laraia B, et al. Coalition building for prevention: Lessons learned from the North Carolina Community-Based Public Health Initiative. *J Public Health Manag Pract.* 1998;4(2):25–36.
66. Vissman AT, Eng E, Aronson RE, et al. What do men who serve as lay health advisors really do?: Immigrant Latino men share their experiences as *Navegantes* to prevent HIV. *AIDS Educ Prev.* 2009;21(3):220–232.
67. Rhodes SD, Kelley C, Simán F, et al. Using community-based participatory research (CBPR) to develop a community-level HIV prevention intervention for Latinas: A local response to a global challenge. *Women Health Issues.* 2012;22(3):293–301.
68. Institute of Medicine. *The Future of Public Health.* Washington, DC: National Academy Press; 1988.
69. Wandersman A. Community science: Bridging the gap between science and practice with community-centered models. *Am J Community Psychol.* 2003;31(3-4):227–242.
70. Hergenrather KC, Rhodes SD. Community-based participatory research: Applications for research in health and disability. In: Knoll T, ed. *Focus on Disability: Trends in Research and Application.* Vol. 2. New York: Nova Science; 2008:59-87.

CBPR RESOURCES

Besides the references cited within this chapter, supplemental resources are listed in this section.

CBPR

- Minkler M, Wallerstein N, eds. *Community-Based Participatory Research for Health: From Process to Outcomes.* 2nd ed. San Francisco, CA: Jossey-Bass; 2008.
- Hergenrather KC, Rhodes SD. Community-based participatory research: Applications for research in health and disability. In Kroll T, ed. *Focus on Disability: Trends in Research and Application.* Vol. 2. New York: Nova Science; 2008:59–87.
- Israel BA, Eng E, Schulz AJ, Parker EA, eds. *Methods for Conducting Community-Based Participatory Research for Health.* San Francisco, CA: Jossey-Bass; 2013.
- Agency for Healthcare Research and Quality. Community-based Participatory Research: Assessing the Evidence. Available at: http://archive.ahrq.gov/downloads/pub/evidence/pdf/cbpr/cbpr.pdf.
- Campus-Community Partnerships for Health. Home Page. Available at: http://depts.washington.edu/ccph/.
- Centers for Disease Control and Prevention. Representing Your Community in Community-based Participatory Research: Differences Made and Measured. Available at: http://www.cdc.gov/pcd/issues/2004/jan/03_0024.htm.

Photovoice

- Hergenrather KC, Rhodes SD, Clark G. Windows to work: Exploring employment seeking behaviors of persons with HIV/AIDS through photovoice. *AIDS Educ Prev.* 2006;18(3):243–258.
- Hergenrather KC, Rhodes SD, Cowan C, Bardhoshi G, Pula S. Photovoice as community-based participatory research: A qualitative review. *Am J Health Behav.* 2009;33(6):686–698.
- Rhodes SD. Visions and voices—HIV in the 21st century: Indigent persons living with HIV/AIDS in the southern USA use photovoice to

communicate meaning. *J Epidemiol Community Health*. 2006;60(10):886.
- Rhodes SD, Hergenrather KC. Recently arrived immigrant Latino men identify community approaches to promote HIV prevention in the Southern USA. *Am J Public Health*. 2007;97(6):984–985.
- Rhodes SD, Hergenrather KC, Griffith D, et al. Sexual and alcohol risk behaviours of immigrant Latino men in the south-eastern USA. *Culture Health Sex*. 2009;11(1):17–34.
- Rhodes SD, Hergenrather KC, Wilkin A, Jolly C. Visions and voices: Indigent persons living with HIV in the southern US use photovoice to create knowledge, develop partnerships, and take action. *Health Promotion Pract*. 2008;9(2):159–169.
- Streng JM, Rhodes SD, Ayala GX, Eng E, Arceo R, Phipps S. Realidad Latina: Latino adolescents, their school, and a university use photovoice to examine and address the influence of immigration. *J Interprofess Care*. 2004;18(4):403–415.
- Wang C. Project: Photovoice involving homeless men and women of Washtenaw County, Michigan. *Health Educ Behav*. 1998;25(1):9–10.
- Wang C. Using photovoice as a participatory assessment and issue selection tool. In: Minkler M, Wallerstein N (eds.), *Community-Based Participatory Research for Health*. San Francisco, CA: Jossey-Bass; 2003:179–196.
- Wang C, Cash JL, Powers LS. Who knows the streets as well as the homeless? Promoting personal and community action through photovoice. *Health Promotion Pract*. 2000;1(1):81–89.

Health Disparities

- Institute of Medicine. *Engaging the Public in the Clinical Research Enterprise: Clinical Research Roundtable Workshop Summary*. Washington, DC: National Academies Press; 2003.
- Wallerstein N. Powerless, empowerment, and health: Implications for health promotion programs. *Am J Health Prom*, 1992;6:197–205.

Qualitative Research

- Patton M, ed. *Qualitative Research and Evaluation Methods*. 3rd ed. Thousand Oaks, CA: Sage; 2002.
- Miles M, Huberman AM. *Qualitative Data Analysis: A Methods Sourcebook*. 3rd ed. Thousand Oaks, CA: Sage; 2013.
- Krueger RA, Casey MA. *Focus Groups: A Practical Guide for Applied Research*. 4th ed. Thousand Oaks, CA: Sage; 2009.
- Morgan DL, Krueger RA. *The Focus Group Kit*. Vols. 1–6. Thousand Oaks, CA: Sage; 1997.

CHAPTER 10

Clinical Investigations

J. Glenn Forister, MS, PA-C

CHAPTER OVERVIEW

Clinical studies are invaluable to health care. This is where laboratory research is translated to patient care. Healthcare organizations are becoming engaged with clinical research to generate income. Many healthcare providers are finding themselves involved with clinical research without much prior experience. This chapter provides an introduction to clinical research.

Learning Objectives

- Define *clinical investigation* and the phases of clinical research.
- Discuss and describe clinical investigation design and methodology.
- Describe subject selection.
- Define and describe *informed consent*, *adverse events*, and *study termination*.

INTRODUCTION

Increasing public demand for new FDA-approved medications and medical devices has generated an increase in clinical research. The overall goal of clinical research is to maintain the safety of the research participant while determining the efficacy of the investigational product. Clinicians are finding themselves more involved in clinical research in roles such as a principal investigator or study coordinator in a research project, whether voluntarily or involuntarily assigned such a role. This chapter provides a basic introduction to the clinical research process by describing the phases of clinical research, discussing subject selection and protection, and describing the informed consent process, adverse events, and study termination.

THE CLINICAL RESEARCH PROCESS

Healthcare providers may be asked to participate in a clinical research study in the role of study coordinator. This may be a request or the role may be assigned by the practice's administrator. Most clinical research studies are conducted in the same manner, whether it is a sponsored pharmaceutical investigation, a medical device study, or benchmark research from an academic institution. Whatever the setting, research processes are somewhat standard.

When conducting any clinical research, the most important aspects are (1) to ensure that the research participants have a complete understanding of the research study, and (2) to protect the participants at all times throughout the study. A specific guideline, known as the International Conference on Harmonisation of Technical Requirements for Registration of Pharmaceuticals for Human Use (ICH) *Guideline for Good Clinical Practice (GCP)*, maintains that every research participant must be completely informed of the study they are about to enter. Being completely informed means understanding the study expectations, potential risks, and potential side effects, as well as how the research site and sponsor (and/or institution) will fully monitor their progress throughout the study. Because healthcare professionals of all types may be asked to assist with a research study in their practice (or even invited to be the study coordinator), the information in this chapter provides a general idea of what to expect when working with most clinical research studies.

Understanding the key personnel roles involved in clinical research is essential. A clinical research study will always identify a principal investigator (PI). The PI is typically a physician who assumes total responsibility for the entire study. The PI is, therefore, responsible for the welfare of the study participants, that is, ensuring that study subjects have been properly informed, have given consent, and have met the study's inclusion and exclusion criteria. The PI also oversees any adverse events (AEs) and manages subsequent outcomes. The PI is responsible for all of the personnel involved in the study: subinvestigators, study coordinator(s), medical technicians, practitioners, and the like. The PI must ensure each person involved is qualified to perform his or her designated role in the study; for instance, an inappropriate assignment of a study responsibility would be having a medical assistant perform a physical exam on a research patient. Therefore, the PI role is a serious responsibility. The PI always answers for any violations that occur at the research site or in the course of the study.

The PI may choose to designate a subinvestigator (sub-I) or coinvestigator to help oversee the research study at the site. A sub-I is especially helpful when a research study is being conducted at satellite clinic locations. The sub-I may be located at a different clinic than the PI and, therefore, can assist in the follow-up of any research participants that are being seen at that particular clinic. Most sub-Is are physicians as well; however, other healthcare professionals or doctoral-level researchers, such as PhDs, can also serve in this role. Sub-Is typically hold some form of medical licensure, and this role involves responsibilities similar to those of the PI. However, the PI retains the sole responsibility for the entire research study and research personnel, including the sub-Is.

The study coordinator is the central person in a research study and is highly involved in the research process. Most study coordinators are registered nurses; however, other healthcare professionals are being asked to assume the role of study coordinator in spite of their busy clinic schedules. The study coordinator's role is vital to the entire project. Most site personnel who are asked to be the study coordinator for a clinical research study are often surprised at the amount of work (or additional work) this role entails. The study coordinator's primary responsibilities include the following:

- Recruiting subjects for the study
- Explaining the research study to the patient and answering any questions
- Reviewing and obtaining the patient's informed consent

- Ensuring all of the study entry procedures have been conducted
- Reviewing the study's inclusion/exclusion criteria with the PI and/or sub-I to verify the patient's eligibility
- Documenting the study visit information on the case report forms (CRFs), either transcribing the data onto paper CRFs or entering them electronically on e-CRFs
- Monitoring the patient's safety and well-being throughout the study by recording any adverse events (AEs), unanticipated adverse events (UAEs), or serious adverse events (SAEs)
- Dispensing, tracking, and storing any study medication or investigational medical device
- Accommodating the sponsor's monitoring visits

If the site does not utilize separate personnel to oversee the regulatory documents (e.g., institutional review board [IRB] submissions and approvals, continuing study renewals, UAE/SAE reporting, etc.), then the study coordinator will assume these responsibilities as well.

Another important role in clinical research is the clinical research associate (CRA), also known as the study monitor. The CRA either is employed by the sponsor or the sponsor-delegated contract research organization or is an employee of the academic institution. The CRA's primary duty is to conduct on-site visits, or *audits*, to ensure the research participants are eligible to participate in the study, are fully protected from harm, and are being treated with the utmost care[1]. The CRA also ensures the site is conducting the research study in compliance with the approved protocol, Food and Drug Administration (FDA) Code of Federal Regulations, and IRB regulations by training the study personnel during the study start-up (site initiation) phase. They also reinforce protocol training and regulatory guidance throughout the study. While on-site, the CRA will examine all of the research participants' medical records as they pertain to the study and review the study CRFs (either paper or electronic) to ensure all data have been captured correctly.

The CRA works closely with the study coordinator to correct any data errors and to resolve any data queries during and after the visit. The CRA usually meets with the PI and/or sub-I to review any issues that were uncovered during the visit. Depending on the type of study and current study status, the CRA may visit a site as often as every 4 weeks or as rarely as once a year. CRA visits can add a layer of work and may seem incredibly burdensome for the study coordinator; however, these visits are completely necessary for the study participants' safety and well-being as well as the overall success of the study.

Written Consent

Once the research site has received IRB approval to begin the study, the site can begin screening and enrolling participants. The first step is always to obtain written informed consent from the patient prior to conducting any study-related procedures. Any designated study personnel can conduct the informed consent process with the potential participant; however, the person conducting the informed consent process must be properly trained in how to conduct the process, as well as be knowledgeable in every aspect of the protocol. Per the ICH E6 Guidelines and FDA Code of Federal Regulations (21 CFR 50), the site is responsible for documenting the informed consent process in the patient's study file. The process entails: (1) allowing the research participant adequate time to read and review the informed consent; (2) discussing the study in detail with the patient; (3) allowing the patient to ask questions and answer any questions to their satisfaction; (4) witnessing the participant's signature/date by cosigning and dating the form; and (5) providing a copy of the informed consent form to the patient while filing the original version in the patient's study file. Additionally, most informed consent procedures include a separate informed consent form regarding the patient's rights that stem from the Health Insurance Portability and Accountability Act of 1996 (HIPAA). The HIPAA section or separate consent form requires the patient to provide his or her signature of approval for the release of medical records and information for the study sponsor or any regulatory agency auditing the study.

Meeting Inclusion and/or Exclusion Criteria

Once the patients' informed consents have been obtained, the study coordinator can then begin to screen each potential study participant, performing the baseline visit procedures to determine whether the patient meets the inclusion/exclusion criteria for the study. The FDA Code of Federal Regulations and the ICH Guidelines explicitly warn against "prequalifying" a patient for a research study (refer to 21 CFR 50 and ICH E6 Guidelines). A site cannot perform any study-related procedures on a potential research candidate prior to obtaining that participant's informed consent. For instance, if the study requires certain lab results or an electrocardiogram (EKG) to be performed to determine eligibility, the research site cannot first draw STAT lab values or perform the EKG to determine whether the results comply with the inclusion criteria, and subsequently enroll the patient in the study. Therefore, the site must obtain the patient's full written consent before determining eligibility. However, some research protocols will allow potential study subjects to be prescreened or prequalified to determine study eligibility. In this case, a designated "prescreen informed consent form," completely separate from the informed consent form for the main portion of the study, is provided. This form must be approved by the IRB before being utilized with any potential patient. The prescreen informed consent form describes prescreening procedures the patient will encounter in detail, and this form clearly states that the patient will be undergoing prescreening for the study to determine eligibility. Whether prescreening or screening, an emphasis must be placed on obtaining the patient's consent in writing. Verbal consent is not allowed in a clinical research study and would be in direct violation of the federal regulations.

Baseline Visit

Baseline visit procedures to determine whether a patient is eligible to participate in a study can vary greatly. Baseline visit procedures typically consist of a medical history, physical exam, and routine lab work. Depending on the study, baseline visit procedures can also consist of a variety of other diagnostic tests. The study coordinator may already have a good idea that the patient is likely to qualify to be enrolled in the study; however, he or she must wait until all of the procedures have been performed and the results obtained to determine eligibility. Once all of the data are available, the next step is to determine whether the patient has met the inclusion and exclusion criteria. To be eligible to participate in a research study, a patient must meet *all* of the inclusion criteria and *none* of the exclusion criteria. If the patient meets just *one* of the exclusion criteria, then the patient is excluded from participating in the study.

During a monitoring visit, the CRA ensures the study subjects were properly enrolled in the study by verifying whether each patient met the inclusion/exclusion criteria. The CRA performs a detailed audit of the study subjects' medical records, paying close attention to the baseline visit procedures that were performed to determine eligibility. If the patient meets all of the inclusion criteria and none of the exclusion criteria, then the patient is determined eligible to participate in the study and, therefore, can continue forward to the next phase. However, if the study's entrance criteria are not met, then the patient is considered a "screen failure" and is immediately withdrawn from further participation in the study. Properly determining study eligibility is as important as the informed consent process. The sponsor, IRB, and FDA always scrutinize these two processes to ensure health and safety. Research participants must be protected and well-informed of their study status at all times during a clinical study.

Randomization

After the eligibility phase, the next phase in a clinical research study is typically *randomization*. The randomization phase determines which study participants will receive the investigational drug or device and which participants will receive a placebo or control. However, not all research studies involve a randomization phase. For instance, some medical device studies do not randomize the participants because the study plan is to have each participant receive some degree of exposure to the investigational medical device. In turn, these study subjects are often considered their own form of control (i.e., Did the device work for them or not?). With some research studies, the study design can become complex regarding the randomization scheme. The sponsor or research institution may want all of the research participants to be exposed to the product being investigated at some point in the study. Therefore, randomization cross-over schemes are often included in the protocol. In this design study, subjects are randomized to either the placebo or active/investigational product group initially and then are crossed over to the opposite group after a certain period. From the study coordinator's perspective, ensuring the randomization has been performed correctly for each patient is another crucial step in the research process.

Follow-up

Following the randomization phase—or baseline visit if no randomization is planned—the research participants usually begin the follow-up visits for the study. The follow-up visit procedures may appear very similar to the baseline visit procedures. The same lab work, x-rays, EKGs, physical exams, and patient questionnaires may be repeated to some extent during these follow-up visits. Once again, it is the study coordinator's job to ensure that all of the follow-up study visit procedures are being conducted. As the first person to receive and review these results, the study coordinator must also be vigilant about the study exam results and/or data generated from these visits. During the follow-up visits, any trends or discrepancies in the patients' results can be detected. For instance, if several of the research participants' lab results indicate that their liver enzymes are abnormally high and are becoming increasingly higher as the study progresses, then the study coordinator can alert the PI and sub-I(s) regarding this trend. Together, the research team can alert the sponsor or the research institution's medical advisor. Therefore, the study coordinator is the protective watchdog over the research participants' health and safety.

Adverse Events

The scenario mentioned in the previous section regarding abnormally increasing liver enzymes is an example of an adverse event (AE). The amount and severity of AEs most often determine whether an investigational drug or device application will be submitted to the FDA for approval. Most pharmaceutical and medical device sponsors, as well as research institutions, require the capture, report, and documentation of AEs to some extent in their research studies. The approved study protocol describes the extent to which AEs will be documented for that particular study. The ICH E6 *Guideline for Good Clinical Practice* (and similarly Code of Federal Regulations 21 CFR 310.305) defines an adverse event as follows:

> . . . *any untoward medical occurrence in a patient or clinical investigation subject administered a pharmaceutical product and that does not necessarily have a causal relationship with this treatment. An AE can, therefore, be any unfavorable and unintended sign (including an abnormal laboratory finding), symptom, or disease temporally associated with the use of a medicinal (investigational) product, whether or not related to the medicinal (investigational) product.*

For example, if a patient returns for the 3-month follow-up visit and reports to the study coordinator that they have had the flu for the past 4 days, this experience is considered an AE. Another type of AE that can occur in a research study is known as a serious adverse event (SAE). The ICH E6 *Guideline for Good Clinical Practice* (and similarly Code of Federal Regulations 21 CFR 312.32) defines an SAE as follows:

> . . . *any untoward medical occurrence that at any dose:*
> - *Results in death*
> - *Is life threatening*
> - *Requires inpatient hospitalization or prolongation of existing hospitalization*

- *Results in persistent or significant disability/incapacity*
- *Produces a congenital anomaly/birth defect.*

Serious adverse events must be reported immediately to the sponsor or research institution responsible for the study. The research site must report the SAE as soon as it becomes aware of the event, no longer than 24 hours from the time the event was initially registered. The sponsor or academic research institution will request that the research team obtain all available information surrounding the event (e.g., hospital records from admission to discharge or the death certificate). The process of collecting, documenting, and reporting AEs and SAEs is much more involved than this chapter covers. Generally, the sponsor reviews the data collection and reporting requirements in depth with the research site personnel during study start-up.

Study Termination

The final phase of a research study is study completion, or study termination. Research participants who have completed all of the required follow-up visits are then dismissed from the study. The procedures for the exit visit can be as extensive as those for the baseline visit. The research team wants to obtain as much data as possible during this visit, knowing that this visit is the last opportunity to collect any additional lab work, EKGs, x-rays, and/or patient questionnaires. Research subjects who have completed the study are rarely asked to come back and complete extra study visits to provide additional information. Study subjects can be withdrawn early or undergo early termination from a research study. The protocol usually provides guidelines and/or potential reasons for a patient's early termination or early withdrawal from the study. The most common reason is the patient no longer wishes to continue participating in the study and, therefore, voluntarily withdraws consent. Other reasons why a patient may be early exited from a study include the following:

- Patient is unwilling or unable to cooperate with study visits or procedures.
- Patient has experienced an AE or SAE.
- Patient relocates to a different area from where the research is being conducted.
- Patient is lost to follow-up (i.e., patient misses study visits and site is unable to contact the patient by phone, email, or certified mail).

IRBs most often want to know the reason(s) why a patient was withdrawn early from the study; therefore, they require the research team to document this information in the study records.

At first glance, the research team may feel that conducting a clinical research study appears to be rather easy. However, most clinicians have never participated in a clinical research project; therefore, they may be unaware of the significant amount of extra time and effort required. A study adds demands and responsibilities to the clinic's normal operations. On the other hand, participating in a clinical research project, or being asked to fulfill a specific role in one, can be a rewarding experience. Becoming involved in a clinical research project, as either a PI, sub-I, or study coordinator, puts practitioners on the cutting edge of a new drug, device, or procedure that could ultimately make a difference in the lives of many patients.

PHASES OF CLINICAL RESEARCH

Clinical research is most often performed to determine the safety and efficacy of a new drug or medical device and/or a new indication for either. Conducting clinical research on a new drug or medical device is extremely expensive. Most pharmaceutical and medical device sponsors spend millions of dollars attempting to receive approval for a single drug or device. The process of developing a new drug or device, conducting clinical research trials, and submitting an application to the FDA typically takes approximately 10 years, with most new drugs or devices never receiving FDA approval.

Clinical research trials involve four phases. Each phase is critical to the overall approval and success of a new drug or medical device. Furthermore, a clinical trial can be halted at any time and during any phase if too many adverse side effects or SAEs occur with the research participants.

Prior to phase I trials, preclinical studies may be conducted on animals to determine whether a new drug or device will be effective. Phase I clinical trials are the initial studies performed to determine the metabolism and pharmacokinetics of a drug (or a device) in humans. Phase I clinical trials are, therefore, considered "first-in-human" research studies. These studies are conducted on a small number of healthy participants (20–100) for a short time, usually for a few days to 1 month. Data regarding side effects associated with increasing doses and evidence of investigational product effectiveness are collected. Phase I studies are used to determine the maximum safe dose that can be tolerated and establishes toxicity.

Once the maximum safe dosage of an investigational product has been determined, the next step in the research trial process is to conduct a phase II clinical trial. A phase II clinical trial is a randomized, controlled study conducted to evaluate the effectiveness and therapeutic range of a drug (or a device) for a particular indication in patients with the disease or condition, as well as to determine common side effects and risks. Phase II research studies are longer than phase I studies, typically lasting a few months to 1 year. During phase II, study participants are randomized to receive either the investigational product or a placebo. Phase II studies involve a larger numbers of research participants (100–300).

After conducting phase II studies, sponsors have an established idea of the therapeutic range of the investigational product as well as the expected side effects. Sponsors then conduct phase III clinical trials to introduce the investigational product to a large number of participants (1000–3000). Phase III studies are expansive clinical trials usually conducted nationally (and even internationally) across multiple research sites. Phase III studies are usually randomized, controlled trials comparing the investigational product to placebo. These trials can be "open label" as well, with the research participants and research team aware of who is receiving the investigational product and who is not. Phase III trials are conducted to gather additional information on the overall benefits and/or risks of the product or device being investigated; they also provide a basis for product labeling. Sponsors prepare to submit their new drug or device application to the FDA for approval at the conclusion of the phase III trials. If the sponsor receives FDA approval for the new drug or device, then a phase IV clinical trial can be conducted.

Phase IV trials are "postmarketing" trials that can be either voluntarily conducted by the investigator or mandated by the FDA as a stipulation for the new drug or device approval. Either way, phase IV clinical trials are conducted to obtain a greater amount of safety and efficacy data in thousands of individuals (i.e., even more than phase II or III). During phase IV studies, the new drug or device is available to the public. Phase IV studies can provide additional information regarding risks, benefits, and optimal use that perhaps did not appear during the phase III studies. Because of the large number of participants and amount of data generated, the FDA recommends that more company-sponsored research involve phase IV clinical trials.

SUMMARY

The overall goal of clinical research is to safely translate laboratory research into applied clinical interventions. The process must be transparent and follow the established national and international guidelines for conducting research on human subjects. It is, therefore, important that all parties understand the purpose and process of the investigation. Each of the steps from IRB protocol approval to the exit visit helps to maintain the integrity of the study and ultimately the results.

REFERENCES

1. Woodlin KE, Schneider JC. *The CRA's Guide to Monitoring Clinical Research.* Boston: Thomson Centerwatch; 2003.

WEBSITES MENTIONED IN THIS CHAPTER

- *ICH E6 Guidelines:* http://www.ich.org/products/guidelines/efficacy/article/efficacy-guidelines.html
- *21 CFR Part 50:* http://www.accessdata.fda.gov/scripts/cdrh/cfdocs/cfcfr/CFRsearch.cfm?CFRPart50
- *21 CFR Part 310:* http://www.access.gpo.gov/nara/cfr/waisidx_03/21cfr310_03.html
- *21 CFR Part 312:* http://www.accessdata.fda.gov/scripts/cdrh/cfdocs/cfcfr/cfrsearch.cfm?cfrpart = 312

# SECTION III

THE RESEARCH PROCESS: ANALYSIS

CHAPTER 11

CHAPTER OVERVIEW

This chapter provides a basic overview of the common statistical techniques used in quantitative studies. This is the first step in the use and understanding of statistics. A large number of books are available on statistics and statistical analysis, and every researcher should have at least one statistical analysis book as a reference. Decisions about data analysis must be made prior to data collection; data analysis planning is part of research methodology. Even those with a basic understanding of statistics will benefit from consulting a statistician about the research design and analysis. Careful attention should be given to the type of research being conducted and the type of data produced by the investigation. Selection of the correct statistical tests results in proper data analysis and greater confidence in the conclusions drawn from the study's results. As a practicing healthcare professional, understanding data analysis is a key part of interpreting medical and research literature.

Data Analysis

Meredith A. Davison, PhD, MPH
Bruce R. Niebuhr, PhD
J. Glenn Forister, MS, PA-C

Learning Objectives

- Define and describe the levels of measurement.
- Define descriptive statistics.
- Define inferential statistics.
- Describe the process for choosing a statistical test.
- Apply common statistical tests to practice data.

INTRODUCTION

Why should clinicians use statistics? Although some healthcare providers earn advanced degrees and engage in health-related research, most are practicing clinicians. All healthcare providers have been exposed to statistical analysis in their education; however, many providers may not see the relevance of statistics in their clinical practice. The basic reason for clinicians to use statistics is to help them understand research articles that help to formulate important decisions for their patients and practice. Healthcare providers are called upon every day to make decisions that are the most cost-efficient and least harmful, and/or comprise the most appropriate treatment plan. These decisions are best made by understanding the medical literature. Frequently, this understanding requires a basic knowledge and appreciation of statistical analysis and inference.

Healthcare providers are not expected to be statisticians. Biostatistics is a specialty unto itself. Consulting a biostatistician is essential for conducting a research study. Regardless of whether a healthcare practitioner ever participates in clinical research, critically analyzing the results of research studies in order to make decisions regarding clinical diagnoses and treatment is an important part of healthcare practice. The following are the primary objectives in evaluating the data analysis of a research study:

- Become familiar with the types of data produced in the study
- Become familiar with the most common statistics in order to read a journal article and grasp its use of statistics and how the study's conclusions flow from the statistical analyses and results
- Understand the rationale behind the selection of statistical analyses and how well specific analyses test the study's hypotheses

In this chapter we explore descriptive statistics and inferential statistics, as well as the styles of results presentation, statistical reference texts, and computer software options. Mathematical and statistical formulas are used sparingly in this chapter. Those involved in research may wish to conduct some data analyses to hone and develop their skills.

LEVELS OF MEASUREMENT

The first step in deciding on the appropriate type of statistical analysis is to determine the level of measurement to be used based on the type of data. The data types are shown in **Table 11-1**. As a general rule of thumb, the higher the level of measurement, the more information can be ascertained from the data. The most basic level of measurement is the nominal level, in which responses are divided into named groups or categories. For example, subjects might be asked to choose the group to which they belong: male or female. The subjects' choices allow the researcher to group subjects by category.

The nominal level of measurement limits the researcher in the type and number of statistical and mathematical analyses. Primarily, only descriptive analysis or summary can be used. These data

Table 11-1 Definitions of Data Types

Data Type	Definition	Example
Nominal data	Data that categorizes	Gender, eye color, race, graduating cohort, practice specialty
Ordinal data	Data defined by an ordering, but the distance between the choices or values is not defined	Likert scales, preference scales, rankings
Continuous data	Data with numeric values; there are two types: interval and ratio.	Numbers
	Interval data: Data with a defined interval between the values, but with no true zero value	Ambient temperature: Zero does not indicate a total lack of temperature; it is a value on a scale. The temperature interval difference between 61°F and 62°F is the same as the interval difference between −61°F and −62°F.
	Ratio data: Data with an absolute zero value, where zero means there is a total absence of what is being measured	Visual acuity, range of motion, height, weight, blood pressure, blood alcohol level

enable the researcher to determine how many subjects fall into each category. For example, in a survey of 100 healthcare professionals, 39 percent were male and 61 percent were female. Some common nominal data types are gender, race, religion, eye color, year in school, and home state. Consider nominal data as information that helps to categorize something or someone.

Ordinal measurement provides an ordering (sometimes ranking) between variables; however, the distance between each variable is not defined. For example, research subjects may be asked to indicate their degree of agreement or disagreement with a series of statements. There is no defined distance between "Agree" and "Strongly Agree" or between "Neutral" and "Disagree." One of the most common forms of ordinal measurement is the Likert scale. The traditional use of the Likert scale is to provide the subject with a statement and ask for the level of agreement or disagreement with that statement. The true Likert scale is a five-point scale with the following terms:

Strongly Agree   Agree   Neutral   Disagree   Strongly Disagree

Although it offers greater possibilities for a more in-depth analysis than nominal measurement, ordinal measurement has limitations with regard to statistical analysis. Several types of ordinal scales exist but each suffers from the lack of uniform distance between units for each respondent. The researcher cannot measure differences with the same amount of precision as interval or ratio data. Many ordinal scales are referred to as verbal frequency scales. These scales use wording such as "always," "sometimes," and "never." Numbers are often used for the responses to ordinal measurements. In essence, vague language such as "sometimes" is assigned a numeric value. One respondent's valuation of "sometimes" may differ from the valuation of another respondent. Both responses, however, are converted to the same number by the researcher using the ordinal scale. Whether these numbers can be analyzed using statistical tests for ratio or interval data is debatable. A statistician can help determine the best method of analysis when utilizing ordinal measurements.

The most sophisticated statistical analyses involve two higher levels of measurement, ratio and interval. With both of these measurements there is an ordering of the points, but the distance between each point on the scale is exactly the same. Ratio measurement differs from interval measurement, however, in that the ratio measurement has an absolute zero. For example, research participants might be asked for the specific number of years since graduating college. A year is a well-defined and understood time interval, with the difference between any consecutive points the same. That is, the difference between 4 years and 5 years is the same as between 65 years and 66 years. A meaningful zero value would exist; therefore, this measurement is a ratio.

One example of an interval scale is ambient temperature. There is a zero value, but the presence of a zero value does not mean total absence of the variable being studied. For example, 0 degrees Fahrenheit (0°F) does not mean the total absence of heat because you can have negative temperatures. Therefore, zero in this case is just one value on the scale.

Continuous data, such as ratio and interval measurements, offer researchers the option of utilizing the highest level of analytical operations. Continuous data also provide researchers with the possibility of using inferential statistics to determine the significance of differences and/or associations between groups and variables.

The four levels of measurement, as well as the appropriate types of statistical analyses to be used with each level, are illustrated in **Figure 11-1**. Keep in mind that the terms *parametric* (normal) and *nonparametric* describe the distribution of the subjects or variables. Also, continuous data always have a normal distribution.

DESCRIPTIVE STATISTICS

A study may yield a large amount of raw data that are organized and summarized by descriptive statistical methods. Summarizing the data is an

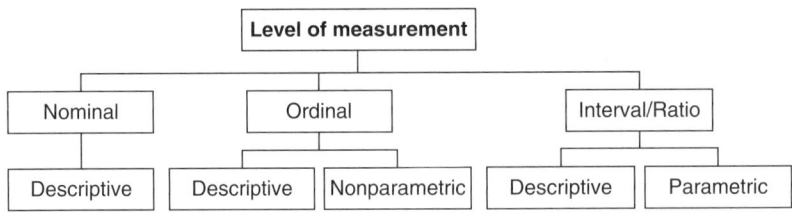

Figure 11-1 Levels of measurement.

essential first step in understanding the results. Then the researcher uses various inferential methods to help test the hypotheses of the study. Descriptive statistics are those processes or analyses that "describe" the sample.

When summarizing data using descriptive methods, the key concepts are *measures of central tendency* and *measures of variability*. In common parlance, measures of central tendency are averages. The most commonly used measures are the *mean*, *median*, and *mode*. The mean is the sum of the scores divided by the total number of scores. The mean can be calculated for only interval or ratio variables. The median is the midpoint of a sequence of ordered variables or the point where half the values are above and half are below. Medians can be calculated for ordinal, interval, or ratio variables. The mode is the most frequently occurring value. It can be determined for variables that are nominal, ordinal, interval, or ratio.

To illustrate the measures of central tendency, consider the following hypothetical data set: The lengths of stay in the cardiac care unit for seven patients following acute myocardial infarction were 3, 12, 5, 7, 5, 8, and 9 days. When performing the statistical calculation for this data set, the data are sorted first from the lowest to the highest numerical value: 3, 5, 5, 7, 8, 9, 12.

> The mode (most frequently occurring score) is 5.
> The median (midpoint of the ordered scores) is 7.
> The mean (sum of the scores divided by the total number of scores) is 3 + 5 + 5 + 7 + 8 + 9 + 12 = 49/7 = 7.

By itself, measures of central tendency can give a misleading view of the data. For example, suppose that the lengths of stay for a second group of five patients were 7, 7, 7, 7, and 7 days, respectively. Similar to the first data set, the mean of this data set is 7. What differs, however, is the variability of the data. In the first group, the length of stay varies from 3 to 12 days. In the second group, everyone had the same length of stay: 7 days.

The three measures of variability most commonly reported in biomedical research are the *range*, *standard deviation*, and *standard error* of the mean. The range, which is the simplest measure, is the difference between the highest and lowest scores. In the first example, the range is 12 − 3 = 9. The range provides an easy "rough cut" of the variability, yet it is of limited value because it does not include all of the data in the computation. As a point of interest, the range of the second example is zero (7 − 7 = 0); this outcome is a statistical anomaly.

The standard deviation (SD) is the key descriptive statistic used to report variability. Mathematically, it is the square root of the variance. The variance is the sum of the squared differences between each score and the mean, divided by the number of scores minus one. The formula for SD is

$$s = \sqrt{\frac{\sum (x - \bar{x})^2}{n - 1}}$$

where x = each score, $\bar{x}$ = the mean, and n = the total number of scores in the sample.

To determine the SD for the first example data set provided, the square root is calculated using the following equation:

$$[(3 - 7)^2 + (5 - 7)^2 + (5 - 7)^2 + (7 - 7)^2 + (8 - 7)^2 + (9 - 7)^2 + (12 - 7)^2]/(7 - 1)$$

This result is the square root of 9, or 3. The SD for this sample data set, therefore, is 3 days. The

SD is the most commonly reported measure of variability.

The standard error of the mean (SEM) is another descriptive statistic. The SEM is the SD divided by the square root of n, and it represents an estimate of the population SD. In the previous example, the SEM is 1.1 (calculated by dividing 3 by the square root of 7).

Although the computation of such basic statistics can be performed with a statistical calculator, using computer software such as Microsoft Excel or SPSS is preferred. The chosen software facilitates computation as well as data management. Additionally, utilizing statistical software minimizes the opportunity for computational error.

INFERENTIAL STATISTICS

Following a descriptive review of the data and determining the level of measurement, the researcher again asks the original question: What is the hypothesis? Most research studies are looking for either a relationship between two or more variables or a difference between the variables. In the study described here, we might be interested in determining whether there is a relationship between a patient's age and the days they spent in the hospital following MI. In this case, we would probably perform a correlation analysis to determine the potential relationship between these variables. Conversely, if we had hypothesized that the length of stay in the hospital cardiac care unit was shorter for patients who had HMO insurance compared to patients with PPO insurance, we would analyze the difference between patients with PPO insurance and patients with HMO insurance. The length of stay in days would be the variable analyzed.

Inferential statistics are used to draw inferences about the results, particularly to test the hypotheses of a study. A researcher studying a problem usually formulates a hypothesis, such as "Aspirin reduces the incidence of colon cancer" or "Problem-based learning produces better clinicians than conventional instruction." Statistical inference, however, is based on testing a null hypothesis. The null forms for the hypotheses given here are "Aspirin has no effect on the incidence of colon cancer" and "There is no difference in the effectiveness of clinicians trained/educated by problem-based learning versus conventional instruction." Therefore, the researcher needs to consider how problem(s) are stated as the study is developed.

In statistical hypothesis testing, the researcher and statistician select a significance level, called alpha (α). By convention, the α level is set at .05 or .01 and is reported without a zero in front of the decimal point ($\alpha < .05$). Remember, the α level is set by the investigator and can be some level other than the one indicated. However, selecting a value greater than .05 should be done with good reason. When the data are analyzed, the statistical test yields a p value, the probability that the observed result could occur by chance if the null hypothesis is true. (The p value is also reported without a zero in front of the decimal point.) If $p < \alpha$, then the researcher rejects the null hypothesis. If $p > \alpha$, then the researcher retains (does not reject) the null hypothesis. If the researcher rejects the null hypothesis, then the researcher is saying that the opposite of the null hypothesis is true. If the researcher retains the null hypothesis, then the researcher is stating that the null hypothesis is true.

Selecting which statistical tests to use is a big question. There are literally hundreds of tests. We cannot even begin to provide information on all of them, or the situations in which they would be used. Decision trees depicting the most common statistical tests are provided in **Figures 11-2** and **11-3** as a reference guide for choosing which test(s) might be appropriate for a particular study. Again, a statistician can provide the best guidance regarding which tests to utilize.

HYPOTHESIS TESTING: NOMINAL DATA

Many medical outcomes are measured on a nominal scale. For instance, one patient has a diagnosis of breast cancer; another patient has a second

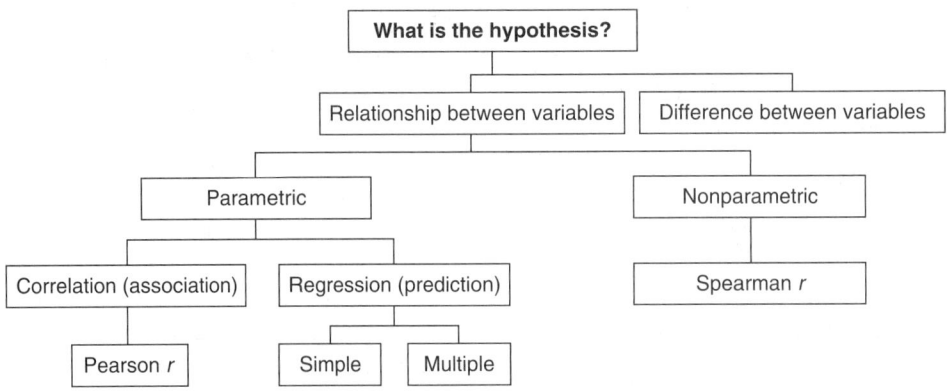

Figure 11–2 Selecting statistical tests based on the hypothesis.

myocardial infarction. Epidemiological studies also yield nominal data—a patient did or did not get the disease. In a study about smoking, the null hypothesis might state, "Smokers are not more likely to have asthma." For this study, with smoking or not smoking as the variables, an appropriate statistical test would be the chi-squared (χ^2) test. (We realize that asthma is a multifactorial disease.) The χ^2 test is simply a way to determine whether an event has occurred more frequently than it would be expected to occur by chance.

The observed χ^2 value is compared to the probability of an event occurring by chance. This is done using a χ^2 distribution table. For example the observed value and degrees of freedom will correspond to a p value on the table. If this value is < .05, the researcher can reject the null hypothesis, concluding there is sufficient evidence that asthma occurs more commonly in individuals who have a smoking history.

Epidemiological studies use nominal data to produce incidence and prevalence rates. For example,

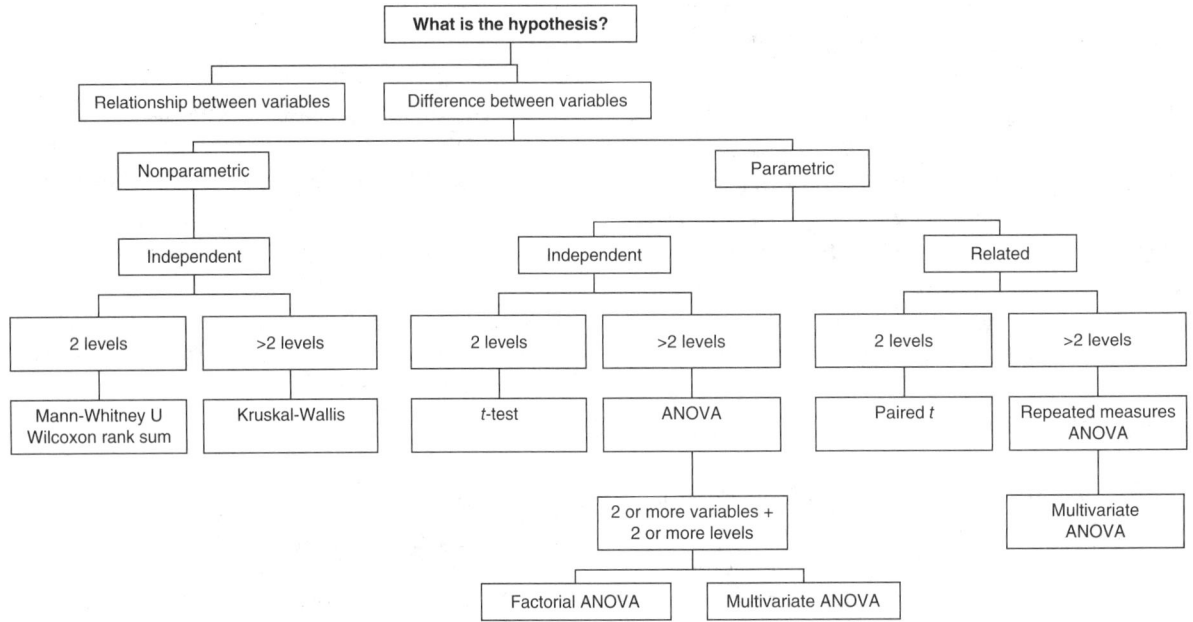

Figure 11–3 How to select the correct statistical procedure.

a study is conducted finding that cigarette smokers are seven times as likely to develop lung cancer or heart disease as those who never smoked. In other words, the relative risk for smokers is 7. Is this risk statistically significant? In this example, a confidence interval is used to test the null hypothesis, which indicates the relative risk = 1 (no added risk of smoking). If the researchers set $\alpha = .05$, then they use a confidence interval of 95 percent. Confidence intervals are reported as percentages. In this case, the confidence interval is found by calculating $[(1 - .05) \times 100\%]$ to give 95 percent. The 95 percent confidence interval for this example is 3.5. This means that the researcher can be 95 percent confident that the actual relative risk is between 3.5 and 10.5 (7 ± 3.5). Because the 95 percent confidence interval does not include the relative risk value of 1, the result is significant at the .05 level. Therefore, the researcher rejects the null hypothesis and concludes that smoking increases the risk of lung cancer or heart disease.

ANALYSIS OF CONTINUOUS DATA: MEASURES OF ASSOCIATION

Determining the association or relationship between two continuous variables (interval or ratio) is a common statistical problem. For instance, what is the relationship between a woman's age and hemoglobin level? What is the relationship between blood sugar level and weight in those who are obese? The measures of association most commonly used are subsumed under the general labels of correlation and regression.

Suppose a clinical educator is concerned about the reliability of an examination on interpreting electrocardiogram (ECG) tracings. Ten students are given a test on Monday, and then are given a parallel test on Tuesday. The exam scores are then correlated. Because the student scores are an interval/ratio variable, the Pearson product moment correlation technique can be used. The result of the statistical manipulation is an r value. This is the correlation coefficient. There are a few different formulas that can be used to manually calculate the correlation coefficient (r); however, the value is typically generated using statistical software. Values of the correlation coefficient (r) vary between -1 (a perfect negative correlation) and $+1$ (a perfect positive correlation). An r value of zero indicates a lack of relationship. The scores on the 2 days are graphed in **Figure 11–4**.

An experienced researcher/statistician would view Figure 11–4 and interpret the correlation as moderate to strong (based on the clustering of the points about a straight line) and as positive (i.e., as Monday's scores increase, so do Tuesday's). The correlation in this example is computed as $r = .88$. Is the result statistically significant? The null hypothesis of no relationship between the two tests' results (the variable), or $r = 0$, is tested at the .05 level of significance. The observed p value is less than .05. The researcher rejects the null hypothesis there is no relationship and concludes there is a significant correlation between the two administrations of the ECG exam, supporting its overall reliability.

Multivariate regression techniques in which relationships among many variables can be examined simultaneously go beyond the simple two-variable correlation. Regression is based on the concept of predicting one variable from another and assigning a probability to these predictions. Complex multisite clinical trials and epidemiological studies are increasingly being conducted utilizing these methods, including discriminant function analysis, factor analysis, path analysis, and logistic regression. In addition, nonparametric correlation techniques

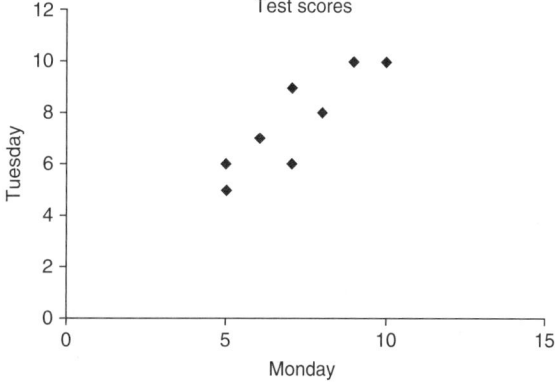

Figure 11–4 Test scores.

exist for ordinal and ranked data. Discussion of these methods, however, is beyond the scope of this text.

ANALYSIS OF INTERVAL/RATIO DATA: COMPARISONS OF GROUPS

The most powerful statistical tests are those that use interval and ratio data from well-designed studies. Ordinal data are often treated as if they are interval data and then are subjected to such tests. The decision as to whether this is acceptable is best left to the statistician. Even if an ordinal value is assigned a number value, the distance between the ordinal values is not defined. A technique known as Rausch analysis can be used with ordinal data, but it is beyond the scope of this basic introduction to completely discuss it.

An example of an appropriate use for analyzing the difference between groups is a research study involving a new antihypertensive drug that is tested against a placebo. Fifty patients are randomized to either treatment or control. After a course of treatment, the diastolic blood pressure is measured. The appropriate statistic to test the null hypothesis is the t-test (sometimes referred to as the student t-test). The researchers set the α level at .05. Statistical analysis produces a t value; in this case, $t = 6.4$. Using t tables yields a p value less than .05, so the researcher rejects the null hypothesis and concludes that the new drug significantly reduces diastolic blood pressure.

The t-test (or student t-test) is perhaps the most commonly used parametric test. It allows for a comparison of the means of two groups. (A paired t-test allows for comparison of the same group at two different times.) The t-test is a special case of a general set of methods collectively known as analysis of variance (ANOVA). Data from complex designs can be analyzed with ANOVA because multiple independent variables, multiple dependent variables, and many subgroups can be tested within a single ANOVA model.

The following example illustrates how to use only one independent variable and one dependent variable. Imagine that a study aims to test the efficacy of over-the-counter pain remedies for nonmigraine headache pain. A total of 25 patients are randomly assigned to one of five drugs in a double-blind manner. The patients are asked to rate their headache pain on a 0–10 scale (where 0 is no pain and 10 is excruciating pain). The null hypothesis is "There is no difference in pain ratings between pain medications." The α level is .05. After 1 month, the results are compiled and summarized. The researcher then performs an ANOVA test that produces an F ratio. The F value is reported with its associated degrees of freedom that are based on the number of comparison groups and the number of subjects. If the F yields a score that has a p value < .05, then the researcher rejects the null hypothesis that there are no significant differences among the drugs. However, which drugs are different from the others? Several multiple comparison procedures are available. A biostatistician can assist in selecting the most appropriate test for the analysis. (F values are found in tables produced with most statistical texts.)

META-ANALYSIS

Many evidence-based medical studies and literature reviews rely on meta-analysis to simultaneously analyze a large number of research studies and determine a conclusion. Meta-analysis can be defined as a process of using statistical integration of the results of several studies to reach an independent conclusion. Meta-analysis is not a singular statistical test or procedure but rather a generalized conceptual approach. The steps to completing a meta-analysis are as follows:

1. Define the hypothesis.
2. Collect the *units of measurement*, that is, the research studies that have been done on the defined topic.
3. Convert the statistics to common values (e.g., z scores, r values, etc.).
4. Compute the measures of central tendency, variability, and prediction from the accumulated data measures.
5. Determine whether the hypothesis is supported.

Meta-analysis has several advantages. It is precise, rigorous, and quantifies decision making about a question. It is also more objective than traditional literature reviews. In a meta-analysis, the inclusion criteria account for the incorporation of multiple related studies, thereby limiting any biases. Additionally, a meta-analysis is replicable, at least in theory. Any reviewer should be able to reach the same conclusion if the same criteria are applied to the same studies. However, disadvantages do exist when conducting a meta-analysis. Because a variety of studies combine different measures of the same variables and statistical techniques in different settings, information about individual differences in the various studies may become lost. Sample size effect may be an issue as well, particularly if some studies have large sample sizes and some have small sample sizes.

CHOOSING A STATISTICAL TEST

When choosing a statistical test, the best option is to consult a statistician. However, a general guideline to *some* statistical testing is detailed here. Choosing the right statistical procedures to test the results of data collection can be a major challenge. Most researchers begin by asking the question: What statistics do I need to make sense of my results?

The statistical tests that are performed should be the most appropriate for the purposes of the study objectives. **Box 11-1** contains a list of research

---

Box 11-1 Uses for Common Statistical Procedures

To summarize data:	Descriptive statistics
To examine the frequency relationship of *one* variable to a theoretical distribution:	Chi-squared test for goodness of fit
To examine the frequency relationship of *two* variables to each other:	Chi-squared test for association
To examine the measured relationship between two variables:	
For ordinal data:	Spearman's rho test
For continuous data:	Pearson's correlation coefficient
To examine the measured relationship of multiple variables:	Multiple regression test
To examine the significance of difference between groups:	
For one group:	t-test
For two independent groups:	
Ordinal data:	Mann-Whitney test
Continuous data:	Independent samples t-test
For two related groups:	
Ordinal data:	Wilcoxon matched pairs test
Continuous data:	Paired samples t-test
For multiple independent groups:	
One independent variable:	One-way ANOVA
Multiple independent variables:	MANOVA
For multiple related groups:	Repeated measures ANOVA

purposes along with some common procedures. Primarily, data are analyzed to summarize them, to identify relationships, and to identify significant differences while controlling confounding variables for all three of these purposes. The results of data analysis allow the researcher to extrapolate his or her findings to a population or group within a population. The choice of statistical tests should be optimal for the type of data to be analyzed and should meet the purposes of that analysis.

Step One

Before selecting statistical tests, the researcher must determine which type of data are being collected: continuous, ordinal, or nominal. Investigations can involve all three or only one type of data. The choice of statistical analysis depends on the type of data collected and how the data are compared.

Step Two

Once the type of data required has been determined, the researcher must decide whether the data are parametric or nonparametric.

- Parametric analyses assume a normal or near-normal distribution exists. For continuous data, a normal or near-normal distribution is always assumed.
- Nonparametric analyses do not assume a normal distribution exists. Nonparametric analyses can be done on data with a normal distribution, but they are not as powerful as parametric tests. Nonparametric tests are typically used for ordinal and nominal data. Continuous data can be converted to nominal or ordinal form. An example would be grouping ages into age ranges.

Step Three

The researcher carefully considers the relationships of the data. Are the results paired or matched?

- Result data are considered paired if the same sample is measured after some intervention (e.g., a treatment of some type).
- Matched samples are those in which the characteristics of the experimental group are matched as closely as possible to a control group.

Step Four

The number and type of variables play a part in the choice of tests: one, two, or more than two (multiple), as well as independent or dependent. There may be no independent variables, one independent variable, or multiple independent variables. Statistical tests are for each dependent variable. There may be more than one dependent variable for each independent variable, but multiple measurements are for each dependent variable only.

Step Five

What is the researcher trying to explain?

1. The relationship between variables

OR

2. The difference between variables

Different tests are used to examine these relationships and differences. (Remember, both can be performed in the same study.)

STATISTICAL TESTS

The following statistical tests are the most commonly used tests in research. These descriptions are designed to provide a starting point and basic concept for the reader to develop an idea of what the tests are and when they should be used. Many more statistical tests are available, and the choice of tests depends on study design and types of data.

Descriptive statistics: The four trends of the sample are mean, mode, median, and range. They are used to describe the sample and sometimes to demonstrate how the sample may reflect a population, if that population's measures of central tendencies (descriptive statistics) are known.

t-test: Tests the difference between two groups' means; can be one-tailed or two-tailed; can be used with paired or unpaired samples. Sometimes called the student *t*-test.

Analysis of variance (ANOVA): Tests the differences among the means of three or more groups for one or more variables.

Analysis of covariance (ANCOVA): A variant of ANOVA that allows adjusting for extraneous, additional, or undesired variables.

Multiple analysis of variance (MANOVA): A variant of ANOVA that allows for the study of multiple dependent variables. If MANOVA results are significant, ANOVA must be done for each variable.

Cochran's Q test: Compares proportions among three or more matched groups.

Duncan range test: A test used after ANOVA to identify means that differ significantly from one another.

Kendall's rank correlation: A test of the linear relationship between two ordinal or continuous variables.

Kruskal-Wallis test: A nonparametric test for significance when using two independent samples. It is comparable to ANOVA, but for rank-ordered data.

Mann-Whitney test: Sometimes called the Mann-Whitney *U*-test; it is the nonparametric equivalent of a *t*-test. Used with ordinal data for two groups.

Multiple regression analysis: Any statistical method that evaluates the results of more than one independent variable on a single dependent variable.

Newman-Keuls test: Tests for significance in multiple post-hoc comparisons.

Pearson's χ^2 test: A test of categorical data for goodness of fit or comparisons of observations.

Pearson's product moment test: A test of the strength of the linear relationship between two interval or ratio (continuous) variables.

Regression analysis: A method of predicting dependent variable variability by one or more independent variables. Most commonly used are simple linear regression and multiple linear regression.

Spearman's rho: A test that demonstrates the degree of relationship between two ordinal variables that may not have a normal distribution.

Tukey test: A test to identify significantly different groups after ANOVA.

Wilcoxon rank sum test: A test of significance for two paired, ordinal data samples.

Tests that can be used with continuous data:

- Descriptive statistics
- *t*-test
- ANOVA
- ANCOVA
- MANOVA
- Duncan range test
- Kendall's rank correlation
- Pearson's product moment test
- Regression analysis
- Multiple regression analysis
- Tukey test

Tests that can be used with ordinal data:

- Descriptive statistics
- Cochran's *Q* test
- Kendall's rank correlation
- Kruskal-Wallis test
- Mann-Whitney test
- Pearson's χ^2 test
- Spearman's rho
- Wilcoxon ranked sum test

Which Test to Use?

The choice of the right statistical test can add power to study findings and provide strong support for outcomes and conclusions. Because so many tests (many more than those listed here) are available, much confusion reigns in the realm of statistical analysis, especially for novice investigators. Many investigators use the tests that are most familiar to them, that is, tests they have used in the past. Understanding what a statistical test can and cannot do is very valuable, but using only one or a few familiar tests for all data analysis can create research limitations.

The number of dependent and independent variables influences the choice of tests more than the category of the data (i.e., nominal, ordinal, continuous). Each *dependent variable* is tested separately, resulting in one big question for the researcher: What do I want to do: summarize, explore relationships, or test for significance of difference?

SUMMARY

In this chapter, we presented the different scales of measurement used in biomedical and educational research. We reviewed differences between descriptive and inferential statistics, including hypothesis testing. Lastly, we introduced the selection of statistical tests. Healthcare professionals participating in research projects need to understand the rationale behind the biostatistician's statistical analyses and how those analyses test the study's hypotheses. The chapter and its Recommended Resources section also provide the basis to perform selected data analyses.

RECOMMENDED RESOURCES

- Cohen P, Cohen J, West SG, Aiken LS. *Applied Multiple Regression/Correlation Analysis for the Behavioral Sciences*. 3rd ed. Mahwah, NJ: Lawrence Erlbaum; 2002.
- Creswell J. *Research Design: Qualitative, Quantitative, and Mixed Methods Approaches*. Thousand Oaks, CA: Sage; 2009.
- Dawson B, Trapp R. *Basic and Clinical Biostatistics*. 4th ed. New York: Lange Medical Books/McGraw-Hill; 2004.
- Glantz, SA. *Primer of Biostatistics*. 6th ed. New York: McGraw-Hill; 2005.
- Glantz SA, Slinker BK. *Primer of Applied Regression and Analysis of Variance*. 2nd ed. New York: McGraw-Hill; 2000.
- Harris M, Taylor G. *Medical and Health Science Statistics Made Easy*. 2nd ed. Sudbury, MA: Jones and Bartlett; 2009.
- Harris R. *ANOVA: An Analysis of Variance Primer*. Itasca, IL: FE Peacock; 1994.
- Jekel, J, Katz, D, Elmore, J, Wild, D. *Epidemiology, Biostatistics, and Preventive Medicine*. 3rd ed. Philadelphia, PA: Saunders Elsevier; 2007.
- Lang TA, Secic M. *How to Report Statistics in Medicine: Annotated Guidelines for Authors, Editors, and Resources*. 2nd ed. Philadelphia, PA: American College of Physicians; 2006.
- Norman GR, Streiner DL. *PDQ Statistics*. 3rd ed. Philadelphia, PA: B.C. Decker; 2003.

Computer Software

Software for statistical analysis is categorized as (1) general purpose data analysis programs with statistical application, (2) complete statistical packages, and (3) special-purpose software for specific applications.

General Purpose Data Analysis Software

Microsoft Excel: Part of Microsoft Office; general purpose software includes several statistical tools. Third-party statistical add-ins are available at http://www.microsoft.com.

Complete Statistical Packages

SAS: SAS, Inc., Cary, NC. A comprehensive package biostatisticians frequently use for large projects. Website: http://www.sas.com

SPSS: SPSS, Inc., Chicago, IL. A comprehensive package frequently used by social science researchers, but also used by some biostatisticians. Website: http://www.spss.com

Stata: StataCorp, LP, College Station, TX. A comprehensive package with excellent graphing capabilities. Website: http://stata.com

Specialized Software

GraphPad Prism: GraphPad Software, Inc., La Jolla, CA. Data analysis software that includes free online quick calculators for various common statistical tests. Website: http://www.graphpad.com. Free calculators available at http://www.graphpad.com/quickcalcs/

SigmaPlot: Systat Software, San Jose, CA. Primarily a graphing package, it includes extensive analysis tools. Website: http://www.sigmaplot.com

Websites

These sites are particularly useful for faculty and students in teaching and learning statistics.

StatLib: A system for distributing statistical software, data sets, and information. Archives of statistical routines and data sets. Maintained at Carnegie-Mellon University. Website: http://lib.stat.cmu.edu

Rice Virtual Lab in Statistics: Excellent simulations and demonstrations. Maintained at Rice University. Website: http://onlinestatbook.com/rvls.html

CHAPTER 12

Exploring Statistics Comparing Differences in Health Care

J. Glenn Forister, MS, PA-C

CHAPTER OVERVIEW

This chapter explores some of the frequently used statistical procedures including the interpretation of parametric tests assessing differences between groups. The statistics used to assess two or more related or independent groups on the basis of single or multiple variables are emphasized. The chapter is restricted to the various forms of the *t*-test and ANOVA because many randomized controlled trials and other clinical studies use these analyses. Although the multivariate versions of the *t*-test and ANOVA are typically excluded from introductory texts, a basic discussion of these procedures has been included. As healthcare researchers explore larger data sets with advanced statistical software, it is likely that readers will encounter such multivariate tests reported in the literature.

Learning Objectives

- Define *test statistic*.
- Describe commonly used statistics that compare groups.
- Compare the null hypothesis of the different forms of the *t*-test and ANOVA.
- Define *noninferior design*.
- Calculate and interpret an effect size.

INTRODUCTION

No single chapter can do justice to the topic of statistical interpretation. However, many articles in the healthcare literature are concerned with comparing the differences between two or more groups. Therefore, it is appropriate to discuss the commonly employed parametric procedures that examine differences, such as *t*-tests and the different forms of ANOVA. These statistical tests may be misunderstood or misinterpreted by health professionals.[1] The purpose of this chapter is to provide a basic understanding of how to assess differences *within* groups and differences *between* groups. Readers should note that other statistical techniques do appear in the healthcare literature; this chapter reviews parametric tests used in one out of three articles published in four of the top medical journals.[2] For some readers, this chapter will be a review; for others, it will be an introduction to some of the essential parametric statistics used to analyze group differences in health care.

COMPARING GROUPS

Study participants are usually divided into groups. Frequently, the goal of medical research is to compare groups of patients in a meaningful way while controlling for random chance. Healthcare professionals need to answer three essential questions about the groups studied:

1. Did something different occur between the groups (usually due to some intervention or treatment)?
2. If something different occurred between the groups, was it due to chance?
3. If something nonrandom occurred between the groups, how large was the effect (was the difference clinically meaningful)?

These questions are answered, in part, by test statistics. The interpretive process may appear complicated initially, but is always related to these three essential questions. The first two questions pertain to the null hypothesis. If something different occurred between the groups, the null hypothesis is rejected. If nothing different occurred between the groups, researchers would fail to reject the null hypothesis. The observed test statistic, such as the t statistic or the F ratio obtained from various computational procedures, is compared to the critical value on the corresponding distribution tables to help answer the first two questions. Assuming the population distribution is normal and variances are equal, each of the test statistics has a known distribution when the null hypothesis is true. Readers should remember, however, that different p values result in different type I error rates. Statistical significance should never be confused with clinical significance. Statistical significance is about the likelihood of observing the results—nothing else. Although calculations for effect size can help answer question three, clinicians ultimately interpret the clinical meaningfulness of study results.

As a reminder, the groups can be unrelated to each other (independent) or related in some way (dependent). The simplest comparison occurs between two groups using one categorical independent variable and one continuous dependent variable. In this case the preferred tests are the independent samples t-test (for independent groups) and the paired t-test (for dependent groups). When more than two groups are studied, the commonly used tests are the one-way ANOVA (for multiple independent groups) and the repeated measures ANOVA (for multiple related groups). Again, each of the tests examines differences between the groups using a single dependent (outcome) variable.

The complexity of test interpretation increases when (1) the groups are categorized using more than one independent variable, (2) the design is mixed (using both independent and repeated measures), or (3) multiple dependent variables are measured. When more than two groups are categorized using more than one independent variable, the one-way ANOVA is replaced by factorial ANOVA.

When multiple dependent variables are measured between two groups, the t-tests are replaced with a procedure called Hotelling's T^2. However, when multiple dependent variables are measured between more than two different groups, the proper procedure is multiple analysis of variance (MANOVA). If the multiple groups are related and measured on more than one dependent variable, a repeated measures MANOVA is used. Each of the tests mentioned thus far will be discussed in the following sections.

t-TEST (STUDENT t-TEST)

The t-test assesses the difference between the means of two unrelated groups or independent samples. The null hypothesis is represented as $H_0: \mu_1 = \mu_2$ and is analogous to saying there is no difference between the group means. This is a statistical test most students remember, but that is not the reason it is called the "student" t-test. The student t-test was given that name because

Gossett, the Guinness Brewery's statistician who published the procedure, used the name "student" to remain anonymous.[3] The test is simply the ratio of the difference between two group means and the standard error of that difference. This ratio is often called the signal-to-noise ratio. This test is useful because it takes sample size into account. The obtained t statistic is calculated using the following formula (usually generated by software):

$$t = \frac{(\text{Mean G1} - \text{Mean G2})}{\sqrt{\frac{S_{G1}^2}{n_{G1}} + \frac{S_{G2}^2}{n_{G2}}}}$$

where

S_{G1}^2 = variance of group 1
n_{G1} = number of subjects in group 1
S_{G2}^2 = variance of group 2
n_{G2} = number of subjects in group 2

The obtained value of t is then compared to the critical value of t found in a table that defines the level of significance on the t distribution. Based on the directional nature of the hypothesized difference between the groups, the critical value is situated in a one-tailed or two-tailed position. If the researcher somehow knows or hypothesizes the results will occur in one direction, a one-tailed test is used. Usually the researcher cannot be certain about the direction of the results. Therefore, a two-tailed test is more commonly used. The tails of the t distribution are represented in **Figure 12–1**.

Some researchers use a one-tailed test to establish noninferiority. The noninferior study design does not attempt to demonstrate a new therapy is better than standard therapy, only that it is *not substantially worse* than standard therapy. In this case, statistical significance is more likely to be achieved because the significance level (.05) is not divided into two directions. Moreover, the null hypothesis in a noninferior design is that the new treatment is worse than the standard therapy. Most health professionals are interested in new therapies that are superior to and more effective than standard therapy. Two-tailed tests are more conservative than one-tailed tests. For this reason, it is important to note whether the *t*-test reported in a clinical trial is one-tailed or two-tailed.

The null hypothesis is more likely to be rejected when (1) mean differences are large, (2) variances are small, and (3) sample sizes are large.[4] However, if the difference between the means is small and the variability within the groups is large, then a smaller number will be divided by a larger number, thus reducing the value of t. In such cases, researchers often fail to reject the null hypothesis, sometimes resulting in a type II error. Furthermore, the power to detect a difference is influenced by the sample size. When using a *t*-test, each group should include a minimum of 15 individuals.[4] The researcher should report the t statistic, the associated *p* value (level of significance), and the degrees of freedom (df). For example, when reporting an intervention group's score was better than the control group's score, the author provides the following: intervention mean, intervention standard

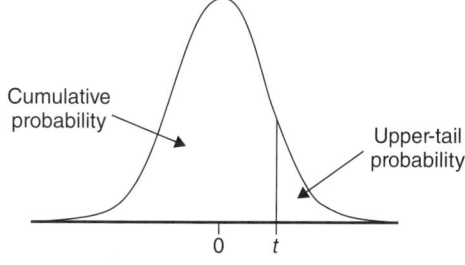

One-tailed test

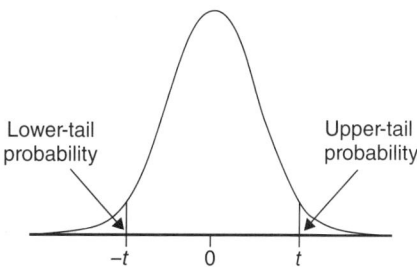

Two-tailed test

Figure 12–1 The t distribution.

deviation (SD), control mean, control SD, df, t = calculated statistic, $p < .05$.

If something nonrandom occurred between the two groups, the next task is to determine if the difference is meaningful. One way to assess the magnitude of the difference is to calculate an effect size. The effect size calculation for the t-test is called Cohen's d (the treatment effect in standard deviation units). The general formula is:

$$d = \frac{\text{Mean}_{G1} - \text{Mean}_{G2}}{SD_{Pooled}}$$

where

$$SD_{Pooled} = \sqrt{\frac{(SD_{G1}^2 + SD_{G2}^2)}{2}}$$

Accepted interpretation guidelines[5] for Cohen's d are presented in **Table 12–1**.

Example

Researchers conducted a study to determine if a group of 30 health professions students exposed to videotaped patient case studies exhibited higher exam scores than an independent group of 32 students exposed to standard lectures. The exam scores of the two groups were compared using the student t-test. The simulation group scored a mean (SD) of 82 (7.45) and the lecture group scored a mean (SD) of 80.5 (7.05). The mean of the simulation group minus the mean of the lecture group = 1.6, $t = .87$, df = 60, $p = .39$.

Because of the small sample size, the 95 percent confidence interval of the difference between the groups ranges from −2.08 to 5.28, indicating the results could go either way when the study is repeated. The p value exceeds .05; therefore, the researchers failed to reject the null hypothesis and concluded the videotaped case studies did not result in better exam performance than the standard lecture. No effect size is calculated when the groups' means are equivalent under the null.

PAIRED t-TEST (MATCHED t-TEST)

The paired t-test is considered more powerful than the independent samples t-test because less variability (noise) is created by the dependent nature of the samples.[4] Usually, two sets of data are collected from the same group of individuals. Often, some form of intervention occurs between the data collection activities. For example, the paired t-test is used in pretreatment–posttreatment study designs examining the same group of patients. The two sets of data in this experimental design may be referred to as two dependent groups. The terminology can be confusing because the word *groups* usually refers to individuals, not data sets; however, in a paired t-test one group of individuals serves as their own controls. The same study participants are treated and assessed to see if the dependent variable changes. The data collected before the intervention can be considered a group and the data collected after the intervention can be considered a group. The null hypothesis is represented as $H_0: \mu_{before} = \mu_{after}$.

As in the student t-test, a ratio of signal-to-noise generates a t statistic. The formula for this ratio is:

$$t = \frac{d}{\sqrt{\frac{\sum d^2 - \frac{\sum d^2}{n}}{n(n-1)}}}$$

Where
  d = difference in paired sources
  n = number of paired scrores

The calculated value of t is compared to the critical value of t, and the researcher either rejects or fails to reject the null hypothesis. The results from paired t-tests will be reported in the same manner as for a t-test. Authors should provide the mean scores before and after the intervention along with standard deviations, the t statistic, and the p value. If the null hypothesis is rejected, the effect size and

Table 12–1 Interpretation of Cohen's d

Effect Size	d
Small	0.20
Medium	0.50
Large	0.80

clinical meaningfulness of the results should be assessed in the same manner as the student *t*-test.

Example

A single group of 44 patients with a first-degree medial collateral ligament tear of the knee were treated with a new cooling gel for pain relief. The investigators assessed the patients' pain scores using a validated numeric rating scale from 1 to 10. Before the gel application, the patients' mean (SD) pain score was 6.4 (1.3). Fifteen minutes after the gel application, the patient's mean (SD) pain score was 5.5 (1.7). The difference in the mean pain score was 0.9 with a 95 percent confidence interval of 0.26 to 1.54, $t = 2.79$, df = 86, $p = .006$.

In this example, the investigators can reject the null hypothesis and calculate a Cohen's *d* (0.59, medium effect size); however, clinicians reviewing the study will ultimately determine if the results are meaningful. For instance, some readers may question the use of ordinal data (the pain scale) in a parametric comparison. Parametric procedures are applied using interval or ratio scaled data. It is, however, common to see ordinal scales for pain and other measured outcomes in the healthcare literature. Readers must decide to accept or reject the results of such analyses. In this example, clinicians may decide to reject the analysis based on the use of ordinal data, or based on the fact that other forms of treatment are more useful than the gel because of greater pain relief achieved over a longer duration. Although the results of the paired *t*-test are statistically significant, readers may require additional evidence that the gel works. For example, the investigators may decide to measure the amount of pain medication used by patients over more than one time interval by employing a repeated measures ANOVA—discussed later in this chapter.

ONE-WAY ANOVA

The one-way ANOVA is an extension of the *t*-test involving more than two groups. This test assesses the relationship between a categorical independent variable and a single continuous dependent variable. The null hypothesis of ANOVA is represented as $H_0: \mu_1 = \mu_2 = \mu_3 \ldots = \mu k$ (where *k* indicates the number of groups). The *t*-tests discussed previously represent a signal-to-noise ratio, with the signal identifying the true difference between the groups and the noise separating the variability within the groups. In ANOVA, the signal-to-noise ratio is the *F* ratio (also called the *F* test). The *F* ratio includes the variance between groups (explained variance, or signal) and the variance within groups (error variance, or noise), therefore, *F* = variance between groups/variance within groups.

$$F = \frac{\text{MS Between}}{\text{MS Within}}$$

The total sums of squares (SST) results from adding the squares of all the deviation scores. In ANOVA, the total sums of squares is partitioned into sums of squares between (effects, SSB) and sums of squares within (error, SSW). The formula is SST = SSB + SSW. This procedure allows investigators to decide how much of the difference in scores is due to treatment and how much of the difference in scores is due to chance. The mean squares (MS) is found by dividing the sums of squares by the degrees of freedom (df). The researcher fails to reject the null hypothesis when the calculated value of *F* does not exceed the critical value of *F* (on the *F* distribution table). See **Figure 12–2**.

Figure 12–3 illustrates how the source table of a one-way ANOVA is constructed for three

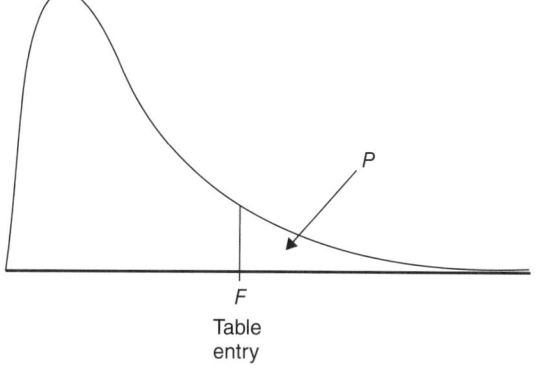

Figure 12–2 The *F* distribution.

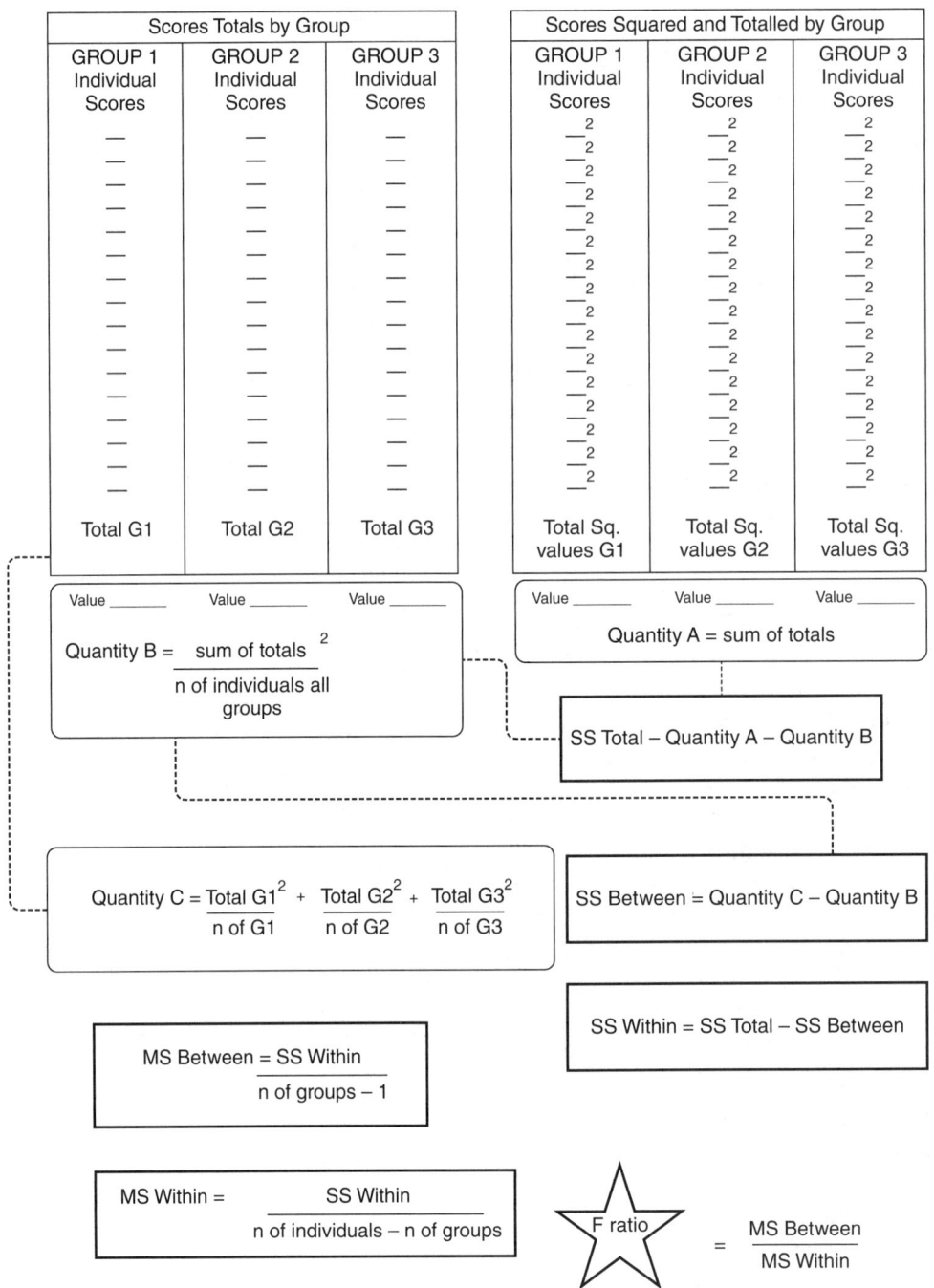

Figure 12-3 One-way ANOVA.

groups. Although statistical software will perform the calculations and produce a source table (see **Table 12-2**), the following steps can be used to manually generate an F ratio:

Step 1: List the groups' raw scores separately in columns.
Step 2: Square each of the individual raw scores to produce another set of columns and sum each

Table 12–2 ANOVA Source Table

Source	Sum of Squares	df	Mean Squares	F	p
Between groups	SSB	Number of groups minus 1	MSB	MSB/MSW	< .05 from the F table
Within groups	SSW = SST − SSB	Number of individuals minus number of groups	MSW		
Total	SST				

column, then produce quantity A by adding the totals.

Step 3: Find the total of all individual raw scores and square the total value, then divide the total by the number of individuals to produce quantity B.

Step 4: Calculate the SST by subtracting B from A.

Step 5: Sum each raw score column, square each sum, and divide each result by the number of individuals in the group.

Step 6: Sum the results from Step 5 to produce quantity C.

Step 7: Calculate the SSB by subtracting B from C.

Step 8: Calculate the SSW by subtracting SSB from SST.

Step 9: Divide SSB by the number of groups minus 1 to generate the mean squares between (MSB).

Step 10: Divide SSW by the number of individuals minus the number of groups to generate the mean squares within (MSW).

Step 11: Calculate the observed F ratio by dividing MSB by MSW. (Compare this value with the critical F on the F table.)

Some published studies using ANOVA will contain the source table; others will not.[3] Although the F ratio allows for hypothesis testing, the interpretation of ANOVA requires further comparisons. Assuming the null hypothesis is rejected, the investigator must determine how the groups differ from each other. The statistical software will generate comparisons—group one with group two, group one with group three, group two with group three, and so forth—with a series of post hoc (after the fact) tests. This process is analogous to *t*-testing but produces the problem of multiple comparisons. Because the likelihood of finding significance by random chance increases with the number of comparisons, the software will adjust the *p* value (significance level), dividing it by the number of comparisons (called the Bonferroni correction).[4] The Bonferroni correction, however, can lead to an increased chance of type II error.[4] Therefore, a multitude of other post hoc tests have been developed with names such as LSD, Tukey, Sidak, and Scheffé. The purpose of these tests is to reduce the chance of a type I error due to multiple comparisons.

Researchers should indicate which post hoc test was used after finding significance in an ANOVA. Once the difference is discovered, the final step is to establish its effect size. Healthcare professionals need to decide if the differences are clinically meaningful. To determine how much of the variance in the dependent variable is explained by the independent variable, a statistic known as eta-squared (η^2) can be calculated from the ANOVA table:

$$\text{eta}^2 = \frac{\text{SSB}}{\text{SST}}$$

Some investigators may report effect size using omega-squared (ω^2). The formula for omega-squared is:

$$\text{omega}^2 = \frac{\text{SSB} - [(k-1)(\text{MSW})]}{\text{SST} + \text{MSW}}$$

Table 12-3 includes the effect size interpretation guidelines[4] for values of eta-squared (η^2) and omega-squared (ω^2).

Table 12–3 Interpretation Guidance for Effect Size Calculations

Effect Size	Eta² (η^2)	Omega² (ω^2)
Small	0.01	0.01
Medium	0.06	0.06
Large	0.14	0.15

Example

Many researchers include a graphical representation of group outcomes related to each other. For example, **Figure 12–4** shows how three different treatments for diabetes affect mean hemoglobin A1C levels. The treatments in this example are (1) usual care, (2) exercise, or (3) dietary counseling. "The p value for the comparison between Group 1 (usual care) and Group 2 (exercise) or Group 3 (diet) was less than 0.05, and the null hypothesis of no difference can be rejected for Group 1 versus Group 2, or Group 3. However, the p value for the comparison of Group 2 to Group 3 was greater than 0.05, so the null hypothesis of no difference could not be rejected."[6] Therefore, the ANOVA distinguished exercise and diet from usual care, but did not find a significant difference in outcome between exercise and diet.

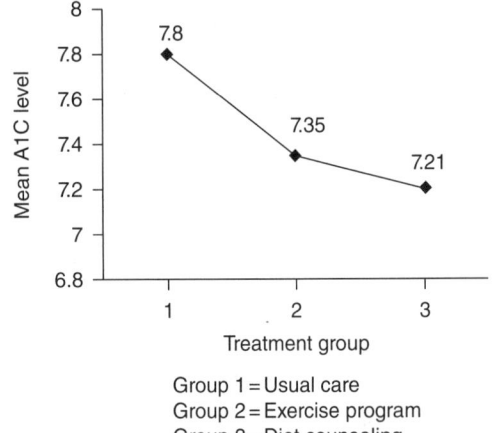

Figure 12–4 Findings from an ANOVA.

FACTORIAL ANOVA

In contrast to the one-way ANOVA, the factorial ANOVA includes more independent variables (called covariates). The procedure allows investigators to test more hypotheses about the ways in which groups may differ. The researcher can check to see if the groups differ based on each independent variable separately. If an independent grouping variable is shown to be significant on its own, the result is called a *main effect*. Sometimes the influence of one independent grouping variable on the dependent variable is conditional on the *interaction* of another independent grouping variable. It is possible for each independent variable to have separate main effects on the dependent variable without any interaction. If an interaction does occur between the covariates, the separate effects are set aside and the effect of one variable is interpreted for each level of the other independent variables. This interactive type of interpretation includes the assessment of *simple main effects*—what occurs as a result of the interaction.

In most cases, the covariate factors are fixed (not random) and are measured at two or more levels. For instance, an investigation of blood pressure medications may include groups treated with different doses of antihypertensive medication. The factor is the dose of medication, and the levels are the dosage categories that divide groups. For example, a new medication for blood pressure could be given in a high dose and a low dose. This single factor (medication) has two levels. If the investigators want to know if the effects of the medication vary by body mass index (BMI), then a second factor (BMI) can be added to the ANOVA. In the one-way ANOVA, the groups would be defined by only a single variable, such as the medication received. In a factorial ANOVA, however, the independent variables can represent differences in treatment along with variables that reflect additional individual differences between the groups. Because the number of comparisons increases compared to one-way ANOVA, the sample size in factorial ANOVA is usually larger than in a one-way ANOVA.

The factorial ANOVA allows investigators to partition the total sums of squares (SST), discussed previously, into more than the two components of a one-way ANOVA (between and error). The factorial ANOVA SST is divided into the model sums of squares and the error sums of squares. The model SS is divided into the SS for factor A, the SS for factor B, and the SS for the combination of factors A and B. Of course, this example is for a two-way factorial ANOVA. When three factors are included, the ANOVA is called a three-way factorial, and so on. In contrast to the one-way ANOVA, multiple F statistics are generated.

When interpreting a significant factorial ANOVA, one looks for significance and assesses the main effects and any interactions. If an interaction is discovered, the *simple main effects* are calculated. If there is no interaction between the factors, then the main effect for each factor is assessed using post hoc multiple comparison tests. Researchers often include graphical representations of the results, including main effects or interactions. **Figure 12-5** expands the previous example and includes different representations of the effects of two factors (medication and BMI), each with three levels, on blood pressure outcomes. The illustration depicts three different hypothetical outcomes: (1) the main effect of medication dose on blood pressure with no BMI effect, (2) the main effect of BMI with no medication dose effect, and (3) the interaction between medication dose and BMI.

When determining the effect size for a factorial ANOVA, researchers use statistical software to calculate omega-squared (ω^2), eta-squared (η^2), or an adjusted value called partial eta-squared,[7] for every significant F statistic. Although the interpretation of factorial ANOVA is more complex, the procedure is frequently preferred to one-way ANOVA because it is useful in comparing groups across a variety of study designs.

REPEATED MEASURES ANOVA

As discussed in the paired *t*-test section, measuring the same set of individuals more than once produces dependent groups of data. In the case of the paired *t*-test, two measurements resulted in two dependent groups of data. When more than two measurements of the same variable are taken from a single group of individuals (especially over time), the result is three or more dependent groups of data. The repeated measures ANOVA is, therefore, an extension of the paired *t*-test. For example, a single group of patients may be subjected to more than two treatments over time, or the treatment response to a single intervention may vary over time. Once again, the participants serve as their own controls, thus reducing error variance and reducing the number of subjects needed. When the researcher seeks to explore differences occurring in individuals over time, the repeated measures ANOVA is the appropriate way to test for significance.

In the one-way ANOVA there are two sources of variability (between groups and within groups). However, in the repeated measures ANOVA the variability is partitioned. The total sum of squares (SST) is divided into the sums of squares between people (SSBP) and the sums of squares within people (SSWP). The SSBP is less interesting than the SSWP. The SSWP reveals how the participants vary around their own mean. The SSWP is partitioned into the sums of squares between treatments and the sums of squares due to random error. The SS between treatments allows for the comparison of the treatment means. This comparison is similar to the between-groups comparison in the one-way ANOVA.

Recall one of the assumptions underlying ANOVA (and other parametric tests) is equal variance. In a repeated measures ANOVA, the equality of variances is determined by something called sphericity. Sphericity of the data is assumed in repeated measures ANOVA. Researchers use a routine called Mauchley's test to check for sphericity and protect against a type I error.[3] If a lack of sphericity is identified, the researcher will make adjustments to protect the alpha level (p value).

The repeated measures ANOVA table (see **Table 12-4**) is assembled in a similar manner as previously demonstrated. The main difference is the labels are changed from between groups and

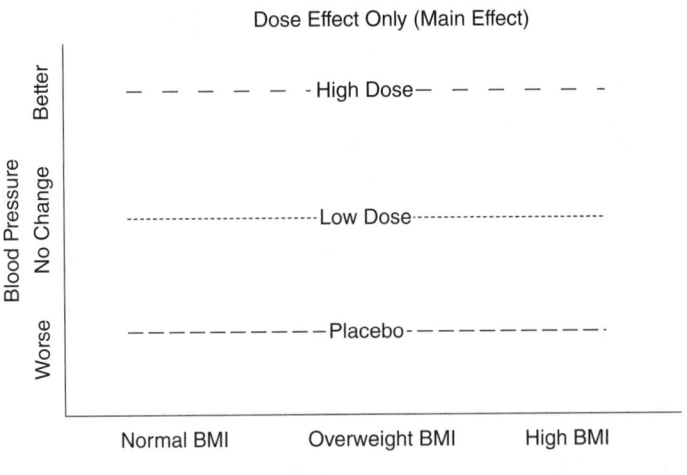
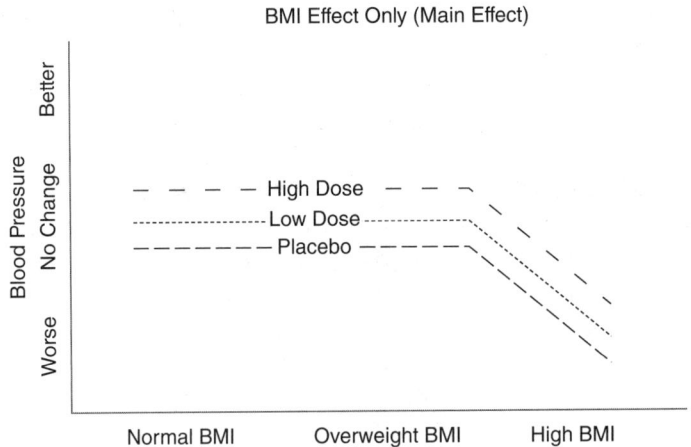
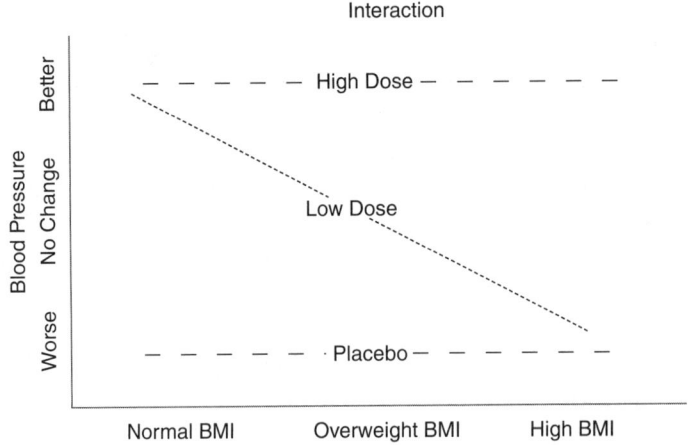

Figure 12–5 Factorial ANOVA.

Table 12-4 Repeated Measures ANOVA

Source	Sum of Squares	df	Mean Squares	F	p
Between persons	SSBP	$(n-1)$	MSBP		
Within persons		$n(k-1)$		$\dfrac{MSBT}{MSE}$	< .05 from the F table
Between treatments	SSBT	$k-1$	MSBT		
Error	SSE	$(n-1)(k-1)$	MSE		
Total	SST	$n-1$			

within groups to between persons and within persons. In addition, the sums of squares within persons are divided into the sums of squares between treatments (SSBT) and the sums of squares error (SSE).

Again, the purpose is to calculate an F ratio and compare it to an established distribution. If a significant F ratio is obtained, then post hoc testing helps to determine what differences have occurred between the individuals' measurements. The effect size can be calculated in the same manner as ANOVA. Partial eta-squared (η^2) or omega-squared (ω^2) interpretation guidelines can be used to assess the magnitude of the differences observed. One drawback of repeated measures ANOVA is the amount of missing data that may accumulate as studies increase in length (as in long-term longitudinal designs). Researchers should consider how to treat missing data in such circumstances. In addition, when the participants receive different treatment conditions during the course of the study, carryover effects from one treatment may influence the results obtained during other treatments.

Example

The following is an example of a repeated measures ANOVA assessing efficacy of treatment over time. A group of patients with chronic venous stasis ulcers received a novel treatment that included electrical stimulation of their wounds over a 2-month period. Measurements of all patient wounds were taken at baseline, 2 weeks, 4 weeks, 6 weeks, and 8 weeks. The patients' wound healing scores were obtained by using a validated wound assessment instrument. The null hypothesis for the repeated measures ANOVA was that wound healing scores would be equal for all of the treatment periods. The p value obtained was < .01, resulting in the rejection of the null hypothesis. Post hoc testing was required to determine how the time intervals differed in relation to wound healing. The investigators determined that the patients' wounds responded between baseline and 4 weeks and then did not change thereafter.

HOTELLING'S T^2

Medical researchers may be interesting in comparing groups using more than one dependent variable. When comparing two groups using multiple outcome measurements, Hotelling's T^2 is used. The test is named after mathematician Harold Hotelling.[8] In contrast to the t-test that compares the difference between two means, Hotelling's T^2 assesses the difference between two *mean vectors*. The null hypothesis is represented as $H_0: \underline{\mu}_1 = \underline{\mu}_2$ and matrix algebra is involved in the calculations. The underscore below the mu symbol indicates the comparison is between mean vectors.

$$\begin{array}{c}\text{The symbol}\\\text{for a vector}\\\text{of means}\end{array} \quad \underline{M} = \begin{bmatrix} \text{mean } v_1 \\ \text{mean } v_2 \\ \text{mean } v_3 \end{bmatrix}$$

$$[\underline{M}G1][\underline{M}G2]$$

The signal-to-noise ratio is created using the between-group difference in mean vectors and the *inverse of the covariance matrix*.[8] It is useful to know that the calculation of the test statistic uses a determinant to represent the value of each matrix. The Hotelling's T^2 is generated algebraically and converted to an F statistic for the purpose of hypothesis testing.

When using Hotelling's T^2, the effect size is determined by something called the Mahalanobis distance (D^2). This statistic is the multivariate version of Cohen's d. The interpretation of the effect is dependent on the number of dependent variables included in the two-group comparison.

Example

In this example, researchers seek to determine if diabetic patients with congestive heart failure (CHF) are different than nondiabetic patients with CHF. The investigators determine that three outcomes of CHF are important: ventricular ejection fraction, serum creatinine, and diastolic blood pressure. The ranges of each of these outcome measures vary; however, the vectors of means for the two groups can be compared using Hotelling's T^2. In this case, the T^2 statistic generated by the computer is 3.52, the F statistic is 1.17, and p is .31. Therefore, the researchers fail to reject the null hypothesis that the vectors of means are equal for the two groups.

MANOVA

The ability to examine group differences in multiple dependent outcome variables concurrently can be valuable. *Multiple analysis of variance (MANOVA)* is a variant of ANOVA that also allows for the study of multiple dependent variables. In this case, the comparison includes more than two groups. Clinicians are often interested in multiple related but differing outcomes. The dependent variables should be related to each other in some way without being redundant. For example, when evaluating the effect of different treatments on pulmonary function, the clinician may be interested in different indices than the forced expiratory volume in 1 second (FEV_1) alone. Using MANOVA, a linear combination of variables including FEV_1, forced vital capacity (FVC), and dyspnea scores can be assessed in lieu of a single metric.

Once again, the comparison of group means is replaced by a comparison of group mean vectors. The null hypothesis is represented as H_0: $\underline{\mu}_1 = \underline{\mu}_2 = \underline{\mu}_3 \ldots = \underline{\mu}k$. Notice the mean symbol in the following equation has a line below it—the notation is for a vector.

$$\begin{array}{c}\text{The symbol}\\\text{for a vector}\\\text{of means}\end{array} \quad \underline{M} = \begin{bmatrix} \text{mean } v_1 \\ \text{mean } v_2 \\ \text{mean } v_3 \end{bmatrix}$$

$$[\underline{M}G1][\underline{M}G2][\underline{M}G3]$$

Like ANOVA, the MANOVA can be constructed using one or more independent grouping variables. Therefore, it is possible to have a one-way MANOVA, a factorial MANOVA, and a mixed MANOVA or repeated measures MANOVA. Most statisticians test for homogeneity of the variance and covariance matrices because these are underlying assumptions in MANOVA. A test called Levene's test checks the null hypothesis that the error variance of the dependent variables among the groups is equal.[3] A test called Box's test checks the null hypothesis that the covariance of the dependent variables is equal.[9] These procedures are simply examples of how statisticians evaluate the equal variance assumption in a multivariate case.

The F value in MANOVA is a multivariate F and can be produced using different named tests of significance. The names to be familiar with are Pillai's trace, Wilks's lambda, Hotelling's trace, and Roy's largest root. Basically, each of these tests will produce an F value with an associated p value to judge whether the results obtained are statistically significant.[9]

If the overall MANOVA results are significant, a separate ANOVA can be completed for each dependent variable, with post hoc testing in each case, for the purpose of interpretation. In addition,

Table 12–5 Source Table for Ventricular Ejection Fraction

Source	SS	df	MS	F	p
Between groups	6762.01833	5	1352.40367	17.47	0.0000
Within groups	524,634.25	6776	77.4253615		
Total	531,396.268	6781			

discriminant function analysis can also be used as an interpretive aid.

Example

Assume the investigators in the CHF example want to compare outcomes among six different causes of CHF, rather than diabetes (as in the Hotelling's T^2 example used previously). Each of the six causes of CHF comprises a separate group. The outcomes of interest are ventricular ejection fraction, serum creatinine, and diastolic blood pressure. The MANOVA will generate a series of F statistics to test the null hypothesis that the vectors of means are equal for the six causal groups. In this example, Wilks's lambda, Pillai's trace, Hotelling's trace, and Roy's largest root all produce F statistics that are significant with p values < .001. Yet, this result only alerts investigators that some differences exist between the groups. After finding significance using the MANOVA, the researchers must perform individual ANOVAs for each of the outcome variables and post hoc testing for any of the ANOVAs that are significant. In this example, the separate ANOVA tables (**Tables 12–5, 12–6, and 12–7**) reveal ventricular ejection fraction is the only outcome that includes a significant difference between groups. (Note the p values for each ANOVA table.)

Because the ANOVA for ventricular ejection fraction is significant, the next step is to look at the associated summary table and post hoc tests (**Table 12–8**).

Visual inspection of the summary table reveals that groups 4 and 5 have lower ejection fractions than the other groups. The post hoc tests such as Bonferroni, Sidak, and Scheffé provide comparison tables (**Table 12–9**) to show which of the comparisons are meaningful.

Table 12–6 Source Table for Serum Creatinine

Source	SS	df	MS	F	p
Between groups	0.266260806	5	0.053252161	0.39	0.8560
Within groups	925.197266	6776	0.136540329		
Total	925.463527	6781			

Table 12–7 Source Table for Diastolic Blood Pressure

Source	SS	df	MS	F	p
Between groups	574.334327	5	114.866865	0.91	0.4756
Within groups	857,943.362	6776	126.708516		
Total	858,517.697	6781			

Table 12–8 Summary Table for Ventricular Ejection

CHF Etiology	Mean Ejection Fraction	SD
1	28.9	8.6
2	29.5	9.2
3	29.5	9.4
4	**26.6**	9.0
5	**25.8**	9.4
6	28.5	9.4
Total	28.5	8.9

Table 12–9 Bonferroni Comparison Table of Ventricular Ejection Fraction by CHF Etiology Group

	Group 1	Group 2	Group 3	Group 4	Group 5
Group 2	0.646295				
Group 3	0.632383	−0.013913			
Group 4	**−2.31245***	**−2.95874***	**−2.94483***		
Group 5	**−3.05831***	**−3.7046***	**−3.69069***	−0.74586	
Group 6	−0.379055	−1.02535	−1.01144	1.93339	2.67925

*The significant p values occur when comparing groups 4 and 5 with groups 1, 2, and 3.

SUMMARY

This chapter reviewed the use of common statistical tests assessing differences between groups. In each case, a signal-to-noise ratio is generated to produce a test statistic that can be compared with a normalized distribution to determine if the differences occurred by chance. This statistical approach to hypothesis testing can be used for various study designs, including simple two-group comparison and complex multivariable, multilevel comparisons. However, hypothesis testing alone is insufficient when reviewing the results of healthcare studies. The researcher must consider the effect size generated by these comparisons. The results should also be contextualized and assessed for clinical meaningfulness.

REFERENCES

1. Altman D. Statistics in medical journals: Some recent trends. *Stat Med.* 2000;19(23):3275–3289. doi: 10.1002/1097-0258(20001215)19:23 < 3275::AID-SIM626 > 3.0.CO;2-M.
2. Harris M, Taylor G, eds. *Medical and Health Science Statistics Made Easy.* 2nd ed. Sudbury, MA: Jones and Bartlett; 2009.
3. Vogt WP, ed. *Dictionary of Statistics and Methodology: A Nontechnical Guide for the Social Sciences.* 3rd ed. Thousand Oaks, CA: Sage; 2005.
4. Coolidge FL, ed. *Statistics: A Gentle Introduction.* 2nd ed. Thousand Oaks, CA: Sage; 2006.
5. Cohen J. Statistical power analysis. *Curr Dir Psychol Sci.* 1992;1(3):98–101.
6. Aparasu RR, Bentley JP, eds. *Principles of Research Design and Drug Literature Evaluation*, Burlington, MA: Jones and Bartlett, 2015.
7. Ferguson C. An effect size primer: A guide for clinicians and researchers. *Prof Psychol Res Pract.* 2009;40(5):532–538. doi: 10.1037/a0015808.
8. Hotelling H. The generalization of student's ratio. *Anna Math Stat.* 1931;2(3):360–378.
9. Meyers LS, Gamst G, Guarino AJ, eds. *Applied Multivariate Research.* 2nd ed. Thousand Oaks, CA: Sage; 2013.

CHAPTER 13

The Results Section

Anthony A. Miller, MEd, PA-C
J. Dennis Blessing, PhD

CHAPTER OVERVIEW

This chapter discusses the results of data analysis. For most manuscripts, the Results section is the shortest and most graphically displayed. It is important that findings, particularly key findings, be presented clearly in a logical fashion. The Results section should consist of the facts and only the facts. Graphs and charts are useful methods for presenting results. The Results section (sometimes referred to as the Findings section) is an important part of a research report; key findings and outcomes of the study are reported there, and this is where the author indicates whether the hypotheses (null hypotheses or research questions) were supported or rejected. All the preceding sections of a research report are designed to build up the reader's anticipation for what is shared in the Results section. Additionally, findings in the Results section should be consistent and correlate well with the preceding Materials and Methods (or Methodology) section.

Learning Objectives

- List and define what information is in the Results section.
- Describe table, graph, and image construction.
- Discuss the importance of the Results section.

INTRODUCTION

The Results section should present only key findings related to the research question, *without* the author's conclusions regarding the meaning and importance of the data, which follows in the Discussion section. The Results section is typically the shortest section of the research manuscript. The section should be written clearly and succinctly, generally in the past tense for experimental or quasi-experimental studies and in the present tense for descriptive studies. For ethical reasons, all of the key findings should be reported, not just those supporting the hypotheses. Information about or descriptions of what was done belong in the preceding Materials and Methods (Methodology or Design) section and should not be included in the Results section.

The reported results must be consistent with the methodology and data analysis. Investigators must be careful to refrain from including any conclusions or opinions in the Results section.

Anything other than the facts could bias a reader's interpretation. The Results section should be neutral in every aspect, allowing readers to form their own conclusions.

The Results section must demonstrate outcomes clearly and in language that will allow readers to make their own conclusions. For example, reporting that the systolic blood pressure decreased on average 10 mm Hg after administration of agent *X* is clearer than reporting that the mean systolic blood pressure was 120 mm Hg after administration of agent *X*.

Ultimately, the Results section is the "meat" of the research report. The results provide the basis for all that follows and, most importantly, the interpretation of meaning. The Results section represents "the major scientific contribution of your study."[1] A common beginners' mistake is reporting raw data rather than summarizing findings. The author's primary task in the Results section is to provide a picture of the data for the reader. The following excerpts provide an example of a poorly written segment in the Results section and a contrasting improved segment:

Facts Without Interpretation

The mean resting pulse rate for the 10 control subjects was 74 ± 4 (SD) compared to the 12 athletes with a mean resting pulse rate of 66 ± 5 beats per minute.

Improved

The mean resting pulse rate was 11% lower in the 12 athletes than the 10 control subjects: 66 ± 5 (SD) versus 74 ± 4 beats per minute, p < .05).

Note that the magnitude of the difference (11%) is reported as well as the probability value indicating that the difference was statistically significant. The first example is ambiguous and leaves it to the reader to determine the meaning of the data, whereas in the second example the author makes clear to the reader what is important about the data.

THE RESULTS SECTION TEXT

The Results section usually begins with a description or profile of the subjects and includes relevant demographics so the reader has a good understanding of how representative the sample was of the population. Numbers, percentages, and central tendency statistics should be used to describe the study sample. An example of this part of the section might read: "Fifty-two percent ($n = 78$) of the healthcare professionals responded to the survey. Twenty questionnaires were returned 'unforwardable.' Of the respondents, 33 were male and 45 were female. The average age was 34 years (SD = ± 6.5)."

After describing the study sample, the researchers report the results of the statistical analysis with sufficient detail to permit the reader to determine that appropriate analyses were conducted and the hypotheses were or were not supported. For descriptive research, frequencies, ranges, and measures of central tendency should be reported. For experimental or quasi-experimental research, the inferential or associational statistics should include the test statistic, the direction, and the level of probability. Confidence intervals and size effects should be reported, adding strength to decisions regarding statistical significance.[2-5]

The word *significant* in discussions of data must be used carefully. *Significant* means "statistically significant" or "clinically significant" when written in the healthcare literature. Some authors see events or numbers of subjects affected as significant because of the event, intervention, treatment, or effect. In the Results section of the manuscript, something is significant only if the result is statistically significant according to the data analysis.

In addition to reporting significance related to hypothesis testing, sufficient information about the statistical test must be provided to allow the reader to understand that the appropriate test was chosen and the preferred method for reporting the statistical test was used.[6] This may be particularly important if a novel approach to analysis was used or if the procedure is considered controversial. It may be appropriate to include such descriptions in the Methodology section. Always assume that readers have a working knowledge of statistics and research design.

Finally, the hypotheses that were supported should be indicated in the Results section, and they should be clearly linked to the null hypotheses or research questions, or to alternate hypotheses where such an explanation is appropriate. At this point, the reasons why the hypotheses were or were not supported are given. Ultimately, the data should speak for themselves.

TABLES AND FIGURES

For the sake of clarity and brevity, tables and figures are used to show research results. Because many researchers use commercially available software for data analysis, the tables and figures are often produced before the author begins writing the text of the Results section. Tables and figures are particularly useful for readers when numerical results are reported. Avoid the temptation of making the topic sentence (first sentence of the paragraph) a reference to a table or figure. For example, "**Table 13-1** presents the means and standard deviations for the control and experimental groups." This is an inappropriate topic sentence and provides no useful information. A better example is "The experimental group showed a 10% improvement in scores over the control group (Table 13-1)."

Many commercial programs (e.g., Microsoft Excel, Harvard Graphics, SPSS) make it fairly easy to create tables and graphs, often without having to re-input data. Because tables and figures are more expensive to reproduce (compared to the body of the text), it is important to use only those graphic elements that are most important to the primary findings. If many numbers, statistics, or other results need to be presented, a well-organized, consolidated table is ideal. Use tables, graphs, and figures wisely.

Tables are used to organize, condense, and list numerical data. Examples include tables that describe the study sample (example shown in Table 13-1), compare groups (example shown in **Table 13-2**), or show correlations (example shown in **Table 13-3**). The types of analyses performed on the research data dictate the format for display in a table. For qualitative or nonexperimental studies, tables are sometimes used to summarize or compare textual information (example shown in **Table 13-4**). For experimental studies, tables like Table 13-1 are used primarily to demonstrate that the independent variables for the control group and experimental group are not significantly different.

Tables should be clear enough to stand alone without explanation in the text. Although tables can be helpful for the organization and display of important findings, they can be confusing if they are not used and/or constructed appropriately. All relevant information for the type of statistic reported (e.g., test statistic, degrees of freedom, probability value, direction, etc. in the case of inferential statistics) must be included. Because readers tend to make comparisons first horizontally from left to right, primary comparisons in tables should be shown horizontally.[7] **Table 13-5** lists additional general guidelines for the use and construction of tables, and **Figure 13-1** shows the elements of a typical table.

Graphs, charts, pictures (including radiographs), computer-generated images, diagrams, flowcharts, drawings, and the like are considered figures. The

Table 13-1 Demographic Profile for PA Class of 2012 (*n* = 20)

	Mean	Median	Low–High	SD
Age	28.10	26.50	23–44	5.44
Previous healthcare experience (months)	21.95	20.50	12–60	10.97
High school GPA	3.09	3.00	2.25–3.90	0.42
Undergraduate GPA	3.36	3.32	3.00–3.90	0.31

Note: GPA = grade point average.

Table 13-2 Comparison of Job Profiles for PA Classes of 2011 and 2012*

Demographic Characteristic	Class of 2011 (n = 12) Frequency	Class of 2011 (n = 12) Percentage	Class of 2012 (n = 18) Frequency	Class of 2012 (n = 18) Percentage
Specialty				
Family medicine	6	50	6	33
Pediatrics	1	8	4	22
General internal medicine	1	8	0	0
Emergency medicine	3	25	2	11
General surgery	1	8	3	17
Other	0	0	2	11
Location				
Urban	5	42	8	44
Suburban	5	42	7	39
Rural	2	17	2	11
Practice type				
Solo	1	8	5	28
Group	4	33	7	39
Hospital	5	42	5	28
Other	2	16	0	0
Unknown	0	0	1	5

*Note: Because of rounding, percentages may not total 100.

variety of types of graphs includes line graphs (example shown in **Figure 13-2**), scatter graphs, histograms (example shown in **Figure 13-3**), bar graphs (example shown in **Figure 13-4**), and pie charts.

Many journals have specific directions for the construction and display of tables, graphs, and figures. When submitting work for publication, be sure to follow the journal's "Instructions for Authors." Editors do not want to spend time

Table 13-3 Intercorrelations Among Educational Outcomes for PA Students (n = 50)

	High School GPA	College GPA	Basic Science GPA	Clinical GPA	Packrat Exam	PANCE
High school GPA	—	0.77**	0.54*	0.36	0.12	0.11
College GPA		—	0.79*	0.23	0.34*	0.17
Basic science GPA			—	0.22	0.27	0.21
Clinical GPA				—	0.56*	0.62*
Packrat exam					—	0.81**
PANCE						—

Note. GPA = grade point average; PANCE = Physician Assistant National Certifying Exam.

*$p < .05$. **$p < .01$.

Table 13–4 Comparisons of Common Cardiac Murmurs

Diagnosis	Location	Timing	Pitch	Quality
Aortic stenosis	Second right intercostal space, sternal border	Midsystolic	Medium	Coarse
Aortic regurgitation	Base, patient seated and leaning forward	Early diastolic	High	Blowing
Mitral stenosis	Apex, patient in left lateral decubitus position	Diastolic	Low	Rumble
Mitral regurgitation	Apex	Holosystolic	High	Blowing

Adapted from Seidel HM, Benedict G, Dains JE, Ball JW. *Mosby's Guide to Physical Examination.* 4th ed. St. Louis, MO: Mosby-Year Book; 1998:467–471.

correcting such items, and failure to follow instructions may result in rejection of the manuscript.

Generally speaking, polygons and histograms are used to plot frequency distributions. Bar graphs are different from histograms in that the columns are separated; these graphs are best used to show comparisons for two or more groups. Bar graphs are frequently used when the independent variables are categorical. When developing graphs (particularly bar graphs), care must be taken to ensure that proportions of the width and height provide an accurate display of the data and are not misleading because of dimensions of the graph. Line graphs are used to show the relationship between two quantitative variables.[8] The intersection of the *x*- and *y*-axes in the lower left-hand corner is typically zero (0). If there is discontinuity in an axis, it should be represented by a pair of diagonal lines (//) to show the missing portion. The dependent variable is generally plotted on the vertical (*y*) axis.

Table 13–5 Guidelines for the Construction of Tables

1. Choose a clear and specific table title so there is no confusion about the contents.
2. Number tables consecutively using Arabic numbers from the beginning of the report and label them accordingly.
3. Use subheadings for the columns and rows. Format cells so the data are clear and easy to read; often alignment on decimals is preferred.
4. Limit your information to include only material related to your descriptive title. For example, do not mix sample demographics with inferential statistics.
5. Do not explain your table in the text; it should speak for itself; however, the table must be identified in the text (e.g., see Table 1).
6. Use table formats that are consistent and that conform to the publisher's guidelines. Check with the publisher in advance or consult the "Instructions to Authors" to determine whether tables and figures should be submitted separately or incorporated within the text.
7. Avoid excessive lines. Generally, vertical lines for columns are not needed, but there should be sufficient space between the columns so the table is easy to read. In addition, tables should be limited to one page.
8. Be sure to include appropriate units of measure (e.g., mg/dL).

Adapted from Wiersma W. *Research Methods in Education: An Introduction.* 7th ed. Needham Heights, MA: Allyn and Bacon; 2000:393–394.

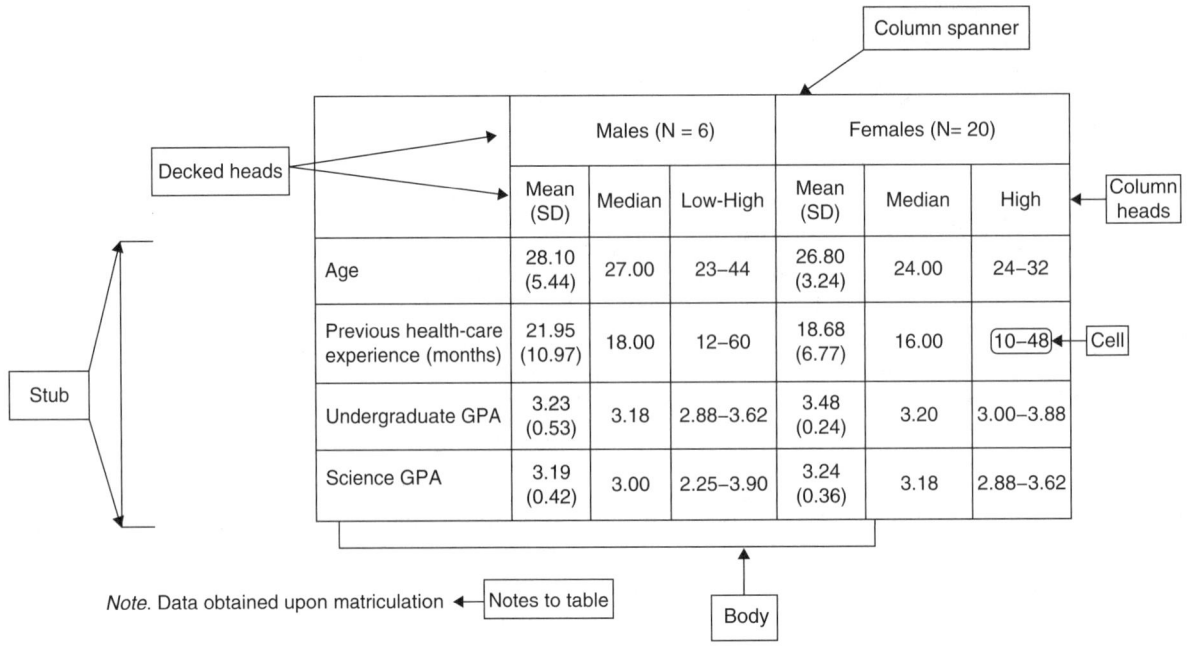

Figure 13–1 Table construction elements.

Many software programs create graphs using color, but most journals reproduce the graphs in black and white. Therefore, it is important to ensure sufficient contrast exists between adjacent bars. Keep in mind that commercial software contains certain features (e.g., three-dimensional bar graphs) that enhance the appearance of the report for a PowerPoint presentation, but may not reproduce well when the size is decreased and colors are converted to black and white. The American Medical Association recommends a shading contrast of at least 30%.[7] In addition to using shading to

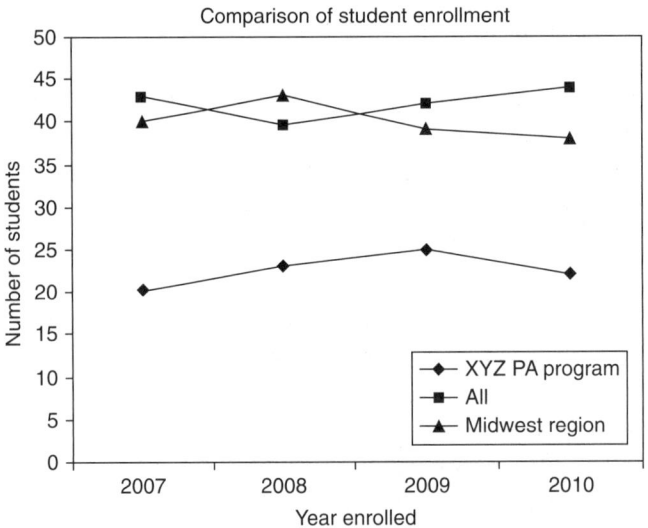

Figure 13–2 Example of a line graph.

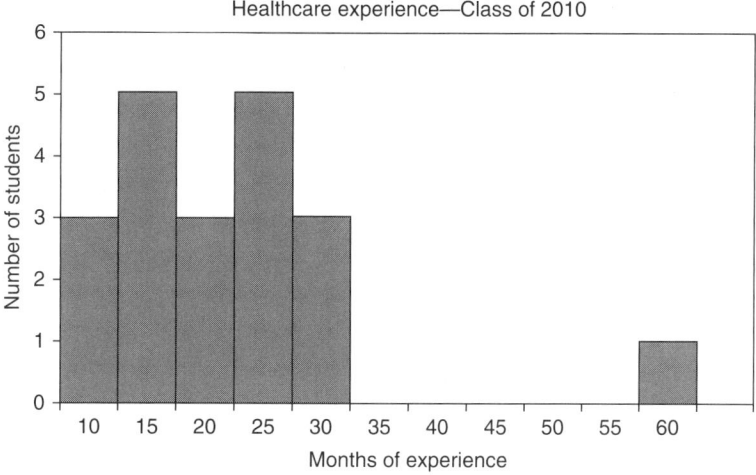

Figure 13–3 Example of a histograph.

distinguish bars or pie chart sections, many commercial programs allow different patterns such as cross-hatching. Pie charts are used to show percentages or proportions of different quantities (e.g., types of students in a cohort) and are used to display results of descriptive research. **Table 13–6** provides a quick review of general guidelines for the construction of graphs.

When presenting results in a paragraph or graphically, it is wise to double check the numbers and data for accuracy. Make sure that graphs present your results clearly. An inadvertent mistake in one number could make readers cautious about all results. More than one error will probably make them ignore everything, even if the conclusions and interpretations are correct.

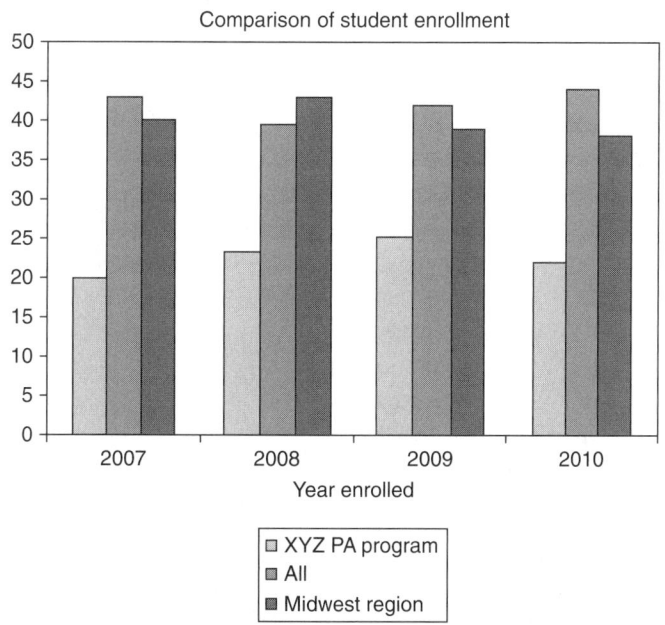

Figure 13–4 Example of a bar graph.

Table 13–6 General Guidelines for Developing Graphs

1. Be sure the graph is labeled as a figure and has a self-explanatory title.
2. Select the proper type of graph based on the data, statistical analysis, and clearest presentation to the reader.
3. Refer to figures in the text and number them consecutively. (Tables and figures are numbered separately.)
4. Be sure there is enough spacing for ease of interpretation and that the grid is scaled proportionately.
5. Check spelling (including caption) and ensure data were entered and plotted correctly.
6. Ensure there is sufficient contrast or pattern difference to clearly separate segments of pie chart or bars on the bar graph. Avoid three-dimensional or other special effects.
7. Check with the publisher for guidance on overall size, font size, resolution, and style specifications.
8. Include legends if necessary, and define abbreviations.
9. Update permission from the copyright holder for reproductions or adaptations from other sources. Be sure the source is noted.
10. For photographs and other illustrations, be sure to mark "TOP" so the publisher has the proper orientation for typesetting and layout. In addition, be sure these items are labeled and identified with your name and article title in case they are separated from the manuscript.

Note: This may not be necessary if the graphic is imbedded in the manuscript.

The big advantage in using figures and tables is that a large amount of data can be presented in a relatively small print space.[9] The number of printed pages is important to publishers. Well-designed figures and tables can display a lot of data in a digestible manner as well as enhance the appearance of a manuscript.

SUMMARY

The Results section of the report is used for presenting the results of the statistical analyses. The section must be clearly written in a concise format. Tables, graphs, and other figures help present data in a way that makes the results easily read, readily understood, and invites interpretation. The Results section also provides the basis for a decision on the rejection or retention of null hypotheses and/or whether research questions were supported or answered. The Results section is free of author (or any other) bias. Think of this section as a place for the factual presentation of the research results. Remember: "the facts and just the facts."

REFERENCES

1. Hofmann AH. *Scientific Writing and Communication: Papers, Proposals and Presentations.* New York: Oxford University Press; 2010:265.
2. Gehlbach SH. *Interpreting the Medical Literature.* 5th ed. New York: McGraw-Hill; 2006:157–159.
3. Sterne JA, Smith GD. Shifting the evidence—What's wrong with significance tests? *BMJ.* 2001;322:226–231.
4. Zeiger M. *Essentials of Writing Biomedical Research Papers.* 2nd ed. New York: McGraw-Hill; 2000:156.
5. Wilkinson L, Task Force on Statistical Inference. Statistical methods in psychology journals: Guidelines and explanations. *Am Psychol.* 1999;54(8):594–604.
6. Creswell JW. *Educational Research: Planning, Conducting, and Evaluating Quantitative and Qualitative Research.* Boston, MA: Pearson; 2012.
7. American Medical Association. *AMA Manual of Style: A Guide for Authors and Editors.* 10th ed. New York: Oxford University Press; 2007:84.
8. American Psychological Association. *Publication Manual of the American Psychological Association.* 6th ed. Washington, DC: American Psychological Association; 2010:151.
9. Bailey DM. *Research for the Health Professional: A Practical Guide.* 2nd ed. Philadelphia, PA: F. A. Davis; 1997:193.

---

*Note that all data portrayed in the tables and figures for this chapter are fictitious and are not intended to represent any actual research study or source. Readers should consult the "Instructions for Authors" in journals to which they intend to submit manuscripts for specific guidelines and requirements.

CHAPTER 14

The Discussion Section

Richard R. Rahr, EdD, PA-C
J. Dennis Blessing, PhD, PA

CHAPTER OVERVIEW

The Discussion section of a manuscript is where the author/investigator is allowed to state interpretations, conclusions, and opinions about the research project and its results. This manuscript section is where the investigator can provide answers to the questions posed in the introduction. Of all the sections of a thesis, dissertation, or manuscript for publication, this section most reflects the author's ability to synthesize experimental results. This is the place where opinions, views, and meaning are presented.[1]

The Discussion section may contain a number of subsections, and may be referred to by different titles, such as summary, implications, interpretations, or recommendations. The section should also include a closing paragraph(s) labeled "Conclusions" or something similar. The section and subsections titles depend on the type of work being produced, as well as local and publication requirements. The author has some discretion on what subsections to include in the Discussion section. This section should center on the importance of the results and their implications and application in patient care, education, or the healthcare professions.[1]

Learning Objectives

- List, describe, and define the components of the Discussion section.
- Define the importance of the Discussion section.
- Define and describe study limitations.
- Define and discuss the importance of the Recommendation section.

INTRODUCTION

The traditional Discussion section of a research report covers the following areas: implications, limitations, discussion, bias considerations, recommendations, and conclusions. A review of several "how-to" research books reveals that similar descriptors, such as summary, interpretation, and analysis, are used in the Discussion section. Even the order of the subsections varies. This chapter focuses on the terms most commonly used in the research literature; however, local or publication requirements may differ.[2]

THE IMPLICATIONS SUBSECTION

In the Implications subsection, the author explores the meaning of the research results. This is the author's opportunity to think critically about the results, draw conclusions, or make inferences; for example, what changes are indicated in clinical practice based on the research findings? What do the results mean to health care and society? Even if there were no statistically significant findings related to the research study's hypotheses or questions, the research effort might still have meaning. One inference from statistically nonsignificant results may be that current practice is supported by the data and results. The recommendations for such studies might well be to make no changes and to continue with the current best knowledge. If the investigation yielded significant results, then an author may take the opportunity to discuss why and what that means in light of what is known. If there are significant findings that have strong implications in practice or in the fund of knowledge, a new approach to the problem or a change in practice may be recommended. Remember, major changes in healthcare practice and theory are seldom based on a single study unless it is a very large, well-designed, and carefully controlled investigation. Meta-analysis, which is the integration and evaluation of several or many independent research studies, is now considered one of the highest levels of research sophistication, particularly for evidence-based practice. Even in evidence-based analysis, however, questions are often raised that require further investigation.[1]

The implications of the study may point out the potential value of a finding or the need for replication or modifications in a subsequent study in order to strengthen the research results or findings. When an investigator believes the results have important implications, those results should be stated in positive terms. Rational arguments based on data and analyses, particularly when contradicting accepted dogma or theory, must be presented clearly.

Here is an example of an implication: Study antibiotic X increased the effective cure rate for osteomyelitis by 25 percent over the currently available drug treatment. If antibiotic X had no major side effects, then it would certainly be recommended for the treatment of osteomyelitis. If an investigator found that giving antibiotic X with the addition of daily treatments in the hyperbaric chamber made no significant difference in the overall treatment outcomes, then the recommendation would be that the additional treatment not be used in tandem. The investigator must explicitly state the implications for clinical treatment based on the findings.

The meaning and limitations of statistical analysis should be considered when stating the implications of the investigation. Here is an example: If the Pearson product moment statistical test is used to measure a variable, and the analysis results in a significant correlation of $r = 0.70$, then this would seem to be a good correlation. However, further analysis using the Pearson's correlation r with a second statistical analysis called the r^2 (the coefficient of determination) returns a result of $r^2 = 0.49$. This second statistic accounts for only 49 percent of the correlation variance. The fact that 51 percent of the research study variance is not explained should cause a conservative interpretation of the implications and recommendation decisions. Any and all discussion must make sense of the statistical analysis and the results.

Ultimately, the Implications subsection is where the author makes the case for the study and its results. Avoid mixing in information or data that do not belong in the subsection. The best critical thinking skills should be used to form the implications with awareness of the current literature in relation to the study results. This is one reason why the methodology is so important. Well-designed and sound methodology allows strong support for the implications. Implications, regardless of type or nature, should have practical and clinical significance and should be clearly supported by the research findings.

THE LIMITATIONS SUBSECTION

The Limitations subsection of the Discussion section is of utmost importance. The study's weaknesses (or limits) must be addressed in the presentation of the research. Problems or limitations should be recognized and pointed out by the researcher so that the overall value of the study can be considered. This explanation may allow those limitations to be avoided if the study is replicated. The researcher may realize, in retrospect, that there were flaws in the methodology.

All studies have limitations. Putting these limitations in front of the reader gives credence to the conclusions and the investigator's understanding of the study. If an investigator realizes the study limitations, then the conclusions include consideration of those limitations. Recognizing and stating the limitations of the work ultimately strengthens the work and its impact.[1]

Authors should clearly state to whom and in what situations the research study's findings or outcomes can be generalized and applied. Again, recognizing and considering limitations is very important in understanding the application or meaning of the study's findings. How well did the sample participants represent the population? The researcher may have inadvertently attracted or recruited only a certain subgroup of the intended population. For example, even though the researcher sought to have a representative sample of both men and women of various age groups, perhaps only women within a certain age range were willing to participate in the study. The findings and conclusions must take this limitation into consideration. Also, can the data from such a study be generalized to the general population? For some investigations, a pilot study may reveal some of these problems (limitations) and help guide the methodology. A well-designed, meticulous study usually has few limitations.

The Limitations subsection should also discuss the randomness of the sample selection and the potential for error in the sampling. Having an experienced researcher as a guide and mentor can assist any investigator in developing a study that is as strong as possible within the ever-present constraints of a practice or educational setting. Consideration must be given to whether an intervening variable or research effect (e.g., the Hawthorne effect) could be responsible for the results.[2]

If limitations are identified or recognized in a research project, investigators must be honest and forthright about those limitations. Such forthrightness gives the researcher, the research project, and its outcomes greater credibility and potential for acceptance. If readers are informed of limitations, other researchers can attempt to avoid these limitations in similar, future studies.

THE DISCUSSION SUBSECTION

The Discussion subsection of the Discussion section is an informative section used to meld together the research report, the interpretation of the results, their implications, and the study's limitations into an objective presentation. In previous parts of the research report there is no room (or justification) for the author's subjective thoughts and insights. The discussion subsection is refreshing in that it allows and encourages authors to give their view of the impact and importance of the research outcomes. This is the author's opportunity to place the study in the ongoing conversation and context of the current literature. The author can interject subjectivity based on previous clinical and research experiences and wisdom (expert opinion). How did the significance or nonsignificance of the data relate to the conceptual framework of the literature that was reviewed? This is where the author gets to answer that question, in their opinion, based on the investigation.

In this subsection, readers expect to be apprised of some practical application of the research findings. The author demonstrates his or her research knowledge and wisdom here. A clinical example could be the matching of patients with providers of the same gender. Is the effectiveness of the encounter perceived to be better by patients? By providers? Again, a number of other factors can influence these perceptions. In the Discussion subsection, all of these factors can be explored in light of the research findings.

In the Discussion subsection, the author may want to discuss the characteristics of survey tools, limitations, generalizations, statistical methods, and bias considerations of the research project. Ultimately, this part of the report is used to critically discuss the study and evaluate research outcomes and their impact. In some formats, the Discussion section is the last subsection of the text.[1]

THE RECOMMENDATIONS SUBSECTION

The Recommendations subsection of the Discussion section usually states the author's ideas on the future research requirements based on the outcomes of the current study. For example, an author may include suggestions to expand the existing research by adding more subjects to the current research plan or to conduct "next step" studies. Other recommendations may include developing a new research design, using a new data collection instrument, or addressing the gaps or weaknesses in the study. Recommendations may include making the study a double-blind crossover model, adding a control group, or suggesting an outside independent investigator repeat the same study to determine if the results can be replicated. The overall purpose of the Recommendations subsection is to alert the reader that additional questions need to be asked and answered. The author should avoid providing so many recommendations that the most important ones are obscured. As elsewhere, the author should strive for relevance, clarity, and brevity in this subsection.[1,2]

THE CONCLUSIONS SUBSECTION

This is usually the last section of the paper, and it is generally brief. The Conclusions subsection of the Discussion section should begin with a brief restatement of the aim(s) of the study and the major research questions or hypotheses. Following that, the author should state the major findings of the study, using a format that can be easily followed. Here is an example:

This study demonstrated that patients who are treated for chronic severe pain with analgesic medication administered around the clock rather than on a PRN schedule had a higher level of functional status. Based on this finding, a major implication might be to change the treatment protocol to a regular schedule rather than PRN medication administration for patients with chronic severe pain.

Clearly stated implications for practice, when backed by sound research findings, help to build evidence-based practice and improve the care of patients.

A high-quality contrast and comparison of the results with the relevant underlying literature is expected. For example, the author can point out that the same or similar research findings have been reported. The author may wish to restate the strong and weak points of the research study; however, redundancy should be avoided unless a point is restated purposefully. The Conclusions subsection also provides the author the opportunity to share personal opinions and experiences that highlight and emphasize the impact of the research study. This should be done carefully; these comments by the author must be clearly related to the current study and should not merely be the author's general opinion. The overall practical value of the information presented in research studies is important in the context of healthcare practice.[2]

The Conclusions subsection is much like a closing abstract, but with a bit more detail than is allowed in the Abstract section. This subsection should provide a complete, but concise, overview of the research study while bringing the Discussion section to a close. In summary, **Table 14-1** presents key elements the Discussion section should include, and **Table 14-2** provides reminders of pitfalls to avoid in this section.[2]

Table 14-1 Key Criteria for the Discussion Section

Clearly state what the research findings contribute to the understanding of the defined problem or question.
Be specific about implications for practice or society.
Describe how the findings fit into the present body of knowledge.
State how the findings support, enhance, or contrast with prior research findings.
If the findings are novel or in contrast to accepted norms, strong support is needed for the interpretations.

Table 14–2 Pitfalls to Avoid in the Discussion Section

Drawing conclusions or formulating implications that cannot be clearly supported by the research findings.

Providing so many recommendations for further study that the most important recommendations are lost.

Having an apologetic tone when describing limitations or study design weaknesses. Be matter of fact.

REFERENCES

1. Bailey DM. *Research for the Health Professional: A Practical Guide.* 2nd ed. Philadelphia, PA: F. A. Davis; 1997.

2. Jenkins S, Price CJ, Straker L. *The Researching Therapist: A Practical Guide to Planning, Performing and Communicating Research.* New York: Churchill Livingston; 1998.

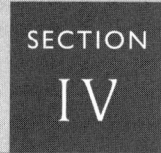

The Research Process: Writing and Interpretation

CHAPTER 15

References

Christine S. Gaspard, MSLS
Katherine A. Prentice, MSIS
Eric Willman, MSIS
Albert Simon, DHSc, MEd, PA-C

CHAPTER OVERVIEW

This chapter reviews common documentation styles used in scholarly and professional writing that apply to thesis, dissertation, and research paper writing. It also examines the process for documenting references using footnotes and the proper construction of bibliographies. Copyright law and fair use doctrine are discussed to provide a basis for the importance of assigning proper credit to sources used in the construction of the research paper. Finally, the chapter considers how the Internet can assist in finding source material for research projects.

Learning Objectives

- Choose a writing style.
- Identify the sources of writing styles.
- Discuss how to evaluate sources of information.
- Describe how to use electronic databases.
- Describe and discuss the importance of proper referencing.
  - Describe how to use elements of reference.
- Define *bibliography*.
  - Describe the types of bibliographies.
- Describe the use of copyrighted material, fair use provisions, public domain, and plagiarism.
  - Define and discuss the penalties for copyright violations.

CHOOSING A WRITING STYLE

Although a variety of styles and formats may be used for writing a research paper, most colleges, universities, and publishers dictate a style that must be followed for constructing a paper (e.g., the layout, bibliography, citation style, etc.). Particular departments or schools within universities often have their own specific style requirements. Many style manuals are available. Before choosing one, authors should investigate the manuscript requirements. Although you may have heard of the Turabian or Modern Language Association (MLA) styles, we focus here on the styles more commonly used within the healthcare professions: the *AMA Manual of Style* (AMA),[1] *Chicago Manual of Style* (CMS),[2] *Uniform Requirements for Manuscripts Submitted to Biomedical Journals* (also known as Vancouver style), and *Publication Manual of the American Psychological Association* (APA).[3] It is important to recognize that some publications may publish their own style manuals with additional requirements. These requirements provided by the journal can be found in the "Information for Authors" or "Instructions to Authors" guidelines usually provided on the publisher's website.

The APA, Chicago, and Vancouver styles are most often employed for writing undergraduate research papers and theses at the graduate level. Dissertation styles may follow one of these or other specific institutional guidelines. It is common for research works and dissertations to be published in the style of the professional or academic journals within that discipline.

Each of these four styles has unique features. The differences that exist in reference styles relate to how the various details (e.g., author's name, etc.) are formatted or which elements are used. For example, APA does not use endnotes or footnotes, whereas AMA, Vancouver, and Chicago do. Beyond these comparisons, there are variations in indentations, punctuation, and format among the four styles. The requirements may appear trivial, but publication and departmental requirements are generally very strict, and manuscripts may be turned down or graded poorly if the style rules are not followed.

The following examples illustrate the differences among these styles. These sample citations show a book by more than one author and a journal article by more than one author.

AMA

1. Hooker RS, Cawley JF, Asprey DP. *Physician Assistants: Policy and Practice*. 3rd ed. Philadelphia, PA: F. A. Davis; 2010.
2. Bloomer RJ, Falvo MJ, Schilling BK, Smith WA. Prior exercise and antioxidant supplementation: Effect on oxidative stress and muscle injury. *J Int Soc Sports Nutr*. 2007;4:9–19.

APA

Hooker, R. S., Cawley, J. F., & Asprey, D. P. (2010). *Physician assistants: Policy and practice* (3rd ed.). Philadelphia, PA: F. A. Davis.

Bloomer, R. J., Falvo, M. J., Schilling, B. K., & Smith, W. A. (2007). Prior exercise and antioxidant supplementation: Effect on oxidative stress and muscle injury. *Journal of the International Society of Sports Nutrition, 4,* 9–19. doi:10.1186/1550-2783-4-9

Vancouver

1. Hooker RS, Cawley JF, Asprey DP. Physician assistants: policy and practice. 3rd ed. Philadelphia: F. A. Davis; 2010.
2. Bloomer RJ, Falvo MJ, Schilling BK, Smith WA. Prior exercise and antioxidant supplementation: effect on oxidative stress and muscle injury. J Int Soc Sports Nutr. 2007 Oct 3;4:9–19.

Chicago

Hooker, Roderick S., James F. Cawley, and David P. Asprey. *Physician Assistants: Policy and Practice*. 3rd ed. Philadelphia: F. A. Davis, 2010.

Bloomer, R. J., M. J. Falvo, B. K. Schilling, and W. A. Smith. "Prior Exercise and Antioxidant Supplementation: Effect on Oxidative Stress and Muscle Injury." *Journal of the International Society of Sports Nutrition* 4 (2007): 9–19.

It is important to follow the style exactly. Writers are advised to consult the appropriate style guides to ensure the proper citation format is followed. Selection of style is largely a matter of convention, tradition, preference, or assignment guidelines.

The APA style is widely used in the social sciences and nursing fields. It offers a format that encompasses parenthetical citations within the text that contain the author's name, year of publication, and page number (when used for direct quotes). A reference list is arranged alphabetically at the end of the paper.

The Vancouver style is one name for the reference style of the *Uniform Requirements for Manuscripts Submitted to Biomedical Journals*, which is widely used in medicine and the healthcare sciences. Vancouver uses an "author–number" citation system from the American National Standards Institute style adopted in the National Library of Medicine's (NLM's) *Citing Medicine*. *Citing Medicine* is not published in a printed book, but it is available online.[4]

The Chicago style is popular with magazines and some other nonscholarly publications. When following the Chicago format, footnote or endnote documentation is used. In this style, the notes are placed on a separate sheet at the end of the document in the order they are cited in the text (i.e., as endnotes) or they are listed numerically at the bottom of each page of text (i.e., as footnotes).

Each style manual contains a comprehensive guide to the documentation of sources and other technical details of publication. These guides can be purchased at bookstores, but many are also available at university and public libraries. Detailed information about most styles is also available on the Web. Although purchasing the style guide is often the easiest way to access the information, sometimes using a secondary or abridged version can meet a researcher's writing needs. For the APA and Chicago styles, a helpful source is the Purdue Online Writing Lab (or OWL) website, Research and Citation Resources.[5] This site provides detailed assistance for writers and includes examples of citations from different sources. Because the Vancouver style is freely available on the Web, the e-book should serve as the "go-to" resource. Remember that synopses provide quick reference for general guidance and are helpful in many situations, but the amount and scope of information they contain may be limited.

DOCUMENTING SOURCES USING REFERENCES AND BIBLIOGRAPHIES

During the research phase, the investigator begins to synthesize his or her thoughts with data, facts, and opinions from research material. All information found in a literature search and other background detail represents the original work of other authors. Whether quoted directly or paraphrased, the use of background sources must be acknowledged with proper documentation. Any background information not known as "general knowledge" in the field should be documented with citations within the text and in a bibliography using the required style. The process of documentation involves creating and sharing a list of all the sources used in the production of your paper. The exact page numbers where the information is found are often required, so good recordkeeping is an advantage when performing a literature search.

Documentation is provided in two major ways:

1. Providing specific documentation either on each page or at the end of a chapter or section, by using in-text citations (i.e., author and date, footnotes, or endnotes).
2. Listing the sources of information used by constructing a bibliography. The bibliography (or reference list) is usually found at the end of the manuscript.

Using Footnotes, Endnotes, and Author–Date Styles

Footnotes and endnotes are parts of a numbered reference style that places the citation number at the end of the relevant content and the bibliographic details at the end of the page, chapter, or paper. Footnotes appear at the bottom of each page. Endnotes may appear at the end of each chapter or at the end of a book (often divided by chapters). Depending on the style that is chosen (e.g., APA), the references may be displayed in parentheses, as author–date citations, or as numbered designators that correspond to a reference list at the end of a text.

Using Bibliographies

Scholarly writing requires the use of a bibliography, that is, a list of works consulted and referenced during background research. Some styles also suggest including all reference materials consulted whether or not they were actually used in the paper. Particularly for dissertation writing, the bibliography encompasses all works available on the subject. For example, some academic departments or thesis committees may prefer terms such as *selected bibliography*, *references*, or *works cited*. The style guide should be consulted for the correct term to use in your research paper.

The bibliography generally follows the endnotes section of the paper (if an endnotes section is used) and is traditionally arranged alphabetically by author unless the style requires a numbered list (AMA). There will be slight differences in bibliographic format depending on the style used. Be sure to consult the specific style guidelines to determine the proper format.

By reviewing your bibliography or reference list, the reader can obtain a sense of the depth and caliber of the research. Clues to research quality include the types of works cited, the dates of publication, and the appropriateness of referenced material. Accurate bibliographies promote scholarly communication by providing readers the information to locate and use the listed works as primary sources themselves.

Two additional variations should be considered when preparing a bibliography. The first is an annotated bibliography, which allows authors' comments to be included with any or all of the listings. The second is to group the entries by source type. In this method, the list is divided into primary and secondary, then published and unpublished sources. Within each category, entries are listed alphabetically. Remember, primary sources are original works such as a book or letter. Secondary sources interpret or analyze content from other sources. Secondary sources can be in many forms, including articles, case studies, or books. Careful consideration of each item is required to determine status as a primary or secondary source.

Bibliographies prepared by other authors can also be useful in conducting background research. Preliminary research produces a collection of articles that contain bibliographies that relate to your research question as well as stand-alone bibliography publications. It is acceptable to use these citations as leads to additional information, but be careful to locate the sources to validate the appropriateness of each entry. It is improper to simply copy the citation list from another article into a bibliography.

COPYRIGHTED MATERIAL, FAIR USE PROVISIONS, PUBLIC DOMAIN, AND PLAGIARISM

Standards of academic conduct require the acknowledgment of all material used in the production of a scholarly work, whether the material was formally copyrighted or not. The copyright status of an item is not actually relevant when preparing your research paper. All materials should be cited, whether under copyright or in the public domain.

The Copyright Act is a comprehensive law that deals with the use of copyrighted material. Under this law, copyrighted material may be used without the permission of the copyright holder for certain specific uses.[6] Although permission from authors of copyrighted materials may be required under certain circumstances, the concept of *fair use* provides for limited use of copyrighted materials. Materials outside of copyright fall within the *public domain* and also can be used without permission, but they must be acknowledged. Generally, the public domain includes material for which the copyright has expired. It is safest to err on the side of caution—assume that all materials are under copyright when preparing research papers or educational materials.

In educational settings, fair use is understood to cover an array of situations that allow the use of copyrighted material without written permission.

However, fair use is a gray area within the law where only guidelines exist, and many instances of disagreement still occur. Research, teaching, and news reporting are included under the fair use umbrella. Consideration of fair use standards can protect writers and instructors from not only plagiarism, but also violating copyright laws. Copyright violation penalties can be very high—up to $150,000 for each willful act—and even unintentional violations can result in fines.[7]

To learn more about copyright, the University of Texas System provides an entire online tutorial on copyright.[8] The Crash Course in Copyright tutorial provides examples from a number of situations and is an important source for writers.[8] Copyright rules tend to change regularly, and legal interpretation sometimes varies by institution.

Certain works, such as those in the public domain, cannot receive the protection of copyright law. The public domain includes facts and other works that lack originality; the clearest example is the telephone book. Government publications also are considered to be in the public domain. There are additional examples of public domain detailed at the website Copyright Term and the Public Domain in the United States from Cornell University.[9] Remember, all works, even public domain items, must be cited in the reference list.

If uncertainty exists concerning whether a work is in the public domain or is copyright protected, legal counsel should be sought prior to publication so infringement of copyright can be avoided. If a work that is not in the public domain is reused in the course of a study, it is necessary to obtain permission from the author and possibly publishing companies. Such use may require that a royalty fee be paid for the right to use that property. The Copyright Clearance Center (http://www.copyright.com) is one broker of license fees that can assist with the copyright permission process.

According to the U.S. Copyright Office, Circular 1 copyright is automatically applied to all works (including computer software and programs) produced after 1978.[10] Some writers prefer extra protection. Writers may choose to have their work registered with the U.S. Copyright Office. Payment and registration paperwork is required when applying for formal copyright. For more information and to find forms online, visit the U.S. Copyright Office website (http://www.copyright.gov).

EVALUATING SOURCES

For most research questions, the problem is not finding enough material, but rather how to determine which sources to utilize. Writers need to evaluate the selected sources for appropriateness and authority. Before the resources are used, they can be assessed by considering the following questions:

- Is the source authoritative?
- Who are the authors of the source, and are they experts in the field?
- Does the academic community regard the authors as credible?
- Does the source represent current theories or trends?
- When was it published?
- Where was the source published?
- Did the work undergo a rigorous peer-review process?

The peer-review process used by some journals is a stringent process of article review before publication. When considering the authority of a publication, it is important to remember that within a peer-reviewed journal, not every item is peer-reviewed. Peer review provides additional confidence the article contains valid arguments and conclusions that result from sound methodology. The use of articles from peer-reviewed sources may carry additional weight and add value to the writing.

In today's Web-based world, all sources should be carefully evaluated. Freely available webpages may not have received the benefit of peer review; they may have been posted by an individual to state an opinion. By considering the questions just listed and carefully evaluating the resources selected, many credibility and validity issues can be avoided.

FINDING REFERENCES USING ELECTRONIC AND INTERNET-BASED SOURCES

It is important to consider how the Web can be used effectively in scholarly research. In the recent past, most research was done using only physical library materials. However, most researchers now begin the search for information using online databases and search engines. Although online sources have not completely supplanted printed materials, no comprehensive research process would be complete without searching both electronic and print sources.

Printed material can be stored in a variety of formats. Many academic and public libraries maintain material in a variety of digital or other technological formats. In addition to digital storage, microfilm and microfiche are still found in many libraries and are still used to provide access to older articles.

Traditional search engines use servers networked together allowing information from around the world to be accessed from any device that can make the online connection. Each search engine uses a different method to find and show results from webpages. Search engines do not usually provide search results from library catalogs and other library resources. Therefore, it is important to find other tools that can access library-provided content. Concurrent searching of multiple library catalogs is available through search engines such as WorldCat (WorldCat.org, http://www.worldcat.org), which allow access to thousands of library catalogs with one search and also can find nearby locations of desired materials.

Some online search tools, such as PubMed for biomedical literature, are tailored to specific subjects. PubMed can be accessed through the National Library of Medicine website (http://www.pubmed.gov). Depending on the area of research, it is wise to become familiar with a variety of search tools because no single search engine can be considered comprehensive or complete.

Each search tool works differently, so it is important to be flexible with search terms and search methods. Keywords, controlled vocabulary, algorithmic relevancy ranking, and good old-fashioned luck all affect your results. Using a variety of subject headings, keywords, and phrases with the Boolean operators AND, OR, and NOT to conduct a comprehensive search can improve results. Although some search tools can correct spelling mistakes, they cannot be relied upon to correct every problem. Misspellings can derail the most well-intentioned search strategies.

Libraries may subscribe to additional proprietary online databases (e.g., CINAHL, Micromedex, DIALOG, Ovid, UpToDate) to find specific content. These subscription search tools are able to narrow down a search with progressively more specific search terms to increase the relevancy of the results. Among the wide variety of library databases, some cater to the general market whereas others are discipline specific. Web search tools such as Google Scholar (http://scholar.google.com) complement results found in library databases. Unlike traditional Google, Google Scholar limits search results to scholarly materials that are more likely to be useful in scientific research and writing.

Web tools can also be leveraged for research projects. Free tools from Google Docs (https://docs.google.com), Skype (http://www.skype.com), Windows Live (http://explore.live.com), Twitter (http://twitter.com), and Wolfram|Alpha (http://wolframalpha.com) offer content, video conferencing, and survey tools; online storage; online collaboration; and more. Subscription services also offer survey tools and video conferencing, but costs vary and should be compared prior to purchase.

Above all, it is important to remember that sources must be cited accurately. Sources should always be evaluated, and only accurate and high-quality content should be included in a serious research project. All original sources cited by an investigator must be read. Using a variety of tools and conducting comprehensive and effective searches give researchers confidence in their results.

SUMMARY

No matter what type of research paper is being produced, the specific style guidelines must be followed meticulously. Bibliography and reference information must be accurate and attributed properly. Avoid plagiarism and double-check details. Good documentation can only serve to strengthen a research paper overall as well as contribute to the validity of its parts, including the literature review, methods, results, and conclusions.

REFERENCES

1. Iverson C, American Medical Association. *AMA Manual of Style: A Guide for Authors and Editors.* 10th ed. New York: Oxford University Press; 2007.
2. University of Chicago Press. *The Chicago Manual of Style.* 15th ed. Chicago: University of Chicago Press; 2003.
3. American Psychological Association. *Publication Manual of the American Psychological Association.* 6th ed. Washington, DC: American Psychological Association; 2010.
4. Patrias K, Wendling DL. *Citing Medicine: The NLM Style Guide for Authors, Editors, and Publishers.* 2nd ed. Washington, DC: National Library of Medicine; 2007. Available at: http://www.nlm.nih.gov/citingmedicine. Accessed June 5, 2014.
5. Purdue University Writing Lab. The Purdue online writing lab (OWL). Available at: http://owl.english.purdue.edu. Accessed June 5, 2014.
6. Library of Congress, Copyright Office. Copyright law of the United States of America and related laws contained in Title 17 of the United States code. 2011. Available at: http://purl.access.gpo.gov/GPO/LPS440. Accessed June 5, 2014.
7. Library of Congress, Copyright Office. Reproduction of copyrighted works by educators and librarians. 2011. Available at: http://www.loc.gov/copyright/circs/circ92.pdf. Accessed June 5, 2014.
8. Harper G, University of Texas System, Office of General Counsel. Copyright crash course. Available at: http://copyright.lib.utexas.edu. Accessed June 5, 2014.
9. Hirtle PB. Copyright term and the public domain in the United States. Available at: http://www.copyright.cornell.edu/resources/publicdomain.cfm. Accessed June 5, 2014.
10. Library of Congress, Copyright Office. Copyright basics. Available at: http://www.copyright.gov/circs/circ1.pdf. Accessed Oct. 13, 2014.

CHAPTER 16

Writing and Publishing in the Health Professions

James F. Cawley, MPH, PA-C, DHL (hon)

CHAPTER OVERVIEW

As clinicians and teachers, being a healthcare professional brings a sense of obligation to contribute to the existing body of research knowledge. This applies to clinical practitioners, students, and faculty in a wide range of healthcare disciplines. The development of skills in writing, formal presentation, and publishing is essential for healthcare professionals as they progress through and develop their careers. Such skills facilitate expansion of multiple career options and further existing knowledge within the professions.

Skills and techniques related to research methods, report writing, and publishing should be part of the educational preparation of all healthcare professionals. Scholarly work is increasingly a requirement for graduation in the healthcare professions. In this chapter, the essential components of a research paper are reviewed in general and the process of writing research papers generated by the various health professions is addressed. Presentations and posters are discussed.

Learning Objectives

- Identify different style manuals.
- List and discuss the processes of publication.
- Describe how to get published.
- Outline and define the elements of a manuscript.
- Define *peer review*, *blinded review*, *authorship*, and *order of authors*.

The process by which research papers are transformed into research publications in the biomedical literature is also discussed. The expansion of clinical investigations and the involvement of more practicing clinicians in the research process requires practitioners to develop publication and presentation skills.

INTRODUCTION

Since the 1600s, thinking and writing have largely been classified into two types: literary and scientific. The literary style has been associated with fiction, rhetoric, and subjectivity, whereas the scientific style has been steeped in fact, plain language, and objectivity. Through the centuries, this division of style increased as the body of scientific knowledge grew; barbs were increasingly exchanged between the two camps of thinkers and writers. By the mid-1800s literature and science often stood as two distinct domains,

Table 16–1 Style Manuals			
Title	**Edition**	**Author or Publisher**	**Year**
American Medical Association Manual of Style	10th	Oxford University Press, New York, NY	2007
The Chicago Manual of Style	16th	University of Chicago Press, Chicago, IL	2010
A Manual of Style	29th	U.S. Government Printing Office, Washington, DC	2000
Modern Language Association Style Manual and Guide to Scholarly Publishing	3rd	Modern Language Association, New York, NY	2008
Publication Manual of the American Psychological Association	6th	American Psychological Association, Washington, DC	2009
Strunk W Jr. & White EB: The Elements of Style	4th	Allyn & Bacon, New York, NY	1999
Turabian KL: A Manual for Writers of Term Papers, Theses, and Dissertations	8th	University of Chicago Press, Chicago, IL	2013
International Committee of Medical Journal Editors: Recommendations for the Conduct, Reporting, Editing, and Publication of Scholarly Work in Medical Journals		Available at: http://www.icmje.org/icmje-recommendations.pdf	2013
National Library of Medicine Recommended Formats for Bibliographic Citation: Supplement: Internet Formats		U.S. Public Health Service, Department of Health and Human Services. Available at: http://www.nlm.nih.gov/pubs/formats/internet2001.pdf	2001

particularly in their respective written work. Although dissension and distance remain between these two broad fields, numerous examples of crossovers have shed light on scientific truths drawing from both domains. During the twentieth and twenty-first centuries, medical thinking and writing and the expression of medical knowledge have been reflected in the evolution of scientific writing.

Every healthcare professional and student should be able to communicate through writing. Effective writing in general and writing for publication are skills to be learned. Scientific writing has its styles and processes. Generally, short, effective sentences with a subject and predicate are better than long, multicomma sentences. Learn to write good declarative statements in an active voice.

STYLE MANUALS

Many resources are available that facilitate the process of preparing research for acceptance as an education capstone and for publication.

Table 16–1 represents a variety of resources that can enhance this process.

Before selecting a particular style manual as a guide, review the journals that offer publishing opportunities pertinent to the research field. The style requirements of the publishing resource (journals or books) must be followed stringently. For most peer-reviewed biomedical publications, two distinct resources contain the most frequently required formatting and guideline protocols. These are the *American Medical Association Manual of Style*[1] and the *Recommendations for the Conduct, Reporting, Editing, and Publication of Scholarly Work in Medical Journals* (formerly known as the *Uniform Requirements for Manuscripts Submitted to Biomedical Journals*), created by the International Committee of Medical Journal Editors.[2]

The *AMA Manual of Style* includes five sections of in-depth instruction on topics including preparing an article for publication, style, terminology, measurement and quantitation, and technical detail. The International Committee of Medical Journal Editors' online documents describe in depth a range of ethical considerations, publishing and editorial issues, manuscript preparation, and reference formatting and usage guidelines. Together, these two resources offer the most commonly used guidelines and requirements for publishing in the peer-reviewed biomedical literature. However, it is always important to consult the "Instructions to Authors" (sometimes referred to as "Information for Authors") section of any publisher to whom a manuscript is submitted because they may include other resources, and preferences vary from journal to journal. There is no substitute for consulting the "Instructions for Authors," which is published by all journals. It is the author's responsibility to submit manuscripts in the required style of target journals. Failure to follow the prescribed style is likely to result in rejection of the manuscript.

The gold standard of style guidelines in the biomedical field is put forth by the International Committee of Medical Journal Editors (ICMJE). The ICMJE has produced multiple editions of what was once known as the *Uniform Requirements for Manuscripts Submitted to Biomedical Journals* (URM), revised and renamed *Recommendations for the Conduct, Reporting, Editing, and Publication of Scholarly Work in Medical Journals* (ICMJE Recommendations) in 2013.[2] The URM was first published in 1978 as a way of standardizing manuscript format and preparation across journals. Over the years, issues in publishing that went well beyond manuscript preparation arose, resulting in the inclusion of sections on editorial policy.

WRITING

All students in healthcare professions should know how to structure a research paper and how to modify it into a publishable article. There are differences between a thesis or dissertation and a published paper. The skills needed to write for publication are also important to the seasoned clinician who has observed an interesting clinical case and seeks to make a contribution to the literature by "writing it up" for publication.

The proper culmination of any scientific research effort in a formal educational setting is the production of a written document reflecting the work that was completed. Recording one's work in a formal style has been and remains the hallmark of scholarly activities.

Scientific papers are the vital currency of academic endeavors and knowledge dissemination. The quality and timeliness of information and its presentation in scholarly papers are determinants of major decision points in central collegiate activities: assignment of student grades, student advancement and graduation, faculty appointment and advancement, tenure decisions, perceptions of professional leadership, national academic reputations, and more. Publishing in prestigious journals with regularity is the expected and rewarded activity in most academic healthcare centers. However, of all the faculty teaching in U.S. colleges and universities, only a small proportion publish regularly.

A healthcare profession's vitality, relevance, and intellectual pedigree are reflected in its literature.[3] When judged by that standard, some of the health professions may be viewed as underachieving. Many believe there is a critical and ongoing need for the healthcare professions to improve contributions to both the general biomedical literature and a specific healthcare profession's literature. One way to obtain this goal is to foster student research and writing with the hope (and aim) of those skills carrying forward into clinical practice.

For faculty members and students of healthcare professions, writing ability and familiarity with publishing in the realm of healthcare science are essential professional skills. These skills, which are critical for success, can be learned by students, perfected by faculty, and appreciated by readers, both professional and lay. Beyond the academic setting, this process can pose a challenge for health professionals. **Table 16–2** provides a list of facts and myths about medical writing that are helpful to the clinician interested

Table 16–2 Medical Writing Facts and Myths
Myth: "I'm a care provider, not a writer."
Fact: Writing is not a career but a necessary skill for medical professionals.
Myth: "I don't have any talent for writing. I've always been bad at it."
Fact: Writing is a skill, not a talent. Medical professionals should learn to write effectively.
Myth: "Writing has nothing to do with science."
Fact: Effective medical writing requires the same qualities found in scientific thought: logic, clarity, organization, and precision.
Myth: "If a piece of writing gets published, it's a good piece of writing."
Fact: Many published medical papers are badly written.
Myth: "Until I have my ideas clearly organized in my head, I shouldn't start writing."
Fact: The best way to clarify thinking is to start writing. Research shows that the act of writing helps clarify and organize thinking and generate ideas.
Myth: "I'll never be eligible for promotion or tenure unless I get a terminal degree. Why should I bother publishing if it won't help my career?"
Fact: Publishing papers in respected peer-reviewed journals has substantial academic value and generates far more career-enhancing opportunities than having a terminal degree and not publishing.

Adapted from St. James D. *Writing and Speaking for Excellence: A Brief Guide for the Medical Professional.* Boston, MA: Jones and Bartlett; 1997:13.

in research. Diana Hacker and Barbara Fister have composed a helpful website that includes examples of papers written in four commonly referenced style manual formats (http://www.dianahacker.com/resdoc/). Additionally, many style manuals now have quick reference links on the Internet; California State University of Los Angeles offers a useful site as a point of departure (http://calstatela.libguides.com/style).

RESEARCH PAPERS

In the healthcare field, as in most other fields, good scientific research papers are the most common form of expression of a scientific finding. Research papers have a clear, well-defined structure. The logical sequence of the research paper's sections (i.e., Introduction or Problem, Review of Literature, Methods, Results, and Discussion) is accepted as the gold standard of the classic research paper structure. This format requires the author(s) to address a given topic answering four basic questions:

1. What is the issue?
2. What methods have been used to investigate the issue?
3. What was found?
4. What are the implications of the findings?

Research papers take several forms, but generally the best form begins by posing a question or identifying a problem. The question may address the need for further research on an issue, propose a new hypothesis, or justify further analysis. The conventional format and approach used in research papers is derived from what Huth calls the concept of critical argument.[4] This idea holds that research papers must convey information in such a way that the reader is convinced the research paper's findings are well considered and ultimately valid.

Critical argument describes text that is coherent and consists of a series of reasons, statements, or facts intended to support or establish a point of view. This tone is "critical" in the sense that it carefully scrutinizes the source of the text's assertions. The "critical argument" is the heart of research writing.

Prose Revision

Research articles published in the biomedical literature typically present new and original information on topics relevant to the primary readership. The accepted scientific standard is that the investigators have applied reasonable standards of methodological rigor and have presented their findings in an accurate, concise, and clearly stated fashion. An extensive review and revision process is required to create an accurate, concise, and clearly stated manuscript. A reader must clearly understand the intent and purpose of a manuscript. Rarely is a first draft of a manuscript accepted for publication. After a paper has been written it must be reviewed, revised, and reread a number of times. A first step toward the revision of a manuscript is to revise for larger segments of content, such as missing or unnecessary information, or erroneous/misplaced content or sequence. The next step is to focus on prose, including sentence length, paragraph length, clauses, phrases, modifiers, and word choices. In revising prose, a seasoned writer seeks to develop fluency. Fluent prose runs along as the reader expects it to run. The reader is not jarred by defects that interrupt the line of thought. Short, simple sentences and a simple structure are best. Once the initial revisions have been made, two people should review the manuscript. One person should be knowledgeable about the subject and scientific writing. The other person should be a general reader. Suggestions gleaned from these reviewers can be used to revise the manuscript again.

Reference Lists

Proper citation of sources of information used in a paper as references is critical. Two reference citation styles are commonly used in academic and biomedical circles. The Vancouver style is a distinctive academic reference citation method where the author(s) and year of publication are cited in the text as they are used. At the end of the paper, these references are listed alphabetically by the first author's last name. This format is typical for graduate school research papers.

The reference citation style used in most medical and health professions journals is the style of the *Recommendations for the Conduct, Reporting, Editing, and Publication of Scholarly Work in Medical Journals* as developed by the International Committee of Medical Journal Editors,[3] and formerly the Council of Biology Editors.[2] This reference format for a journal article takes the following form:

Author(s). Title. Journal. Year; Volume: Pages.

Here is an example:

Hanson RL, Pettitt DJ, Bennett PH, et al. Familial relationships between obesity and NIDDM. Diabetes. 1995;44:418–422.

Consistency is one of the most important aspects of reference citation in an academic paper. Reference citation style and policies are typically included in the "Instructions for Authors" section published in journals. References cited should include only those documents that are readily available. You, as the author, should have access to every reference, either electronically or in hard copy. A good dictum to remember is "If you can't put your hands on it, don't cite it."

Special formats and/or requirements exist for monographs, government publications, informal documents, Internet sources, and personal communications. Here are some additional points about references:

- Recent literature sources are now available on the Internet on PubMed.
- Textbook citations should be rare.
- Garbled, incomplete, or nonfunctional references, particularly Internet citations, will disturb your readers (and editors).
- Citations from Internet sources such as Wikipedia, WebMD, Medscape, and the like are *not* acceptable.
- References from subscription services (e.g., MDConsult, UpToDate, etc.) are not acceptable.

Authors should refrain from citing a "personal communication" unless it provides essential information not available from a public source, in which case the name of the person and date of communication should be cited in parentheses in the text, not in the references section. It is always important for authors to obtain written permission and confirmation of accuracy from the source of a personal communication.

Some, but not all, journals check the accuracy of all reference citations; thus, citation errors are not uncommon in the published version of articles. To minimize such errors, references should be verified using either an electronic bibliographic source, such as PubMed, or print copies from original sources. Authors are responsible for checking the accuracy of all references including checking sources for information about retractions. References should be numbered or listed consecutively in the order in which they are first mentioned in the text. Identify references in text, tables, and legends by Arabic numerals in parentheses. References cited only in tables or figure legends should be numbered in accordance with the sequence established by the first identification in the text of the particular table or figure. The titles of journals should be noted according to the style used for MEDLINE (http://www.ncbi.nlm.nih.gov/nlmcatalog/journals).[2]

References drawn from Internet sources for use in academic papers have created an ongoing controversy on the frontier of scientific communication. Internet sources are becoming a leading category of reference information used by authors in presenting a paper or defending a thesis. Internet sources allow authors to obtain information that should be accurate and current. For example, in a paper on the topic of healthcare professionals in surgery, an essential "factoid" included in the first paragraph of this paper might be the current number of providers working in a particular field of surgery. In the past, published information would have been consulted to obtain that information, which would be, by its very nature, dated. Presently, consulting an Internet source is more likely to yield the most current data available.

The controversy for Internet resources is to be sure of the source of the information. Many Internet sites appear to be authoritarian, but they are not. Some might support products of questionable value, and some might convey individual opinions, which lack the science to support contentions. Investigators must be sure of the scientific value and trustworthiness of all sites.

Citation of Internet Sources

Many, but not all, online sources have value. Some Internet sources are unreliable and have questionable credibility. It is now common practice to include Internet references in peer-reviewed medical and healthcare literature. Internet reference sources can and should be permitted with the following ground rules:

- The Internet source is not a personal Internet site (e.g., an individual home page).
- Any person can readily access the Internet site and obtain the same information cited by the author.
- The citation contains as much specific information as possible.
- The date of access is always included.

The following examples of Internet citations are from the American Medical Association's *AMA Manual of Style: A Guide for Authors and Editors*, 10th ed.

1. Rosenthal S, Chen R, Hadler S. The safety of acellular pertussis vaccine [abstract]. *Arch Pediatr Adoles Med* [serial online]. 1996;150:457-460. Available at: http://www.ama-assn.org/sci-pubs/journals/archive/ajdc/vol_150/no_5/abstract/htm. Accessed November 10, 1996.
2. Gostin LO. Drug use and HIV/AIDS [*JAMA* HIV/AIDS Web site]. June 1, 1996. Available at: http://www.ama-assn.org/special/hiv/ethics. Accessed June 26, 1997.

Additional care must be taken to ensure that information or texts acquired from Internet sources are properly acknowledged. According to Glass and Flanagin, there are four types of plagiarism:

1. *Direct plagiarism:* Verbatim lifting of passages without enclosing the borrowed material in quotation marks and crediting the original author.
2. *Mosaic:* Borrowing the ideas and opinions from an original source and a few verbatim words or phrases without crediting the original author. In this case, the plagiarist intertwines his or her own ideas and opinions with those of the original author, creating a "confused, plagiarized mass."
3. *Paraphrase:* Restating a phrase or passage, providing the same meaning but in a different form without attribution to the original author.
4. *Insufficient acknowledgment:* Noting the original source of only part of what is borrowed or failing to cite the source material in such a way that a reader will know what is original and what is borrowed.[5]

A key rule is to provide any and all information needed to allow the reader to go to the same Internet site and review the same information cited by the author. This cardinal rule also applies to published reference sources. The second rule is completeness; follow a sequence of author(s) (individual[s] or an organization), work title, site, latest date, Web address, pages (if applicable), and any other specifics that allow the reader to access the site. If the reader is unable to verify citations in an article, doubts about the validity of your efforts may arise.

Electronic Journals

Most medical journals are now published in electronic as well as print versions, and some are published only in electronic form. A number of e-journals are listed among MEDLINE titles. The principles of print and electronic publishing are identical, and the recommendations of the ICMJE apply equally to both. Electronic publishing provides opportunities for versioning and raises issues about link stability and content preservation. There are three e-journal approaches:

- Journals that are completely electronic with no regular print version;
- Journals that are titled the same in both the print and electronic versions, but each publishes some unique content;
- Journals with both print and electronic versions that publish the same content.

APPROACHES TO PUBLICATION

A potential writer, such as a new graduate from a healthcare profession program, an experienced clinician, or a faculty member, may take a wide range of approaches toward entering the world of the published. For many clinicians, the first effort at publication may be somewhat easier and have a greater chance at success if a manuscript other than an original research article is submitted. As publication efforts progress, the alternative options may be considered. Beginning with something other than an original research manuscript offers a new author experience in dealing with journals, editors, and the review process. A good place to start is sending query letters to the publishing editors of journals you wish to consider as potential targets.

A query letter is an appropriate method for determining interest in a research paper, a commentary, or an opinion article among biomedical editors. Responses to a one-page query letter can be used to gauge the interest of a particular journal in publishing an article on a certain topic. Addressed to the editors of one or more potential target journals, a query letter should pique the editor's interest by asking, "Would you consider a submission on [your topic here]?" Avoid forcing the editor to make an immediate decision; recognize that no editor will commit to a publication decision before seeing the final manuscript and obtaining at least one other review. If they are not interested in your topic, you and the journal can save a lot of time and effort by establishing this up front. Query letters should be sent to a number of target journals. However, the manuscript should be submitted to only one journal at a time. If the manuscript is turned down for publication, it can be submitted to another journal.

BEST CHOICES FOR NEW WRITERS

To become familiar with the process of manuscript submission and peer review, it may help to start small and consider beginning with case reports, review articles, book reviews, or letters to the editor. They are listed in the descending order of their perceived value and importance in peer-reviewed publications, but all are good starting points for less-experienced writers. Each of the categories has different content and requirements, but the rigor of preparation is typically less than that required for an original research article. These options are described in more detail in the following sections. On the opposite end of the spectrum, editorials, book chapter authorship, and textbook editor roles are typically reserved for subject matter experts and invited senior academicians.

Original Articles

In terms of academic currency, original articles are typically valued more highly according to the importance of their content, their relevance for promotion and tenure of the author, and establishing the author's professional reputation. Original articles are not required to be data-driven clinical projects of "bench science" or laboratory origin. They may instead reflect policy analysis, utilization patterns, cost–benefit analyses, and a host of other relevant topics that contribute to advancing the knowledge base of the healthcare professions. The key is they are original pieces of work that represent an original investigation or approach.

Clinical Review Articles

The clinical review is one of the most common types of papers that appear in healthcare literature. This reflects, in large part, the need for practicing clinicians to obtain an easy-to-read, concise summary of a particular health condition or disease. Review articles cite current theory and clinical practice for specific diseases and conditions, but they do not consist of original research on the disease or condition conducted by the author(s). Typical section headings of a clinical review article include Introduction, Etiology, Pathophysiology, Clinical Manifestations, Diagnostic Imaging/Laboratory Findings, Diagnosis, Treatment, Prognosis, Health Promotion/Disease Prevention, and Recommendations.[6]

Systematic Reviews

A more sophisticated clinical review format is the systematic review, in which a far-reaching survey of the existing literature on a given topic is performed, analyzed, and presented. Systematic reviews essentially comprise a detailed literature review of all retrievable studies on a given topic; they attempt to identify, appraise, select, and synthesize all available high-quality research evidence relevant to that question. Systematic reviews often use statistical methods (meta-analyses) to combine results of the eligible studies, or they may score the levels of evidence depending on the methodology used when they pool similar data from a number of studies. Systematic reviews are more extensive and transparent than traditional literature reviews and depend heavily on current bibliographic retrieval services (e.g., PubMed) as critical sources.

Case Reports

Case reports, once a staple of clinical literature, and for that matter the format of many academic teaching exercises and presentations, remain an important type of paper appearing in biomedical journals.[2] Case reports are typically detailed, illustrated clinical descriptions of individual occurrences of disease. Over the past 20 years, however, case reports have become less frequent in biomedical literature and tend to convey little new information. Biomedical journals usually publish clinical research trials, but case reports may provide important information. Those that merit publication include case histories that are unique, or nearly unique, and cases of a new disease or an unexpected association (such as an outlier case or one with unexpected therapeutic events). They may represent notable early clinical observations that herald new diseases. Case studies still appear in the healthcare literature and offer practicing clinicians an opportunity to share interesting and informative cases.

Editorials

The editorial section of journals is often the most revealing and, occasionally, the most controversial section of the journal. At times, an editorial in a major biomedical journal is an invited comment on a paper appearing in the same issue. Editors may choose to invite subject experts to compare and contrast their opinions with the paper and other related studies. Articles that have the potential for substantial impact on a disease or society are often complemented with an invited editorial, as are articles that endorse a significant departure from the traditional method of treating a disease or condition. Editorials can be personal opinion pieces that address issues and controversy in society, medicine, and the profession. Editorials sometimes present minority opinions on professional trends and directions. Editorials can be submitted by anyone, but journals may have policies that govern what can be addressed in an editorial. Generally, the editor of the journal makes the decision on whether to publish an editorial.

Position Papers: A Variant of the Editorial

Many highly respected journals are owned by professional societies, and these often contain official statements and position papers produced by the organization. Some journals choose to publish occasional "point–counterpoint" position papers on controversial topics. Although such articles typically do not contribute new data to an issue, the questions they pose often result in the development of new studies or new ways to approach an ill-defined issue. Position papers may attempt to influence readers, members, or those outside of the profession or professional society.

Position papers sometimes deal with therapeutic or clinical issues. They are usually the result of reviews by experts who then recommend a course of action. It is common for standards of care to emerge from such positions or expert opinion.

Book Reviews

Book reviews are common departmental features of biomedical journals. In some journals, particularly those in the field of the history of medicine, book reviews comprise a large portion of the content. An effective and engaging book review begins when the reviewer, an individual well versed in the field, asks the following questions: Is this book needed? Does it add a new perspective to the topic? Is it a helpful addition to the clinician's library? Reviews of books are commissioned by the editor or the department editor and are thus usually invited publications. Book reviews may or may not count as "significant publications" by institutional promotion and tenure committees. However, doing a book review is a valid publishing opportunity and a good exercise for aspiring researchers and authors.

Letters to the Editor

For readers, the well-written, informed, pointed response to a previously appearing article can be among the most interesting sections of a journal. Letters to the editor often include frank challenges to published findings. The real and personal risk of publishing any work in a peer-reviewed journal is that writers open themselves to public and professional criticism and occasional humiliation when their work is challenged or refuted by experts on the topic. For other writers and aspiring authors, however, a letter to the editor may represent an entry channel to publication and further contributions. If they appear in a major medical journal, letters to the editor count as a "major publication" as indexed in Index Medicus. Letters to the editor should directly address a recently published paper and/or provide new information. Letters are usually limited to 500 words or fewer, and journals typically restrict the number of times letters to the editor by a given author can be published. Typically, if a published work is challenged or commented upon in some way, the original author is allowed a counter-response.

Abstracts and Posters

Abstracts and poster presentations are excellent opportunities to present research in a peer-reviewed forum. National meetings of healthcare professional organizations typically offer an excellent opportunity for poster and abstract presentations. The American Academy of Physician Assistants (AAPA) is a helpful resource, for example, and offers guidelines, which are included in the following section (used by permission).

Frequently Asked Questions

Q. What is a poster?

A. A poster is a method commonly used to present research in the biomedical sciences; it is actually a bulletin board that displays one or several large pieces of paper. A poster provides an opportunity to publish a very short article and discuss it with your peers at a conference. It is a static, visual medium used to communicate ideas and messages. When research is presented on a poster, the content of the poster should be focused on generating active discussion of the research. A great poster is readable, legible, well organized, and succinct. The Science and Engineering Library at University at Buffalo, The State University of New York has excellent web resources to help you create an effective poster (http://libweb.lib.buffalo.edu/guide/guide.asp?ID = 155).

Q. Does it have to be original research?

A. No, although original research is the sine qua non for poster presentations, other types of research or scholarly activity are welcome. Appropriate research results from a survey, an interventional study, a secondary data analysis, an epidemiologic study, a cost–benefit analysis, an evaluation of a diagnostic test, or something else. Interesting case studies, patient vignettes, and innovative practice techniques are also welcomed. Posters that have been presented at other professional meetings within the past 12 months are typically eligible for submission. Students are strongly encouraged to present research done in the program. Faculty are encouraged to present their educational research, innovative curricular designs, or case studies.

Q. Is the process competitive?

A. There is no competition to get your abstracts approved per se. In most cases, if the guidelines are followed and quality work is presented, the abstract is accepted. In general, originality of the work, adequacy of the data, and clarity of expression are the determining factors for selection. Specific selection criteria vary for each category as listed below.

- *Original research*
  - *Is the purpose or the objective clearly stated? Is the scope of the topic too broad or too narrow?*
  - *Is the description of the materials and methods understandable? Are the data collection and experimental techniques adequate for the study?*
  - *Are the analytical procedures used adequately described? Is the research design appropriate for the data collected and the subject of the study?*
  - *Are the results presented in sufficient detail to support the conclusions? Do they follow from the data and analysis?*
  - *Are the interpretations sound?*
  - *Is the conclusion clear?*
  - *Is the information presented important? Are there practical implications of the information? Is the information new? Is the research original?*
- *Clinical report or case study*
  - *Is the information presented clearly and understandably?*
  - *Is the information presented applicable?*
  - *Is the information clinically important, relevant, and significant?*
- *Previously presented poster*
  - *Is the information appropriate?*
  - *Does it satisfy the criteria previously given for original research?*
- *Educational research or interventions*
  - *Is the abstract thoughtful, organized, and clear?*
  - *Is an innovative method presented that is original and effective?*
  - *Are measurable outcomes presented?*
  - *Does the project impact special populations?*
  - *Does the project have value to other health professions' educators and their professions?*

Q. Do you have an example of what a poster looks like?

A. The University of North Carolina provides an example of the principles of poster design and summarizes the abstract review process at http://gradschool.unc.edu/student/poster-tips.html.

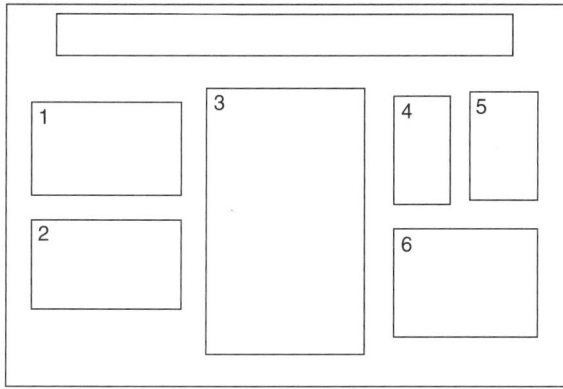 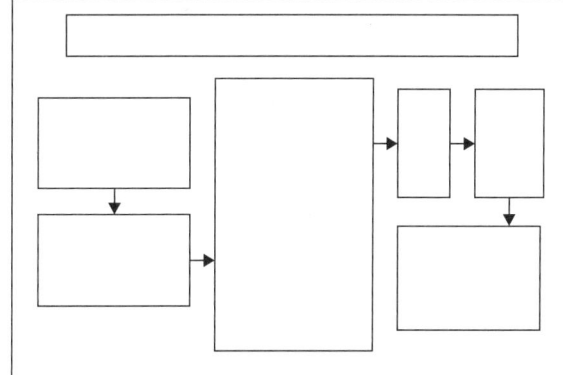

Figure 16–1 Example of poster formats.

Posters

The poster display board is 8 feet wide by 4 feet tall with a 1-inch metal border. The background material is a neutral-color cloth. **Figure 16–1** demonstrates the look of a classic original research poster. The top banner should include the title, author names, and their affiliations. The poster should read from top left to bottom right. The title should be legible from 8 feet away and the remaining words from 4 or 5 feet away.

Look at Figure 16–1 for examples. Keep in mind these important tips:

- Keep it simple.
  - Present only enough information to support your conclusions.
  - Eight poster panels are the maximum for effective presentation.
- Use graphs, charts, and figures to emphasize the key points; less text is better.
  - A good ratio is 20% text, 40% graphics, and 40% open space.
  - Don't use all capital letters; they are much harder to read.
- Above all, be clear, concise, and organized.

ELEMENTS OF THE RESEARCH PAPER

Tables

Tables are an essential component, the hallmark, of the Results section. As ideal vehicles for summaries of numerical and categorical data, tables are often far better than text for conveying this type of information. A table typically includes columns, rows, fields, titles, footnotes, and display trends. A table should stand alone and be readily understood without referring to the text, and each table should present at least one key result. Collectively, tables contain the vital findings of the investigation or study and represent the essence of an original research paper.

Effective tables should be constructed with a purpose in mind. Use of mutually exclusive categories is desirable, and the number of rows and columns should be kept to the minimum needed to convey the results. The use of several small tables is more effective than one large, complex table. Tables should be referred to in the text of your manuscript and placed within the text near that reference.

Illustrations and Figures

Illustrations and figures provide features central to the research paper: evidence, efficiency, and emphasis. The quality typically required for publication suggests that illustrations are best when prepared by professional graphic artists. As with tables, figures and illustrations should be referred to in the text at the appropriate point.

Titles

The title of a research study in any form is important, particularly when it is published. The title may be the reason people are attracted to your work and introduces to readers what has been published. There are two types of titles: indicative (what the paper addresses) or informative (describes briefly the paper's specific message). The title should be accurate, succinct, and effective. Clinicians must triage through a voluminous and growing number of biomedical journal articles to determine which ones should be read; the first (and usually only) part read by most readers is the title. Word selection for the title is, perhaps, one of the most critical parts of the paper because it is the principal determining factor in the reader's decision to read the paper. The title should arouse enough curiosity that the article is further examined. Creating a catchy title is an editorial art form.

In the review and/or editing process, authors should not be disappointed or defensive if the title submitted with the manuscript is changed (i.e., it is often changed substantially). Editors are experienced at determining what title best catches the readership's eye for their particular journal.

ORAL PRESENTATIONS

Many professional meetings provide opportunities for participants to orally present their research. A common method is a 10-minute presentation followed by a 5-minute question-and-answer session. This is an excellent opportunity to present work in progress or the results of a finished project or study. The most frequently used product for digital presentation of data is Microsoft PowerPoint. Numerous self-paced PowerPoint training courses are available from Microsoft online (http://office.microsoft.com). Additionally, entering "PowerPoint presentations" on Internet search engines results in more than a million hits on sites that offer additional instruction or assistance.

Becoming a good speaker and presenter requires experience, effort, and practice. A beginning speaker has only effort and practice at hand. The experience comes from making oral presentations. A first-time speaker or presenter can expect to be nervous. As audience size grows, so does the level of anxiety. These are normal responses and feelings; even veteran speakers get "butterflies" from time to time. Two key ways to overcome initial fears are (1) to know your material and (2) to practice, practice, and practice some more. Two common traps plague all presenters. The first is reading the visual presentation. This pitfall should be avoided carefully. If all a presenter does is read a visual presentation, there is no need for an oral presentation. There are very few audiences that cannot read. In general, use notes or key words to guide the delivery of material. The second common mistake many first-time speakers make is they have practiced to the point of reciting a memorized piece of work. Never recite. Good speakers retain some spontaneity and emotion in their voices, and they talk to the audience. Humor can add a lot to a presentation, but it must be appropriate for the audience, the material, and the speaker.

The last key aspect of being a good speaker and presenter is to respect the time frame allowed for your presentation. Practice helps frame a time period, but it is never the same as being in front of an audience. It is better to end a presentation a bit early than to run over the allotted time. One way to avoid running over is to allow some time for questions at the end of a presentation. In some venues, directions specify the allowance of a set time period for questions. Generally, 5 minutes is a reasonable time for questions. Much depends on the length and subject matter of your presentation. A plus point for always allowing time for questions is that if you run a few minutes long in presentation, the only thing lost is the question period. If you are short of your allowed time, it gives you a longer period to field questions.

Becoming a good presenter requires work. The more experience a presenter has, the less effort and practice necessary to do the presentation itself. Beginning presenters and speakers may benefit from participating in formats and venues that have short 10- to 15-minute periods or panels and co-presentations. Opportunities that involve small audiences are also conducive to gaining needed experience.

GRADUATE PROJECTS/PAPERS IN THE HEALTHCARE PROFESSIONS

During the 1990s, as more educational programs on healthcare professions either began by, or converted to, awarding master's degrees, and later clinical doctoral degrees, theses or dissertation requirements became more common. A final graduate paper typically requires extensive modification, usually a specifically tailored reduction in length, to be a suitable candidate for peer-reviewed publication. The academic format needs to be modified to fit the format required by a specific journal. Editors and editorial board members are expert at determining whether a master's thesis or doctoral dissertation has been reworked to fit the specifications of a journal. Adding early publications to one's resume is likely to enhance employment opportunities and professional advancement. Some healthcare professions' publications do not accept manuscripts from students as a matter of policy, due to the high overall rejection rate of unsolicited manuscripts. If a graduate project is worthy of consideration for publication, then a query letter should be sent to either a member of the editorial board or the editor of a target journal. Acquiring their guidance in advance can increase the chances for publication.

Writing the Paper

Huth proposed a writing system that utilizes a process in which one writes a first draft, places it aside for a couple of days, rereads it, and then begins the second draft (rewrite). This iterative–reiterative process is continued until the paper is finished.[6] Authors should consider sharing the paper with a friend who has critical writing and editing skills. Colleagues with content expertise should also be consulted. It may take as many as 20 or more drafts and rewrites until a final product is achieved. Quality is the aim, and a great deal of effort is needed.

Working with Editors

Writers and editors have historically shared an uneasy alliance. According to Arthur Plotnik in *The Elements of Editing*, editors are foot soldiers in the eternal war between raw talent and the people who process that talent.[7] As long as writers write primarily to advance themselves and editors edit to satisfy readers, there will never be a lasting peace. Writers know their particular subject; editors know their audience. A well-known truism is that knowledge of the subject does not necessarily translate into good writing, and good writing does not necessarily correlate with good editing. The editor may determine that a writer's style does not correlate with the journal's requirements or quality standards. Embrace the editorial review process. All writers need a good editor's touch.

When conflicts of interest arise in the editing process, the readership, not the writer, receives first consideration. This is where the writer must have thick skin. Some of the writing is always changed in the editorial process. Manuscript content is the writer's province, but the form is the editor's specialty. Many manuscripts must be revised a number of times. Each revision is reviewed, and the changes made to meet required or recommended improvements may need further work. Like other biomedical journals, journals in the health professions are typically expensive to operate, and editors are required to make the most efficient use of their printed pages. **Figure 16-2** shows the stages of publication.

BASIC STEPS IN PUBLICATION

How is the right journal chosen as a target for a manuscript's publication? Different journals feature different types of formats: original reports, special articles, short papers, editorials (usually invited), clinical notes, and letters to the editor. Initially, the format of the paper should consider the choice of venue and format. If this decision is difficult or problematic, one of the journal's editors or editorial board members may provide clarification. Is the topic of the proposed paper within the journal's scope? Is the topic represented frequently or only rarely? Does the target journal offer the best match of audience with your topic? What formats does the journal accept? Determine who cares

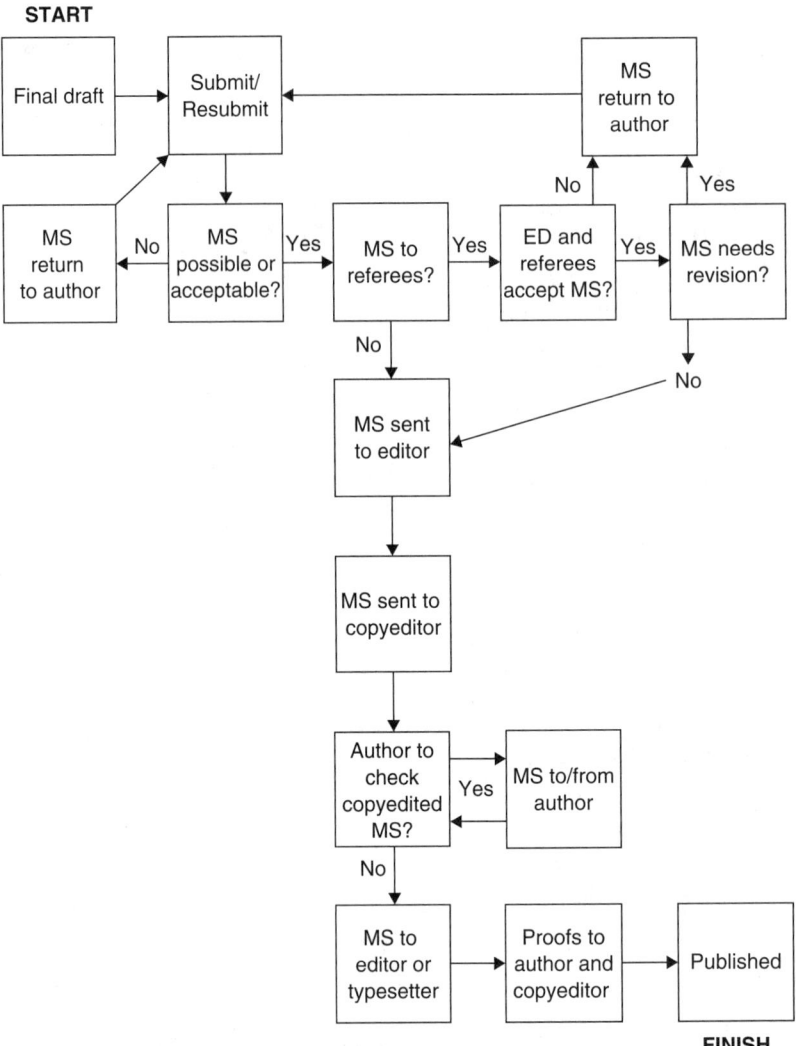

Figure 16–2 The manuscript process.

about the message of your paper. Is it best suited for a clinical specialty journal or a general medical journal? Is it best suited for clinicians, educators, researchers, or all of these groups?

Duties of a Potential Author

Based on the topic of the paper, several journals may be publishing candidates. Begin with the most recently published issue of a target journal and carefully read each back issue for at least the past year, then review the last few years' publications. Ensure that an article on the same topic has not been published recently. If it has, determine whether the paper merely rehashes existing information or adds new information. In assessing the suitability of a paper for a particular journal, these guidelines should be followed:

- Read the journal's "Statement of Editorial Purpose."
- Review the journal's editorial board membership.

- Consult the annually published list of peer reviewers.
- Read the journal's most recent "Information for Authors" statement.
- Evaluate the journal's publishing style regarding article format and requirements for tables, charts, abstracts, footnotes, citations, and references.

By performing these tasks, the author can determine in advance whether the project fits a specific journal or if it needs to be modified in certain ways. Has the relevant work of leaders, members of the journal's editorial board, and peer reviewers been reviewed and cited? This aspect of writing is often referred to as "chanting the names of the ancestors." At least one editorial board member and one or more peer reviewers review each provisionally accepted manuscript. If their relevant work is not cited, the paper may be deemed incomplete.

Communicate with the Connected

Dialogue with editors, editorial board members, peer reviewers, or subject matter experts on the research topic is extremely helpful in the publishing process. After a target journal has been chosen, send a proposed outline of the manuscript to determine preliminary interest. Getting from the "unsolicited" to the "solicited" side of the journal's editors is a challenging but worthwhile task to pursue. These are the "connected" people in the publishing realm.

Request Reprints of Previously Published Articles

Every peer-reviewed journal lists the contact person (usually the first author) for article reprints. One way to begin a relationship with professionals is to review their body of work and write a letter stating how much you enjoyed his or her work, combined with a few cogent observations. This individual may end up reviewing your manuscript, or may eventually become a collaborator.

Requirements and Resources for Writers

Writers must develop a thick skin to persevere through the paper's revision, possible or repeated rejection, and the eventual publishing process. Writers must be meticulous in their work.

Students in healthcare professions attempting to meet graduate-degree paper requirements must have access to biomedical literature databases. Basic requirements include access to medical literature databases, preferably accessible electronically via the Internet. Academic reference librarians can be wonderful friends; they can make the literature review and reference retrieval process much less intimidating. Writing also requires uninterrupted time, with ready access to reference and resource material, including reference documents, a personal computer, and other favorite writing aids. Time for writing must be scheduled on a regular and predictable basis. Close the door if necessary, or write from home if that option exists.

The Peer-Review Process

To evaluate the accuracy of submitted manuscripts, most reputable biomedical journals employ the peer-review process. This process typically involves sending the manuscripts to two or three individuals, selected by the editor, who are in a position to judge the value of the work. In more selective journals, only a few submissions ever make it to the peer-review process. These journals often have full-time editorial positions that are filled by healthcare professionals (e.g., physicians and other clinicians) who have developed skills in medical writing and editing. This is the case at journals such as the *New England Journal of Medicine*, *Journal of the American Medical Association*, *Annals of Surgery*, and *Annals of Internal Medicine*, among many others.

Manuscripts submitted to journals are privileged communications that are authors' private, confidential property, and authors may be harmed by premature disclosure of any or all of the manuscript's details. Reviewers, therefore, should keep manuscripts and the information they contain strictly confidential. Reviewers should not publicly discuss authors' work and must not appropriate authors' ideas before the manuscript is published. Reviewers are expected to respond promptly to requests to review and to submit reviews within the agreed-upon time. Reviewers' comments should be constructive, honest, and polite. Reviewers should declare their conflicts of interest and recuse themselves from the peer-review process if a conflict exists.[2]

On receipt, most reputable journals conduct an initial internal review of the manuscript. The editor or an associate editor reads the manuscript and determines its eligibility for peer review. If it is determined to be a candidate for publication, the manuscript is then sent to peer reviewers from various related fields. Often, peer reviewers are editorial board members and/or editorial consultants who perform these services for the journal on a regular basis.

The peer-review process is regarded as an extension of the basic principles of science and scholarship. Peer review has existed for more than 200 years and has achieved nearly universal application for assessing research reports before publication. Peer review is considered a critical quality control. Yet despite this widespread utilization, the process has been shown to have flaws, and relatively little is known with regard to the quality and utility of the information that is eventually published.[8,9]

Blinded Review

Journals vary in their policies about masking, or hiding, the names and affiliations of authors when the article is sent to reviewers. Most, but not all, biomedical journals mask the identities of authors. A question regarding the value of the peer-review process is the potential of a reviewer being familiar with the author's identity, which creates a bias. In several disciplines, only a few investigators are involved in a particular field of research, and the identities of authors may be easily recognized by peers. This is the Achilles' heel of the peer-review process that has led some journals to adopt the policy of unblinded review.

The Publishing Decision

Possible outcomes of the peer-review process include the following:

- Acceptance
- Minor revisions required
- Major revisions required
- Outright rejection

The response from the editor typically consists of a cover letter summarizing the reviewers' comments, recommendations, and the blinded reviewers' evaluation sheets. Always pay close attention to recommended suggestions, changes, or critiques. Address all concerns expressed by the reviewers, including data inconsistencies and errors, even if you disagree with them. It is not unusual for authors to disagree with peer reviewers. When the case is well made by the author to retain the original version, the section of the manuscript in question may remain unchanged. Rejection letters with a copy of the submitted manuscript should be reviewed and saved. Some rejection letters are carefully worded invitations to resubmit. Rejection is part of the process. All successful authors have a history of rejection, and none should take it personally. The manuscript may be resubmitted after completing all of the required revisions and addressing all of the concerns of the editor and reviewers.

Submitting the Final Manuscript

Assuming the final version of the manuscript meets all publishing requirements, the packet is then sent to the journal, including the requisite number of manuscript copies. Be aware that the specific format of the title page may vary by journal (e.g., whether or not an abstract is required as part of the manuscript). The final packet should also be accompanied by a cover letter that summarizes the basic rationale for the paper. The cover letter must also include an author attestation statement that neither the paper, nor its essential substance, is presently under consideration by another journal and has not appeared elsewhere (e.g., in another journal). This statement must be fully acknowledged and signed by all authors indicating that the work is their own and has not been published or submitted elsewhere.

Authors must follow precisely the "Instructions to Authors" of the particular journal to which they are submitting. The final draft submission should be flawless. This becomes very important when work is submitted to a journal in which there is significant competition for space. If an editor must choose between two manuscripts of relatively equal importance, then the one that requires the least amount of corrective action from the editorial staff is more likely to be accepted.

The next step is the receipt of the page proofs. Be prepared for a rapid turnaround requirement; as few as 24 hours is not unusual. This requires an author to drop everything to address the proofs and return them for final typesetting.

Realize that the copyright protection is assigned to the journal that accepts the work; in reality, it is no longer the author's paper. If some of the data must eventually be included in another manuscript (e.g., a published table), permission must be secured from the publisher, regardless of authorship.

Conflicts of Interest, Disclosures, and Institutional Review Board (IRB) Approval

It is standard operating procedure for peer-reviewed healthcare professions journals to include requirements for full disclosure on any real or perceived conflict of interest with the manuscript content, affiliated sponsors and organizations, or coauthors. This also includes disclosure of any investment or financial interest or funding associated with any product or organization referred to in the manuscript. Additionally, federal law requires any research involving human subjects be reviewed and approved by a designated and approved institutional or regional institutional review board (IRB) prior to commencing any research. It is not fully appreciated within the health professions communities that this includes *all* human subject research, regardless of whether the project includes federal funding. Any research including medical and administrative record data, leftover tissues, health services research, survey, behavioral, biomedical, or any other healthcare research is included in this requirement. Even if the research seems likely to be exempt from IRB approval (e.g., an anonymous survey that is optional to complete), evidence of an IRB-approved exemption must be acquired for biomedical journals to consider the work for publication. Many uninformed researchers have been frustrated when they completed a project and discovered after the fact that IRB approval was necessary, rendering their research unacceptable for publication. This standard applies to research in all healthcare professions.

Authorship

The corresponding and/or first author must carefully select coauthors as the research or project ideas are developed. Adding colleagues or friends who contribute little to the work is inappropriate and serves to alienate the coauthors who perform the work. A coauthor should have generated at least part of the intellectual content of the paper as well as had a part in writing the paper, including reviewing it for possible revision or revising its intellectual content. A coauthor should be able to publicly defend all of the content of the paper in the scientific community.

Criteria for Authorship

In the development of a manuscript, it is important to apply criteria to determine who should qualify as an author. The ICMJE recommends authorship be based on the following four criteria:

1. Substantial contributions to the conception or design of the work; or the acquisition, analysis, or interpretation of data for the work, *and*
2. Drafting the work or revising it critically for important intellectual content, *and*
3. Final approval of the version to be published, *and*

4. Agreement to be accountable for all aspects of the work in ensuring that questions related to the accuracy or integrity of any part of the work are appropriately investigated and resolved.

The ICMJE further indicates that "in addition to being accountable for the parts of the work he or she has done, an author should be able to identify which coauthors are responsible for specific other parts of the work."[2]

Before a researcher agrees to collaborate, it is wise to know the work habits, reliability, and temperaments of potential coauthors. Are they committed to deadlines? Do they return calls and provide information in a timely manner? Do they do what they say they will do? All of these issues matter when it comes to coauthoring manuscripts. The more coauthors included, the more difficult it becomes to reach consensus about and satisfaction with the paper. It is important to agree up front about work responsibilities and authorship order. The overall responsibility of the manuscript always rests with the first author.

Assignment and determination of authorship on papers submitted to biomedical journals has undergone significant evolution in recent years. Now a greater sense of accountability for the intellectual contributions of authors is the norm. Authorship of a paper submitted to a biomedical journal indicates that the individual has invested substantial intellectual effort in the conceptualization and writing of the manuscript. To qualify as a coauthor, an individual should fulfill the following criteria[10]:

- Participated in the work sufficiently to take public responsibility for all or part of the content
- Made substantial contributions to the intellectual content of the paper in one or more of the following categories:
  - Conception and design
  - Acquisition of data
  - Analysis and interpretation of data
  - Drafting of the manuscript
  - Critical revision of the manuscript for substantive intellectual content
- Statistical analysis
- Obtaining funding
- Administrative, technical, or material support

Today, the most reputable medical journals require authors to sign a form attesting to their input into the paper and verifying their qualification for authorship designation.

Group authorship sometimes presents problems, particularly with citations. Group authorship is the listing of the name of a group in place of the names of individual authors. Modified group authorship, in which individual names are listed followed by the name of the group, is also used. Group authorship is most often associated with studies involving many investigators (e.g., multicenter clinical trials or genomics) because it allows investigators to share credit equally.

PubMed is the National Library of Medicine's (NLM's) bibliographic database, with citations dating back to 1966. In the past, the NLM did not include group authors in the MEDLINE author field; rather, the group name was included as an add-on to the title. The NLM now lists group authors under a separate "collective name" field. The Science Citation Index (SCI) is a scientific and biomedical bibliographic database used to track citations to individual articles. Instead of listing the research group in the author field in its source listing, SCI lists either all individual names in the group or the writing committee members' names in the order they are listed in the article.

SOME CHALLENGES FOR HEALTH PROFESSIONS PUBLICATIONS

Over the past 40 years, the healthcare professions have seen journals come and go and, in the main, have had difficulty in gaining recognition beyond their professional readership. Part of the problem is the very specialized interest of clinicians for, primarily, clinical review–type articles. Most clinicians are employed full-time and, therefore, do not have the time nor direct incentive to write and publish medical articles. Those that do, primarily educators, are relatively small in number and tend to write on educational and curricular topics and not on clinical matters. Clinicians in the health professions seek material of a clinical nature that will help them to remain current on advancements in medical care and make them more effective in serving their patients.

Thus, many healthcare professionals who might otherwise seek to write and publish are forced to compete with physicians and other biomedical scientists in the biomedical world who are academics, clinical researchers, or basic science researchers, and have the resources and incentives to write and publish. Healthcare professionals usually are not trained to be writers and/or scholars but instead are prepared to be clinicians. Most are in no position to produce original biomedical studies and research products sought by journals. As a result, the healthcare professions literature has tended to focus primarily on concise and current clinical review articles, that is, papers that summarize a specific clinical problem and outline recommended management. Although this focus tends to serve the needs of the primary audience, it does not contain original research material. As a consequence, journals specific to the healthcare professions fail to have a readership beyond their own profession. This may change as more students gain research experience as a component of their education, as more health professions educators become involved with research, and as more and more clinicians participate in research as part of their practice.

Medical Journals

Many healthcare professionals, both clinicians and academics, commonly publish papers in biomedical journals. Those in the nonphysician healthcare professions (PAs, NPs, CNMs, PTs, etc.) at times publish in journals that are aimed primarily toward physician audiences, such as the *New England Journal of Medicine*, *Journal of the American Medical Association*, *The Lancet*, and *British Medical Journal*, as well as leading specialty journals such as the *Annals of Internal Medicine*, *Annals of Family Medicine*, *Health Affairs*, and *Annals of Surgery*.

The modern medical publishing business is an intensely competitive enterprise. Virtually all biomedical journals are dependent on their sponsors (professional societies and commercial publishers) for their viability. The business operations of these ventures in turn depend, most of the time, exclusively on advertising revenue. This fact of life (that biomedical publications depend on revenues from advertisers) requires editors and editorial boards to balance scientific direction and standards and journal content with the requirements of those who are "paying the freight" in the operation of the publication.

The vast number of publications in biomedicine are essentially businesses. Publishing medical journals is an expensive venture. Publishers of various biomedical journals comprise the following:

- Professional organizations that sponsor and produce a journal identified as their official journal
- Proprietary publishing firms
- Philanthropic organizations, including journals such as *Health Affairs*, a health policy resource subsidized by Project Hope, or the *Milbank Memorial Fund Quarterly*

MANUSCRIPT FLAWS THAT PREVENT PUBLICATION

Authors fall prey to several pitfalls in the preparation and submission of manuscripts to biomedical journals (**Table 16-3**). Editors and reviewers are always looking for reasons to be skeptical regarding the worthiness of a manuscript for publication. Although the reasons for rejections are extensive, the author should bear in mind the following common scenarios:

- The topic is inappropriate for a specific journal. The manuscript is a sound piece of investigation, description, or opinion and is presented in a suitable format, but the topic is not appropriate for a particular journal.

Table 16-3 Reasons for Manuscript Rejection

Excessive use of philosophy
Loose organizational style
Material not sufficiently important
Information not easily generalized
Unclear what methods were used
Results described in an unclear way
Statistics used incorrectly
Sample size inadequate
Conclusions unwarranted
Results not compared with similar studies
Inadequate period of observation, use, or evaluation of method
Inadequate review of the literature

Adapted from Geyman JP, Bass MJ. Communication of results of research. *J Fam Prac.* 1978; 7(1):120.

In some cases, these papers may represent previously rejected or recycled manuscripts that the author(s) did not bother to reconfigure in the required format for that journal.

- The use of imperfect style and "crazy-quilt" fonts. A manuscript containing imperfect style that has differing sections with differing fonts and font sizes indicates that it may be a "cut-and-paste" effort, one that is recycling the work of others or an uncoordinated collaboration among authors that has not been properly edited. Manuscripts with these types of sloppy narrative reveal inattention to detail and a nonsystematic structure. Editors regard such papers as a waste of time because it appears the authors have not put forth the proper effort to prepare the manuscript to specifications.
- "Cut-and-paste" citations were used. Cut-and-paste citations lifted verbatim from reference sources are ill advised. If a citation is not physically available, then do not quote it. Do not be surprised if editors or reviewers ask for verification, particularly if the citation looks suspicious. If this verification falls short, it raises questions of plagiarism, and the paper will be summarily rejected.
- Tables and/or text were used without permission. Give credit where credit is due. If a table from someone else's work is copied or modified for use, acknowledge the source. The required permission may need to be presented to the publisher.
- Errors in mathematical calculations occurred (bad math). Be aware that the journal will calculate any math included in the manuscript, such as percentages in a table. It is always recommended authors double-check their data, including the math in tables.
- The same material was used to publish several articles. Editors are well acquainted with the tendency of authors to partition their work into "least publishable units," a phenomenon also known as "salami science." In this case, a data set is split into smaller subsets, each with a narrow focus, in an effort to publish as many papers as possible from one core data set. Examples include submitting single-center reports from multicenter studies and short-duration reports from long-duration studies. The dangers of repetitive publication of the same material are many. An old or recycled paper must be sufficiently updated or have new data added to justify publication.
- Citation or reference inaccuracies were found. Authors are obligated to double-check the accuracy of all citations within their work. Citation error is a serious problem in biomedical publications. One study of peer-reviewed surgical journals found a 48 percent citation error rate, casting doubt in many cases that original reference sources were reviewed by the authors.[9]

ON WRITING AND PUBLISHING

Writing is difficult and time-consuming work. Authors must fundamentally calculate the questions of "Why write a paper if it does not stand a reasonable chance of being published?" and

"What do I have to say?" Dr. John Billings, founder of the National Library of Medicine, espoused four primary rules for the aspiring author:

1. Have something to say.
2. Say it.
3. Stop as soon as you have said it.
4. Give the paper a proper title.

Strive to Write Clearly

Clear thinking leads to clear writing. George Orwell said, "Good prose is like a windowpane; that is, what you have to say should not be obscured by how you say it."[11] Prose is bad when readers need to stop and look at it again to understand its message. The central message of a book written by a long-time editor of *JAMA* was embodied in its title, *Why Not Say It Clearly?*.[12] Interestingly, this book appeared during a time when biomedical writing was criticized by, among others, the late Michael Crichton (a well-known author and film and television producer), who was then a recent medical school graduate, as being deliberately "obfuscatory." Writing clearly means using words with the greatest degree of accuracy in transmitting what you wish to communicate to others.

A STEP-BY-STEP APPROACH TO PUBLISHING A MANUSCRIPT

The essential steps in the process of publishing a paper in the biomedical literature are as follows:

1. Determine the central message of the paper.
2. Decide whether the paper is worth writing.
3. Identify the appropriate audience for the paper.
4. Select the target journal.
5. Search the literature.
6. Determine authorship and an expected timetable.
7. Assemble the sources and materials needed to write the paper.
8. Develop a structure for the paper; make a detailed outline.
9. Write the first draft, conforming it to the journal's requirements for manuscripts.
10. Revise the first draft and cycle through several more drafts; add appropriate tables, graphs, and illustrations.
11. Finalize the manuscript; complete all sections.
12. Obtain comments and critiques from selected "personal consultants."
13. Submit the article to the selected journal in the required format; include a formal cover letter with the appropriate disclaimer.
14. Promptly respond and revise the manuscript as indicated in the editor's communication; respond to all author queries.
15. Resubmit the corrected manuscript; proof the final typescript; assign copyright.

SUMMARY

After deciding to attempt to publish a paper that results from a research study, several key steps should be considered. These include making sure the paper is a quality effort and the writing is clear and concise. Authors must carefully select the journal or journals that may be interested in the type of work that has been produced. The editor may be contacted about his or her interests. The "Instructions to the Author" should be followed explicitly. If the journal is interested, cooperate on revisions and suggestions for the paper. This process takes time and patience, sometimes up to 1 year. There may be many reasons for the rejection of a submission; rejection is not personal. In fact, for those who seek to publish often, rejection is part of life. Remember that the work has value in the experience gained in the process of scientific inquiry. If research is an ongoing part of a healthcare professional's life, publication success will eventually occur with perseverance.

REFERENCES

1. American Medical Association. *AMA Manual of Style: A Guide for Authors and Editors.* 10th ed. Chicago, IL: Oxford University Press; 2007. Available at:

http://www.amamanualofstyle.com/oso/public/index.html. Accessed October 13, 2014.
2. International Committee of Medical Journal Editors. Recommendations for the conduct, reporting, editing, and publication of scholarly work in medical journals. December 2013. Available at: http://www.icmje.org/icmje-recommendations.pdf. Accessed October 13, 2014.
3. Kole, LA, Currey R. Writing to be published—Why and how (and when). *J Am Acad Phys Assist.* 1999;12(3):92, 93, 96.
4. Huth EJ. *Writing and Publishing in Medicine.* 3rd ed. Baltimore, MD: Williams and Wilkins; 1998.
5. Glass RM, Flanigan A. Communication, biomedical II. Scientific publication. In: Reich WT, ed. *Encyclopedia of Bioethics.* 2nd ed. New York: Macmillan; 1995.
6. Huth EJ. *Scientific Style and Format: The Council of Biology Editors Manual for Authors, Editors, and Publishers.* 6th ed. Cambridge, England: Council of Biology Editors; 1994.
7. Plotnick, A. *The Elements of Editing: A Modern Guide for Editors and Journalists.* New York: MacMillan; 1982.
8. Wagner E, Jefferson T. *The Shortcomings of Peer Review.* West Sussex, UK: Lear; 2001;14:257–263.
9. Lock S. *A Difficult Balance: Editorial Peer Review in Medicine.* London, England: Nuffield Provincial Hospitals Trust; 1985.
10. *Journal of the American Medical Association.* Authorship responsibility, conflicts of interest and funding, and copyright transfer/publishing agreement. Available at http://www.ala.org/acrl/sites/ala.org.acrl/files/content/issues/scholcomm/docs/copyright_exercise_jama_agreement.pdf. Accessed October 13, 2014.
11. Orwell G. Why I Write. In *A Collection of Essays.* New York: 1954, p 320.
12. King L. *Why Not Say It Clearly?* Boston, MA: Little, Brown; 1978.

ADDITIONAL RESOURCES ON MEDICAL/ACADEMIC WRITING

Day RA, Gastel B. *How to Write and Publish A Scientific Paper.* 6th ed. Westport, CT: Greenwood Press; 2006.
Henson KT. *Writing for Publication—Road to Academic Advancement.* Boston: Allyn & Bacon; 2005.
Katz MJ. *From Research to Manuscript: A Guide to Scientific Writing.* New York: Springer; 2005.
Strunk W Jr., White EB. *Elements of Style.* 4th ed. Boston: Allyn & Bacon; 1999. Also online at http://www.bartleby.com/141.

ACKNOWLEDGEMENTS

The author extends appreciation to P. Eugene Jones, PhD, PA-C; Roderick S. Hooker, PhD, MBA, PA; Leslie Kole, PA-C; J. Dennis Blessing, PhD, PA-C; and Arnold "Bud" Relman, MD for inspiration, encouragement, and collaboration over many years.

CHAPTER 17

Interpreting the Literature

J. Glenn Forister, MS, PA-C
J. Dennis Blessing, PhD, PA

CHAPTER OVERVIEW

More than 2 million biomedical articles are published in medical, health, and professional journals each year.[1] For most clinicians, wading through even a small number of journals or articles can be daunting. Medline indexed 1,116,710 articles in 2013.[2] The challenge is to not only stay abreast of current changes in practice, but also to be able to meet the expectations of the informed healthcare consumer.

Healthcare professionals must be able to interpret the scientific and medical literature quickly and completely to meet the challenges of applying new information and meeting the needs of patients. The role of textbooks is to provide a good foundation, but current literature is the key to modern practice. Reading journals remains a source of current information for many clinicians.

Ultimately, an important question for every clinician is: What is important to my patients and my practice? Answering that question is the key to providing contemporary and effective care. Part of the answer lies in developing skills that critically examine the literature to answer those questions. This chapter provides guidance to clinicians who are interested in a systematic approach when interpreting the literature.

Learning Objectives

- Identify professional journals for a healthcare profession.
- Define the key elements in the interpretation of the literature.
- Identify, list, and discuss the steps in evaluating the medical literature.
  - What questions should be explored in the interpretation?
    - Is the problem identified and defined?
    - Is the design appropriate?
    - Are the analyses appropriate for the design and data?
    - Is the conclusion based on the results?
- Develop an understanding of the general approach to reading and interpreting the healthcare literature.

INTRODUCTION

Interpreting the medical literature is a process of integrating, synthesizing, and summarizing information obtained from different sources into a recommendation for application in practice. The intent is to apply the best knowledge available to make the best choice for the circumstances encountered in clinical practice. Summaries of this information, known as integrative literature, come in many forms: systematic reviews, overviews, meta-analyses, practice guidelines, decision analyses, and cost-effectiveness analyses.

The concept of evidence-based medicine is expanding, and the extraction of evidence from the literature into practice, although logical, presents some challenges. Busy clinicians must develop skills that allow them to become critical consumers of select literature and decide what applies to their patients. This process comprises "the application of the best available evidence to patient care."[2] As skills in interpreting the literature are developed, it is important to remember patient care is at the heart of the procedure. Being patient-centered enhances the implementation of correct patient care decisions.

Literature interpretation is a skill that must be learned, practiced, and applied. As more healthcare research articles are reviewed, the results can sometimes be confusing, conflicting, and confounding. Given the advent of evidence-based medicine, systematic reviews, and meta-analyses, it is no wonder clinicians often become more confused by the literature rather than enlightened. Clinicians must develop interpretation skills over time. If the literature is not continually read and effectively analyzed, clinical practices will become stale and even possibly incorrect.

The more immersed in research healthcare practitioners are, the greater their ability to synthesize and utilize the literature. However, becoming an expert in interpreting the medical literature takes years of experience, as well as a broad understanding of processes, statistical designs, and analyses. This chapter helps begin a solid foundation and reference point from which an understanding of medical literature can be built.

To conduct a research project, the researcher must have some understanding of what the research problem is and what has occurred in the area of interest. This particularly pertains to obtaining the maximum benefit from the literature search. For example, healthcare students may wonder if they are entering a profession that will be the right career for them in the long run. The problem is they do not know much about this subject and may not be sure where to go for the answers. The answer to this question can be researched as the degree of "satisfaction"; that is, is the chosen profession a satisfying one? If someone is entering a profession where job satisfaction is low and attrition is high, then the profession's practitioners are not well served. Reviewing the literature on job satisfaction can help a student determine whether a chosen profession is satisfying to others who are on the same path.

The literature search is often a quest for theory building. It also helps the researcher discover what research has been done and how it could be done better or differently. The scholar's research should say something new or validate existing work, while it connects with research that already has been reported. Literature provides a basis for a foundation in theory and topics of concern. How the literature is interpreted influences the overall research process. Understanding how to interpret the literature helps the practitioner develop a knowledge base as well as the ability to make the case for a new investigation.

Interpretation of the literature takes on greater importance when it involves the care of others. Misinterpretations can lead to significant errors in healthcare practice. This chapter is based on several resources[3,4] and the authors' experience to provide a general guide for how to interpret the medical literature.

INTERPRETING THE LITERATURE

First Things First

The first step to literature interpretation is to read enough background information on the subject in order to understand as many aspects as possible of the issue being studied. Most healthcare professionals and students have developed some literature interpretation skills by reading or studying various resources in their fields. A rudimentary step in literature interpretation is to understand certain terms used in research (e.g., percentages, means, validity, limitations, probability, subjects, and population). Recognizing the meaning and significance of research terms becomes easier as the ability to interpret the literature progresses. Furthermore, incorporating such terms in the context of research also becomes easier as experience is gained from understanding the literature. One useful suggestion is to *never* let a term go undefined while reviewing the literature, especially if the material is important to the clinician's own research projects, clinical practice, or patient care. Another suggestion is to develop a bibliography of useful references. Historically, many researchers have simply made copies of important articles and kept them in their file cabinets. Because so many articles are retrievable, storing electronic documents on a computer hard drive may be all that is needed. Many journal articles are now available online and can be quickly accessed.

The Scientific Method

Understanding the literature can be a challenge because the research is dynamic and fueled by new technology. The principles of the scientific method are integral to the literature process (searching and interpreting) because an emphasis is placed on gaining knowledge from the rigorous process of systematic observation, analysis, and reasoning.

Schematically, all concepts must pass through the scientific method corridor. This process adds value and becomes part of one's fundamental knowledge. Therefore, the literature search must include and incorporate scientific observation and data collection. The formal process of acquiring scientific knowledge, whether through reviewing the literature or recording observations, must be conducted in a logical and reproducible manner. In essence, this means any competent clinician could replicate the literature search and reach the same conclusions. A researcher incorporates the scientific method into his or her project by defining each step as follows:

1. *Problem:* A precise statement of what knowledge was sought and why it was sought
2. *Question:* A single sentence that asks a question related to the problem
3. *Method:* The plan of how the research was done and how the knowledge was gained
4. *Results:* Unequivocal statements of the knowledge that was gained
5. *Interpretation:* Application of the knowledge gained

How the results of this process are interpreted is key to understanding how the results will be utilized to provide better care for patients. Recognizing the steps of sound scientific investigation, as well as applying scientific concepts, will help the clinician interpret the results in a meaningful manner.

Questions to Ask (and Answer)

Whether interpreting the literature for application in practice or gathering data for a research project, part of the task and challenge of reviewing literature is to assess what has been published on the topic of interest. **Table 17-1** outlines a set of questions to be asked and answered before making any assumption about the literature.

Ultimately, this method of literature inquiry or evaluation eventually becomes second nature as it is practiced. Writing down answers to these questions while evaluating an article reinforces the steps toward becoming a critical evaluator of literature. New questions may emerge as well during this process.

Although many of these questions are self-explanatory, additional clarification may be needed to ensure thought processes are consistent and clear. While reviewing various information sources, new thoughts on evaluating the literature tend to emerge. Such thoughts and concepts precipitate the development of an individual research style and process. Only through scrutiny, analysis, and replication can consumers of the literature ask the right questions, challenge the answers, and find answers to more questions. The scientific process and the information that results from that process are then validated. This process defines the cumulative development of scientific knowledge.

SIGNIFICANT QUESTIONS TO ASK WHEN EVALUATING THE LITERATURE

1. *What is the source (journal) of the article?*
   The reputation of a source can be as important as a citation. Journals that tend

Table 17–1 Questions to Ask and Answer

1. What is the source (journal) of the article?
2. Was the publication peer reviewed?
3. Who are the authors and what are their affiliations?
4. What (or who) is the main subject of the study?
5. What problem(s) were investigated?
6. What is the purpose or rationale for the study?
7. Who or what constituted the sample or population?
8. What was the design of the study?
9. What statistical analyses were used?
10. What are the results?
11. Are the results clear?
12. Did the results answer the identified questions?
13. Do the results seem valid?
14. Are the interpretations (conclusions) of the results consistent with the study design and analysis?
15. Are the results consistent with findings from similar studies?
16. What do the results mean to medicine and health care, and you and your patients?
17. Can the results be applied to your research or clinical practice?

to have the highest subscription rate typically have a higher degree of prestige. The top journals in a specific discipline are most often cited due to their solid reputation in the medical community. For clinical articles, these include the *Journal of the American Medical Association* (*JAMA*), *New England Journal of Medicine*, and *Lancet*. However, other lesser-known journals also publish high-quality work. Each journal is ranked according to citation rates. Although lower-ranked journals can publish sound scientific articles and higher ranked journals can publish articles of poor quality, the ranking system is a helpful measure of quality.[3] Each publisher has a set of standards related to manuscript acceptance. Journals with high submission rates and low acceptance rates are often considered stronger sources than those with low submission rates and high acceptance rates. In addition, the journal's impact factor can be an important metric when comparing the relative value of a journal title within its field. The Journal Citation Reports at ISI Web of Knowledge is a database that can be utilized to research this information.

2. *Was the publication peer reviewed?*
Peer review is a process of manuscript critique by someone familiar with the same body of literature that the author is submitting. Since the 1950s, the majority of scientific manuscripts submitted for publication undergo a peer-review process. This review is intended to critically evaluate a manuscript, so the reader is offered some confidence that the resulting publication has been scrutinized for soundness, valid results, and conclusions that fit the findings. Journals are ranked by their scientific merit and readership. Readership often rests on the journal's ability to provide new and important information that can be confidently accepted. However, not every article in a peer-reviewed journal is necessarily subjected to the peer review process. Many journals have special sections or features that have a different manner of review or oversight. An article

can be in a peer-reviewed journal, but undergo a different process than peer review.

3. *Who are the authors and what are their affiliations?*
   The reputation of the author(s) can be important, particularly for controversial findings. Experts in a particular field may know many of the contributors to their body of literature. For the person just entering the field, time is needed to familiarize him- or herself with subjects and the important names. To help feel confident about the literature you are reviewing, you may have to do some homework on the reporting media and the authors, particularly if the literature concerns important discoveries or contributions. You may recognize the work of some authors and the reputation they bring to the literature. On the other hand, a note of caution is needed before accepting every finding regardless of the source or author.

   The author's affiliation can have some influence in the consideration of a reported study. Certain institutions and universities tend to be centers of excellence in particular areas of science and learning. These institutions tend to attract a body of scientists and writers expanding work in a specific area. Being aware of this aspect of the research helps the reader understand the authors' perspective and what may have influenced their work environment. It also helps the reader to understand why the investigators are studying these particular problems in the first place.

4. *What (or who) is the main subject of the study?*
   The answer to this question may be the same, or similar to, the problem investigated. Depending on the type of investigation, the main subject could be different from the problem. For example, in a study of student test-taking performance, the subjects of the study are the students; however, the problem investigated could be how the students study for tests, how they act during tests, and/or what they remember after the test. In health care, the subject of a research study could be cholesterol, but the problem investigated could be cholesterol's response to some intervention.

5. *What problem(s) were investigated?*
   The answer to this question should be self-evident from the text. The research problem is the issue or topic of focus. For example, perhaps a healthcare professional knows little about the career patterns of female EMT-Paramedics. The problem presented is the difficulty in predicting how long various types of EMT-Ps will remain in the workforce. Healthcare economists and labor experts need to address these questions for the purpose of education or implementation of health policies. The research question is always a narrower aspect of the research problem. The hypothesis is a method of addressing a research question. Research questions and hypotheses should be clearly stated and linked to the problems being investigated. Also, any assumptions made by the investigators should be assessed. Assumptions can confound and influence the study and report.

6. *What is the purpose or rationale for the study?*
   This question is the "why" of the study. Why was it done? What purpose did it serve? Was it an important problem? In research, many questions can be asked; however, for research literature to be valid, the questions should serve a useful purpose with sound rationale for its undertaking.

7. *Who or what constituted the sample or population?*
   Sample size is often critical for population research. Who or what was studied and how many were in the sample or subsamples studied should be clear. It is important to understand this aspect of the study, especially in terms of applying the results in a healthcare setting or with patients. The number of subjects studied can affect outcomes: too small a number may not be representative or may miss a pertinent factor; too large a number may minimize some important or key findings. To extrapolate data and apply them outside a study, the characteristics of the sample must be evident and comparable to the population from which the sample is selected. However, what may be true for one group of individuals may not be true for another, so results should always be considered cautiously.

8. *What was the design of the study?*
   Often the design of the study is critical to the outcome. The methods should be described in enough detail to allow the reader to make conclusions about the results and applications. Each study design is susceptible to limitations, threats to validity, threats to statistical analysis, and threats to conclusions. Even the fundamentally sound randomized assignment, double-blind studies have limitations. Clinicians should become familiar with the limitations of the various types of studies and look for biases in study design, because these flaws may affect conclusions and interpretation of the results.

9. *What statistical analyses were used?*
   Were the appropriate data analyses performed for the data type and study design? A statistics book is a very useful resource; it may also be a good idea to consult a statistician. Statistics can be confusing, and even experienced researchers make mistakes. Observe closely how the data were analyzed. Do the data and statistical analyses make sense? Sometimes reviewing the statistics may be helpful in understanding the results and conclusions.

10. *What are the results?*
    The results should be reported as unambiguously as possible. Two researchers undertaking the same study should report their findings in similar ways without any subjective interpretation. Determine whether the results of the study seem consistent with the study design and the analyses used. Do the data make sense and are the results consistent with current knowledge? Analysis results that indicate extremes should be examined closely.

11. *Are the results clear?*
    Do the results have meaning to the intent of the study? Are they understandable? Are they consistent with the methods and analyses proposed? When results are not clear, either the study was conducted in a confusing manner or the statistical methods used may simply be unfamiliar to the reader.

12. *Did the results answer the identified questions?*
    The results may not be expected, but that does not necessarily mean they are wrong. If the methodological process was conducted correctly, then the results should stand alone and the majority of readers should draw similar conclusions. Results should answer the questions posed earlier in the study. Although the answers often lead to more questions, the primary research questions should be addressed in the Results section.

13. *Do the results seem valid?*
    Validity is at the heart of most studies. Validity is defined as making common sense and being persuasive to the reader.

The major categories of validity are internal and external validity. If a research study has been performed correctly without errors, then the study is considered to be internally valid. If the study represents the realities found in the general population, then it is considered externally valid.

Face validity simply means that the results of a study can be taken at face value. Because of vagueness and subjectivity, psychometricians abandoned this concept a long time ago. However, when reading an article, one may get a sense that something does not seem right, especially if the reader is very knowledgeable about the topic. This represents a problem with face validity.

Construct validity assesses the degree to which the measure relates to other variables as expected within a system or theory. In contrast, content validity is the extent to which the method of measurement includes all of the major elements relevant to the construct being measured.

14. *Are the interpretations (conclusions) of the results consistent with the study design and analysis?*
Here, the authors of the article make the correct conclusion about the data. However, this area can be open to personal bias and misinterpretation. The reader, therefore, has to determine whether the conclusions are consistent with the type of information provided by the study design.

15. *Are the results consistent with findings from similar studies?*
One should have a sense of the problem, either from previous literature reviews or one's own clinical experience. Studies that deviate greatly from what is already known should be examined with caution. However, this deviation does not mean the study is wrong. Occasionally, new discoveries emerge from unexpected or unanticipated results.

16. *What do the results mean to medicine and health care, and you and your patients?*
This question may be the most important one the clinician can ask. What do these results mean to your practice and to the people for whom you provide care? For medicine and health care, it is important to examine the validity of an intervention to make sure it is applicable to the patient population. The risks and benefits of an intervention study should be clearly understood, as well as what the results mean to the patients' overall well-being.

17. *Can the results be applied to your research or clinical practice?* This is a practical question. The results may be valid and important, but you must consider whether or not you can replicate them in your setting.

EVIDENCE-BASED MEDICINE: A NEW WAY OF LOOKING AT THE MEDICAL LITERATURE

A general assumption has developed that if something claims to be "evidence-based" it is the guiding light for practice. However, the key to evidence-based medicine is the applicability to patient care. The evidence-based concept does not replace clinical experience and/or expertise. Evidence-based research should bridge the gap between rigorous research and clinical investigations for the clinician, ultimately for the patients' benefit. Evidence-based outcomes can come from research studies or from the synthesis of existing data and outcomes (e.g., meta-analysis). Regardless, the "evidence" must still be interpreted or evaluated as it relates to the needs of patients.

Friedland et al.[4] have developed a straightforward approach to evaluating evidence-based medicine. This five-step approach is presented in **Table 17–2**.

Although this is a concise approach, it does not eliminate the need to ask and answer the previous questions. The table outlines a process that

Table 17–2 A Five-Step Study Guide for Evidence-Based Medicine

Step	Question to Ask	Evaluation Points
Step 1	Do I want to evaluate the study?	Is it interesting, novel, relevant?
Step 2	What are the research question, study design, study findings?	What are the populations studied, variables, study design, results, outcomes, findings, and/or conclusions?
Step 3	Are the findings believable?	Do the subjects and variables represent the research question? Are the findings attributable to chance, biases, or confounding variables? Are the findings believable in the context of existing knowledge?
Step 4	What are the important findings?	Are the findings clinically relevant?
Step 5	Will the study help my patients?	Are the subjects similar to my patients? Are the interventions applicable to my patients? Will the findings/outcomes result in an overall benefit for my patients?

Adapted from Friedland DB, Go AS, Davoren JB, Shlipak MG, Bent SW, Subak LL, Mendelson T. *Evidence-Based Medicine: A Framework for Clinical Practice*. New York: Lange Medical Books/McGraw-Hill; 1998:145–246.

is a part of a larger evaluation and interpretation scheme of medical literature.

Two statistical calculations can be very useful when interpreting the results from a randomized, controlled trial of a new therapy. These two calculations are the number needed to treat (NNT) and the 95 percent confidence interval (CI). Each of these calculations is used for different types of data. Remember, it is important to be aware of the type of data reported by the literature being reviewed.

The NNT calculation is used when the article being reviewed contains categorical results (e.g., improved versus unimproved) and two groups (e.g., treatment and control). The NNT is intuitive and helps clinicians communicate the expected outcome of a selected therapy. The 95% CI calculation is used to compare the means (i.e., the central tendency) and standard deviations (i.e., variability) of a continuous measure (e.g., blood pressure) between two sample groups (e.g., treatment and control). The 95% CI determines the potential range of possible values present in the overall population based on the sampling scheme used in the study. Sometimes the calculated CIs overlap. This overlap is an indication that the treatment studied may be no different than the placebo or control treatment when it is used in a population larger than the study's sample.

To calculate the NNT, some basic rates are first calculated and applied, as shown in the formulas in **Table 17–3**. Here are the steps:

1. Calculate the experimental event rate (EER).
2. Calculate the control event rate (CER).
3. Calculate the absolute risk reduction (ARR).
4. Express the ARR as a proportion and divide into 1.

The NNT to produce the intended clinical outcome can then be assessed. Be aware that the formula changes depending on the outcome being measured (i.e., a reduction in bad events or an increase in good events).

Many papers include the 95% CI of the mean in the publication. When it is not given, it is important to perform a quick calculation. To calculate the 95% CI for a mean when using a continuous measure, the mean, standard deviation, and number of subjects must be known for each group. If any of this information is missing or if the outcome

Table 17–3 Calculating Event Rates (ER), Absolute Risk Reduction (ARR), and Number Needed to Treat (NNT)

	Control	Experimental
Event	a	b
No event	c	d
Totals	a + c	b + d
Event rate	Control event rate CER = a/(a + c)	Experimental event rate EER = b/(b + d)
Measure	The experiment reduces the bad event.	The experiment increases the good event.
Relative risk reduction	(CER − EER)/CER	(EER − CER)/CER
Absolute risk reduction	CER − EER	EER − CER
Number needed to treat	1/ARR	1/ARR

measure does not contain continuous data, then the calculation cannot be performed (**Figures 17–1** and **17–2**).

Here are the steps:

1. Calculate the standard error (i.e., the standard deviation divided by the square root of the number of subjects in the sample).
2. Determine the constant from a table if the number of subjects is < 60; otherwise, use the constant 1.96.
3. Multiply the constant (usually 1.96) times the standard error from step 1.
4. Add the result from step 3 to the mean of the sample to get the upper confidence limit.
5. Subtract the result from step 3 from the mean to get the lower confidence limit.
6. Perform these steps for both the control and experimental groups to see if the limits from each group overlap.

If the confidence limits overlap, then no difference in the treatments is likely to occur when they are administered to a larger target population.

The last consideration in the interpretation of evidence-based literature is the level of evidence (**Table 17–4**). When studies are analyzed for best evidence, a rating system is used. This evidence rating can be a guide for clinicians regarding the strength of the evidence and its source.

In addition to the evidence-level rating, qualifiers are also used to describe the source of the evidence (**Table 17–5**).

Another presentation format for evidence-based medicine is the POEM or Patient Oriented Evidence

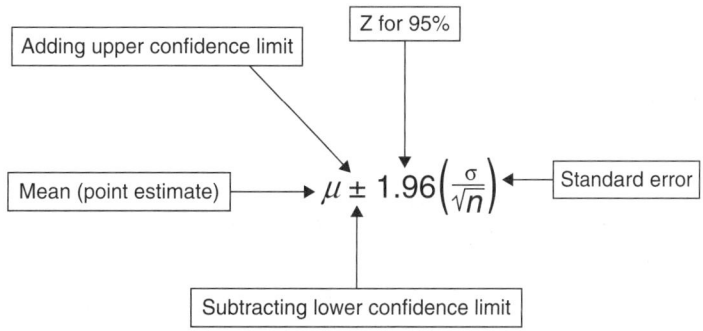

Figure 17–1 Formula for 95% confidence interval of the sample mean for $n > 60$.

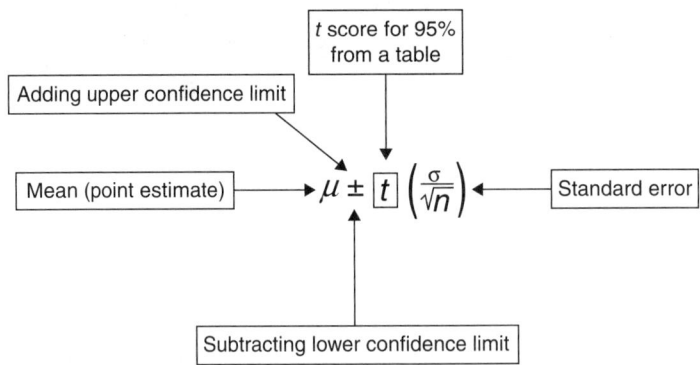

Figure 17–2 Formula for 95% confidence interval of a small sample.

Table 17–4 Levels of Evidence

Level	Description
A	High-quality evidence that considers all important outcomes: randomized controlled trials (RCTs), well-done systematic reviews of RCTs, meta-analyses, systematic reviews using comprehensive search strategies
B	Well-designed, nonrandomized clinical trials: systematic reviews of studies other than RCTs with appropriate search strategies and well-substantiated conclusions, lower-quality RCTs, cohort studies, case-control studies with nonbiased subject selection and consistent findings, quality retrospective studies, certain uncontrolled studies, well-designed epidemiologic studies with compelling findings
C	Consensus or expert opinion

Data from Siwek J, Gourley ML, Slawson DC, Shaughnessy AF. How to write an evidence-based clinical review article. *Am Fam Physician.* 2002;65(2):251–258.

Table 17–5 Level of Evidence Modifiers

Modifier	Description
1	Nonrandomized clinical trial
2	Systematic review of nonrandomized clinical trial
3	Lower quality of randomized clinical trial
4	Clinical cohort study
5	Case control study
6	Retrospective study
7	Uncontrolled study
8	Epidemiologic study

Data from Siwek J, Gourley ML, Slawson DC, Shaughnessy AF. How to write an evidence-based clinical review article. *Am Fam Physician.* 2002;65(2):251–258.

that Matters. The POEM is a commercially available format in which the evidence-based medical literature is reviewed and summarized.[5] The intent of the POEM format is to present evidence-based results in a concise and easily readable way that is applicable in clinical practice. A number of journals have a POEM section or a POEM feature. These types of summaries are very helpful, but for those interventions or outcomes that affect patients, the original work should always be reviewed.

A GENERAL APPROACH TO READING THE LITERATURE

Asking all the right questions, going through all these steps, and reading as much as possible are still very time consuming. Many resources are available that can be easily accessed. Still, the amount of information available is overwhelming. With more than 2 million biomedical publications per year,[1] developing an approach to reviewing the current medical literature is an important professional skill. However, no single approach works in every situation. A general approach follows, but it may be modified in many ways.

1. Identify the journals that are pertinent to the specialty of interest.
2. Develop a strategy for reviewing those journals.
3. Set aside a specific time each week when journals can be reviewed. (Allow ample uninterrupted time for reading and review.)
4. Identify those articles of interest by their title or by reading their abstracts.
5. Make a quick review of the tables and figures.
6. Make a decision to read the article.
7. Apply the techniques for interpreting the article.
8. Apply the results to your practice.

SUMMARY

Interpreting the literature involves synthesizing information from different medical, healthcare, and scientific studies and integrating pertinent outcomes into the healthcare practice. Healthcare professionals must develop a sound process for reviewing and evaluating medical literature. Skilled interpretation of the medical literature incorporates up-to-date information that benefits a practice and its patients. Professionals who fail to stay abreast of the medical literature may quickly fall behind and lose competency. As evidence-based analyses increase, so does the pressure for practice trends to follow that evidence. However, evidence must be balanced with clinical experience and expertise to support the highest likelihood of improved patient outcomes.

REFERENCES

1. Arndt KA. Information excess in medicine: Overview, relevance to dermatology, and strategies for coping. *Arch Dermatol.* 1992;128(9):1249–1256.
2. Medline. Medline search results. Available at: http://www.ncbi.nlm.nih.gov/pubmed?term=2013%5Bpdat%5D&cmd=detailssearch. Accessed October 13, 2014.
3. Sackett DL, Richardson WS, Rosenberg, Haynes RB. *Evidence-Based Medicine: How to Practice and Teach EBM.* New York: Churchill Livingstone; 1997.
4. Friedland DB, Go AS, Davoren JB, Shlipak MG, Bent SW, Subak LL, Mendelson T. *Evidence-Based Medicine: A Framework for Clinical Practice.* New York: Lange Medical Books/McGraw-Hill; 1998:145–246.
5. Essential Evidence Plus Web site. Available at: http://www.essentialevidenceplus.com/. Accessed October 13, 2014.

APPENDIX

APPENDIX OVERVIEW

Research is not free or inexpensive. In fact, research is a large enterprise in many universities, colleges, and schools. For many researchers, finding funding is as much a part of the process as the research itself. Grant support is one funding method that is available from many sources, from the federal government to foundations. This appendix was developed as an introduction and outline for students and healthcare professionals seeking small or nongovernmental grants.[1]

Funding Research: Grants

J. Dennis Blessing, PhD
William D. Hendricson, MA, MS

INTRODUCTION

Every research project costs something. The cost can be low for small projects that do not require a lot of resources, or very expensive requiring salaries, supplies, consultants, overhead, and more. Grants can be a method of funding all or part of a research project. For students, the most likely source for grant funding is their institution or their health profession's organizations and foundations. Funding may be hard to locate and require a number of steps to gain, but lack of effort will not provide anything.

The first challenge is to find an agency that will offer a grant. An Internet search will yield a large number of possibilities, probably more than anyone will ever be able to explore. Limit searches by the objective or subject of the project. If the project involves a certain condition, search for organizations that revolve around or involve that condition. For example, if a project involves diabetes, a good place to begin is the American Diabetes Association. If the project involves a specific health profession, then look at the professional organization's website for possible support. Never waste time applying for grants with any organization that does not have a relationship, interest, or involvement with the objectives of a project. Make contact with the organization and briefly describe a project to ascertain if it is the type of project for which funding could be obtained. Some key considerations:

- What is the overall purpose or mission of the grant program? What is its significance?
- Does the organization provide grants to support higher education, specifically healthcare professions education or student projects?
- What types of projects does the foundation support? Are student projects eligible for support?
- Are there any specific restrictions on who can receive grants?
- Is the funding range adequate to meet the project needs?
- What is the application process, including deadlines?
- Most importantly, who is the person identified as the grant program director for the foundation? This is the person to contact.

WHAT TO DO

1. Contact the grant program director. Discuss your concept to ascertain if the funding organization will fund the type of project you want to do.
2. Follow grant directions exactly. Be clear, compelling, and convincing (the three Cs of grant writing).
3. Describe the project in its entirety. The following questions should be addressed in the required format for the grant:
    a. What problem will be addressed, and in what population? The problem statement should identify an unknown, a phenomenon that is not understood, or something that has been problematic to accomplish. Address a gap in knowledge. What is the project's significance?
    b. What is the purpose of the project? What, specifically, is proposed?
    c. What research question(s) will the project answer? *or* What hypothesis will be tested?
    d. What methods will be used to answer these questions or test the hypothesis? Will the methods provide the needed data?
    e. What outcomes will be measured (i.e., what data will be collected)? Does the analysis include the proper tests for the type of data collected? What do the statistical tests to be done tell the investigator?
    f. What will be learned if the project is conducted (i.e., what is the benefit)? How will the gap in knowledge be addressed?

USEFUL TIPS WHEN APPLYING FOR A GRANT

1. Be concise and use common, direct language. Be specific. Do not waste words. Do not try to impress reviewers by using "big" words.
2. Stay on target. Address only the project and its aims, goals, or objectives. Do not drift off the subject. Give the who, what, when, where, and how of the project.
3. Stay within the grant format for page or section lengths. The grantor's requirements must be met.
4. Develop a realistic and accurate budget. Be able to justify all expenses. Use grant money only as specified in the budget.
5. Be prepared to negotiate with the grantor.
6. If the grant is awarded, know the deadlines and meet them.

CONCLUSION

Grants can be a method to cover the costs of a research project. The information in this appendix is very limited. A lot of information about grant writing is available. Use it to help in your efforts to acquire grants.

REFERENCE

1. Hendricson WD, Blessing JD. Funding the research: Grants. In: Blessing JD, Forister JG, eds. *Introduction to Research and Medical Literature for Health Professionals.* 3rd ed. Burlington, MA: Jones & Bartlett Learning; 2013:46–86.

Glossary

a priori: By reasoning from self-evident facts (literally "before").

absolute value: The value of a number regardless of its sign.

abstract: The summary of a study in clear and concise terms. Usually limited to 100 to 250 words.

accuracy: The extent to which a scale correctly represents the amount or classification of a variable.

alpha (α): Level of significance or cutoff point used to determine whether the samples being tested are members of the same population or of different populations. Alpha is commonly set at .05, .01, or .001.

analysis of covariance (ANCOVA): A method of removing pretreatment variations (as measured by the control variable) from the posttreatment means (criterion variable) before testing the significance of the posttreatment differences among the groups. Analysis of covariance provides a basis for ruling out pretreatment differences when the interest is in testing posttreatment differences.

analysis of variance (ANOVA): A statistical method that tests the difference between two or more means when studying groups. Independent variables are nominal (categorical) values and dependent variables are interval values. Asks whether the squared variation of the case scores around their treatment means (*within*) is greater than the squared variation of the means themselves around the grand mean (*between*). These two totals are expressed as a ratio. Comparison of variances reflects different sources of variability, that is, *within* versus *between*.

analysis of variance, one-way: Only one independent variable is manipulated. See *analysis of variance (ANOVA)*.

anonymity: Condition in which subjects' identities cannot be linked to their individual responses.

applied research: Research designed to answer practical questions.

associated keywords: A set of words used as identifiers of the topic area.

assumptions: Statements taken for granted or considered true, even though they have not been scientifically tested.

attributes: Characteristics of persons or things (e.g., age, eye color).

attrition: The loss of participants during the course of a study. Attrition can introduce bias by changing the composition of the sample initially drawn, particularly if more subjects are lost from one group than another.

average: An ambiguous term generally suggesting typical or normal. The *mean, median,* and *mode* are specific examples of mathematical averages.

baseline measure: The measurement of the dependent variable before the introduction of an experimental intervention.

basic research: Discovery research that seeks to add knowledge or support or refute theories.

beneficence: The principle that one should do good and, above all, do no harm.

beta (β) coefficient: Standardized regression coefficient that allows comparison of relative importance of variables in regression analysis.

bias: That quality of a measurement device that tends to result in a misrepresentation of what is being measured in a particular direction. For example, the questionnaire item "Don't you agree that your physician is doing a good job?" is biased because it encourages favorable responses.

bibliography: A list of source materials or references that are used or consulted in the preparation of a work. The references of the bibliography are usually cited in the text.

bivariate correlation: An analysis technique that measures the extent of the linear relationship between two variables.

case study design: Intensive exploration of a single unit of study, such as a person, family, group, community, or institution.

causal relationship: Relationship between two variables where one variable (independent variable) is thought to cause or determine the presence of the other variable (dependent variable). Three criteria must be satisfied: (1) the cause precedes the effect in time, (2) the two variables are empirically correlated with one another, and (3) the observed correlation between the two variables cannot be explained away as being due to the influence of some third variable.

central limit theorem: A theorem stating that even when statistics, such as means, come from a population with a skewed (asymmetrical) distribution, the sampling distribution developed from multiple means obtained from that skewed population tends to fit the pattern of the normal curve.

central tendency: A statistical index of a typical set of scores that comes from the center of the distribution of scores. The three most common indices of central tendency are the mean, median, and mode.

chi-squared (χ^2): A test to assess whether observed frequencies of nominal data differ from expected frequencies. A nonsignificant value indicates the classes are independent. A significant value indicates an association. Range is zero to infinity.

citation: The reference to an authority or author of a document.

code book: A document used in data processing and analysis that tells the location of different data items in a data file and the meanings of the codes used to represent different attributes of variables. Often a notebook, this document lists all methods used so another researcher could duplicate the work.

coding: The process of transforming qualitative data into numerical symbols. Often done for computer input prior to analysis.

coercion: To compel someone by threat of harm or excessive reward to do something they would not ordinarily undertake (e.g., obtaining participants for dangerous research projects by offering large sums of money).

Cohen's kappa: See *kappa coefficient*.

cohort study: A study in which some specific group is studied over time, although data may be collected from different members in each set of observations (e.g., a study of the clinical practice of physician assistants who graduated in 1976, to whom questionnaires were sent every 5 years).

comparative descriptive design: Used to describe differences in variables in two or more groups in a natural setting.

comparison group: Commonly known as the *control group*; a group not receiving a treatment, reward, or intervention.

concept: A term that abstractly describes and names an object or phenomenon, thus providing it with a separate identity or meaning.

conceptual definition: A definition that provides a variable or concept with a theoretical meaning and is established through concept analysis.

conceptual framework: A set of highly abstract, related constructs that broadly explains phenomena of interest, expresses assumptions, and reflects a philosophical stance.

conclusions: Opinion or interpretation of the results or meaning of a study.

confidence interval: The range of values within which a population parameter is estimated to lie.

confidence level: The estimated probability that a population parameter lies within a given confidence interval.

confidentiality: Management of data in research so subjects' identities are not linked with their responses. This differs from *anonymity*, in which the subjects' identities are not known.

confirmability: The ability of researchers to accomplish or reproduce the results of a qualitative study.

confounding variable: An uncontrolled variable that may compete with a manipulated variable for interpretive priority. Makes a clear interpretation of the results of a study difficult or impossible.

consent form: A form used to document a subject's agreement to participate in a study.

construct (pronounced with emphasis on first syllable): An image, an idea, or a theory that has some general meaning that is not directly observable.

construct validity: The degree to which a measure relates to other variables as expected within a system of theoretical relationships. In other words, construct validity is based on the logical relationship among variables (e.g., patients who report they are satisfied with their physician assistant are more likely to comply with treatment).

content analysis: Qualitative analysis technique to classify words in a text into a few categories chosen because of their theoretical importance.

content validity: The extent to which the method of measurement includes all the major elements relevant to the construct being measured.

contingency tables: Cross-tabulation tables that allow visual comparison of summary data output related to two variables within a sample.

control: Rules imposed by the researcher to decrease the possibility of error and increase the probability that the study's findings are an accurate reflection of reality.

control group: A group of subjects to whom *no* experimental stimulus, treatment, or intervention is administered and who should resemble the experimental group in all other respects (also known as *comparison group*).

convenience sampling: Simply entering available subjects into the study until the desired sample size is reached (also known as *accidental sampling*).

copy editor: The person who makes corrections on a manuscript to achieve consistency in style, word usage, and spelling, following the appropriate publication guidelines.

correlation: A consistent relationship between two variables such that one variable can be predicted from knowledge of the other. With a *positive correlation*, both variables increase together, that is, a positive value increase. Positive does not mean good, beneficial, advantageous, or better. With a *negative correlation*, one increases when the other decreases or one variable is high and the other is low. Negative does not mean bad, adverse, worse, or least.

correlation analysis: Statistical procedure conducted to determine the direction (positive or negative) and magnitude (strength) of the relationship between two variables.

correlation coefficient (r): A statistic that shows the degree of relationship between two or more variables.

correlation matrix: A table that presents variable correlation coefficients. Basically a visual representation of the relationships of two or more variables.

correlational research: Systematic investigation of relationships between two or more variables to explain the nature of relationships in the world and not to examine cause and effect.

cost–benefit analysis: Economic technique that examines costs and benefits of alternative ways of using resources to determine which way produces the greatest net benefit, assessed in monetary terms.

cost-effectiveness analysis: Type of outcomes research that compares costs and benefits of different ways of accomplishing a clinical goal (e.g., diagnosing a condition, treating an illness, or providing a service). The goal is to identify the strategy that achieves the desired result for the least cost.

covariance: The measure of effect by two or more variables.

covariate analysis: See *analysis of covariance (ANCOVA)*.

covert data collection: Collection of research data without the subjects being aware that data are being collected.

credibility: A term used in qualitative research meaning that the study is performed in an appropriate and rigorous manner.

critical analysis of studies: Minute examination of the merits, faults, meaning, and significance of studies.

cross-tabulation: A determination of the number of cases occurring when simultaneous consideration is given to the values of two or more variables, such as sex (male/female) cross-tabulated with smoking status (smoker/nonsmoker). The results are presented in a table format according to the values of the variables.

crossover design: Experimental design in which more than one type of treatment is administered to each subject; the treatments are provided sequentially, rather than concurrently, and comparisons are made of the effects of the different treatments on the same subject.

data: The reports of observations of variables.

data coding sheet: A form for organizing and recording data for rapid entry into a computer.

data collection: Precise, systematic gathering of information relevant to the research purpose or the specific objectives, questions, or hypotheses of a study.

data entry: The process of entering data (usually in coded form) into an input medium.

data triangulation: Collection of data from multiple sources in the same study.

deception: Misinforming subjects for research purposes.

decision theory: Theory that is inductive in nature and is based on assumptions associated with the theoretical normal curve. The theory is applied when testing for differences between groups with the expectation that all of the groups are members of the same population.

deduction: The logical model in which specific expectations of hypotheses are developed on the basis of general principles.

deductive research: Moving from prior hypotheses to observation or empirical research, other than discovery research.

degrees of freedom (df): Equal to the sum of the two sample sizes, minus the value 2 ($n_1 + n_2 - 2$). The different rows in the t table, each showing a different value of df, accommodate the changes in the sampling distribution of t because the sizes of samples may vary.

demographic variables: Characteristics or attributes of the subjects that are collected to describe the sample.

dependability: In qualitative research, the confidence in the data collection methods (analogous to reliability in traditional research terminology).

dependent variable: A phenomenon that is affected by the researcher's manipulation of an independent variable.

description: The precise measurement and reporting of the characteristics of a population or phenomenon under study.

descriptive correlational design: Used to describe variables and examine relationships that exist in a situation.

descriptive method: A research plan undertaken to define the characteristics and/or relationships of variables, based on systematic observation of these variables.

descriptive statistics: Calculated values that represent certain overall characteristics of a body of data.

design: Blueprint for conducting a study that maximizes control over factors that could interfere with the validity of the findings.

diary: A written record of a subject's observations and feelings, collected by the researcher for analysis.

dichotomous variable: A variable that places subjects into two groups (e.g., male/female).

directional hypothesis: A hypothesis that states the specific nature of the interaction or relationship between two or more variables.

discriminant analysis: A form of regression analysis used to place a variable in a linear combination with other measurements.

dispersion: The distribution of values around some central value, such as an average. The range is a simple example of a measure of dispersion.

disproportionate stratified sampling: A sampling strategy wherein the researcher samples different proportions of subjects from different strata in the population to ensure adequate representation of subjects from strata that are comparatively smaller.

distribution: A collection of measurements usually viewed in terms of the frequency with which observations are assigned to each category or point on a measurement scale.

double-blind experiment: An experiment in which neither the subjects nor those who administer the treatment know who is in the experimental group or control group.

editor: The person in charge of a research publication who decides which articles are to be published, manages the overall production of the publication, and heads the editorial staff.

effect size: A statistical expression of the magnitude of the difference between two variables, or the magnitude of the difference between two groups, with regard to some attribute of interest.

epistemology: The science of knowing; a branch of philosophy that investigates the origin, nature, methods, and limits of human knowledge.

ethical principles: Principles of respect for persons, beneficence, and justice relevant to the conduct of research.

ethics: The values or guidelines that should govern decisions in research or medicine. The social obligation the researcher has to his or her subjects.

ethnographic research: A qualitative research methodology for investigating cultures. This method involves collecting, describing, and analyzing the data to develop a theory of cultural behavior.

evaluation research: Research that has as its objective the description and evaluation of some existing social policy or program (oriented towards program research). Differs from applied and basic research.

exclusion criteria: Sampling requirements identified by the researcher that eliminate or exclude an element or subject from being in a sample

experimental group: The subjects who are exposed to an experimental treatment or intervention.

experimental method: A research plan undertaken to test relationships among variables based on systematic observation of variables that are manipulated by the researcher.

experimenter effects: A source of bias in experimental research in which subjects react to personal attributes of the experimenter or pick up cues about what the experimenter is seeking and modify their behavior accordingly.

external validity: The degree to which the results of a study generalize to the population. The process of testing the validity of a measure, such as an index or scale, which is conducted by examining its relationship to other, presumed indicators of the same variable.

extraneous variable: A variable, other than the independent variable, that may exert effect on the subject or variable being studied.

F: Designation letter for the value derived from an F test.

F ratio: A statistical value used in analysis of variance and other statistical methods.

F table: A table of values that represent the percentage points of the F distribution.

F test: A test for comparing two or more means: the ratio of variance between groups divided by the variance within groups (error). As the number of observations in each sample (n) increases, the critical value of F increases; smaller differences between the variances of the samples will become significant because variations tend to level out as the proportion of the population sampled increases.

fatigue effect: When a subject becomes tired or bored with a study.

feasibility study: A study of whether a research project can or should be performed, as determined by examining the time and money commitment; the researcher's expertise; the availability of subjects, facilities, and equipment; the cooperation of others; and ethical considerations.

field research: A form of research that consists of observations made in uncontrolled, real-life situations that are often not easily reduced to numbers.

findings: The translated and interpreted results of a study.

focus group interview: An interview in which the respondents are a group of individuals with some trait in common who are assembled to answer questions on a given topic.

forced choice: Response set using a scale that has an even number of choices, such as four or six, so that respondents cannot choose an uncertain or neutral response.

frequency distribution: A description of the number of times the various attributes of a variable are observed in a sample.

generalizability: The quality of a research finding that justifies the inference that it represents something more than the specific observations on which it was based. Sometimes this involves the generalization of findings from a sample to a population.

Hawthorne effect: A term coined in reference to a series of productivity studies at the Hawthorne plant of the Western Electric Company (Chicago). The researchers discovered that their presence affected the behavior of the workers being studied. The term now refers to any impact of research on the subject of study.

heterogeneous: Having a wide variety of characteristics; the use of heterogeneous subjects reduces the risk of bias in studies not using random sampling.

history effect: The effect of an event unrelated to the planned study that occurs during the time of the study and could influence the responses of subjects.

hypothesis: A provisional theory set forth to explain some class of phenomena, either accepted as a guide to future investigation (working hypothesis) or assumed for the sake of argument and testing. A statement to be tested in a study. An expectation about the nature of things derived from a theory.

hypothesis testing: The determination of whether the expectations that a hypothesis represents are, indeed, found to exist in the real world.

inclusion criteria: Sampling requirements identified by the researcher that must be present for the element or subject to be included in the sample.

independent variable: A phenomenon that is manipulated by the researcher and is predicted to have an effect on another phenomenon. A variable whose values are *not* problematic in an analysis but are taken simply as given. An *independent variable* is presumed to cause or determine a *dependent variable*.

indicator: A thing or person that indicates and therefore can serve as a proxy for a concept.

indirect measurement: Measurement of indicators or attributes of an abstract concept rather than of the abstraction itself.

induction: The logical model in which general principles are developed from specific observations.

inductive research: Any form of reasoning in which the conclusion, though supported by the premises, does not necessarily follow them. Research as discovery is used to develop or generate hypotheses. Inductive research is used to move from observation to development of hypotheses.

inferential statistics: Statistical methods that make it possible to draw tentative conclusions about a population based on observations of a sample selected from that population and furthermore make a probability statement about those conclusions to aid in their evaluation; inferential methods include sampling theory, hypothesis testing, and parameter estimation.

informed consent: The process used to inform subjects of the risks, benefits, and goals of research studies.

institutional review: A process of examining study proposals for ethical concerns by a committee representing an institution.

internal validity: The extent to which the individual items comprising a composite measure are correlated with the measure itself.

interrater reliability: The degree of consistency between two raters who are independently assigning ratings to a variable or attribute being investigated.

interrupted time series design: A study design involving the collection of data at different points in time, as contrasted with a cross-sectional study. Also known as *longitudinal study*.

interval scale: Interval measure; the assignment of numbers to identify ordered relations of some characteristic. The interval scale is arbitrarily assigned and at equal intervals but has no zero point.

interview: Structured or unstructured verbal communication between a researcher and a subject, during which information is obtained for a study.

kappa coefficient (k): A statistical measure of interrater agreement. Also referred to as Cohen's kappa.

key terms: See *associated keywords*.

level of significance: In the context of tests of statistical significance, the degree of likelihood that an observed, empirical relationship could be attributable to sampling error. For example, a relationship is significant at the .05 level if the likelihood of its being only a function of sampling error is no greater than 5 out of 100.

Likert scale: A type of composite measurement in survey questionnaires. Likert items use response categories such as strongly agree, agree, disagree, and strongly disagree. Pronounced Lick-ert.

limits of confidence: A term used in constructing confidence-interval estimates of parameter values to specify confidence that the interval includes the parameter value; using procedures for constructing a 95 percent confidence interval, for instance, you would enclose the true parameter value within its limits on 95 percent of such attempts. The higher the level of confidence, the wider the interval.

literature review: A review of prior relevant literature that serves as the basis or beginning point for a research endeavor.

longitudinal study: A study design involving the collection of data at different points in time

Mann-Whitney *U* test: A nonparametric hypothesis-testing procedure used to decide whether two given independent samples could have arisen by chance from identically distributed populations; a test for comparing two populations based on independent random samples from each.

MANOVA (multivariate analysis of variance): A general term for analysis using two or more independent variables.

matrix: A two-dimensional organization; each dimension is composed of several positions or alternatives. Any particular "score" is a combination of the two dimensions.

mean (M): The sum of the scores in a distribution of a population or collection of things divided by the number of scores. In common usage, the average.

measurement: A scheme for the assignment of numbers or symbols to specify different characteristics of a variable. Characteristics include validity, accuracy, precision, and reliability.

measurement error: A deviation from accurate or correct measurement. *Random error* is as likely to occur in one direction as the other around the mean. *Bias* is systematic error that tends to occur regularly in one direction, owing to faulty procedure or measurement technique.

measures of central tendency: Statistical procedures (mean, median, mode) for determining the center of a distribution of scores or a typical value.

median: The midpoint or midscore in a distribution. The middle number in a sequence of numbers.

member checking: A technique used in qualitative research to establish credibility. Study participants are asked to verify the accuracy of data collection and/or interpretation.

meta-analysis: The statistical integration of the results of a number of independent studies.

methodological triangulation: The use of two or more research methods or procedures in a study.

mode: The most frequent score in a distribution.

mortality: Subjects who are lost to a study or drop out from the study or a group. It does not necessarily mean the death of the subject.

multiple-factor analysis of variance (or multivariate analysis): A statistical model for testing the consequences of manipulating two or more independent variables in a single research design. Each independent variable (factor) will have two or more levels. The F ratio is the statistic used to conduct the appropriate hypothesis tests in multiple-factor designs. Specific techniques include factor analysis, multiple correlations, multiple regression, and path analysis.

multivariate analysis: The analysis of the simultaneous relationships among several variables. Examining simultaneously the effects of age, sex, and social class of patients seen by different providers would be an example of multivariate analysis. Specific techniques include factor analysis, multiple correlation, multiple regression, and path analysis.

multivariate analysis of variance (MANOVA): Extension of the basic analysis of variance design to include more than one dependent variable.

narrative review: When the reviewer reads and thinks about a collection of relevant studies and then writes a narrative account of whether the hypothesis under consideration seems to be supported by the evidence.

natural setting: Field settings or uncontrolled, real-life situations examined in research.

needs assessment: Questions concerned with discovering the nature and extent of a particular social problem to determine the most appropriate type of response.

negative case analysis: A technique used by qualitative researchers to enhance credibility by seeking out aberrant examples or data that do not initially fit.

nominal scale: Designation of subclasses by assigning numbers or symbols that represent unique characteristics. It is the weakest level of measurement because it denotes the least information about observations (e.g., eye color: Blue = 1; Brown = 2).

nondirectional hypothesis: A hypothesis stating that a relationship exists but not predicting the exact nature of the relationship.

nonparametric statistics: Tests that do not directly incorporate estimates pertaining to population characteristics. Examples are chi-squared, log-linear models, and Wilcoxon matched-pairs signed ranks tests.

nonprobability sampling: A sample selected in some fashion other than those suggested by probability theory.

nonsampling error: Imperfections of data quality that result from factors other than sampling error, such as misunderstanding of questions by respondents, erroneous recording by interviewers and coders, or keypunch errors.

normal distribution curve: The characteristic values and frequencies of a variable based on empirical observations that are predicted to follow a specific graphic curve.

null hypothesis: A statement that statistical differences or relationships have occurred for no reason other than the laws of chance operating in an unrestricted manner. The null hypothesis is sometimes stated instead of or in addition to the hypothesis. It is a form of the hypothesis stated in a negative manner.

objectivity: A characteristic of the scientific method; the condition in which to the greatest extent possible the researcher's values and biases do not interfere with the study of the problem.

one-tailed test: A directional hypothesis test that incorporates a rejection region in only one tail of the probability curve used for a given statistic. In setting up a directional hypothesis, the researcher must be very confident beforehand that there is no reason to expect differences in an opposite direction. Used only when there is very good reason to make a directional prediction.

ordinal scale: The assignment of numbers or symbols to identify ordered relations of some characteristic, the order having unspecified intervals. Ordinal scales do not represent the magnitude of differences, only order or ranking.

outcomes research: Method developed to examine the end results of patient care; the strategies used are a departure from traditional scientific endeavors and incorporate evaluation research, epidemiology, and economic theory perspectives.

outliers: Extreme scores, which can change the mean and violate homogeneity of variance.

P value: The probability value level used to accept or reject a study value as significant or nonsignificant. For instance, $p < .05$. Thus, if researchers report that a difference was "significant at the $p < .05$ level," they are saying the probability of the outcome was less than 5 percent due to chance.

paired sample: Two matched groups that are studied before and after the same intervention. Also used to describe a single group that undergoes the same measurement before and after some intervention. Also known as a matched sample.

paradigm: A way of looking at a natural phenomenon that encompasses a set of philosophical assumptions and that guides the approach to inquiry.

parameter: A characteristic of a population or sample.

parametric test: Statistical test that requires interval data and the assumption of a normally distributed population.

participant observation: A data collection method used by some qualitative researchers who embed themselves in the environment and activities of the study's participants. See *field research*.

Pearson's *r* or Pearson's product-moment correlation coefficient: A parametric test used to determine the relationship between variables.

peer debriefing: A technique used in qualitative research to enhance credibility. Peer debriefers are knowledgeable colleagues who help the investigator deal with emotions, test working hypotheses, and resolve ethical dilemmas.

persistent observation: A technique used by qualitative researchers to enhance credibility, exemplified by researchers who strive for deeper meaning over time or from probing.

phenomenon: Any object or event, the characteristics of which can be observed. Plural is *phenomena*.

pilot study: A smaller version of a proposed study conducted to develop or refine the methodology, such as the treatment, instrument, or data collection process.

population: The total number of members (or persons) in a defined group.

population distribution: The frequency with which observations in a population would be assigned or expected.

population mean: The estimate of a population mean (average) based on the mean of the sample and normal distribution.

poster session: Visual presentation of studies at a professional gathering, using pictures, tables, and illustrations on a display board.

power: The probability that a statistical test will detect a significant difference that exists.

power analysis: Analysis used to determine the risk of a type II error, so the study can be modified to decrease the risk if necessary.

practice effect: Improvement of subject performance due to increased familiarity with the experimental protocol.

precision: The exactness of the measure used in an observation or description of an attribute.

prediction: The ability to estimate the probability of a specific outcome in a given situation.

predictive validity: The degree to which an instrument can predict some criterion observed at a future time.

principal investigator: In a research grant, the individual who has primary responsibility for administering the grant and interacting with the funding agency.

probability sample: The general term for a sample selected in accord with probability theory, typically involving some random-selection mechanism. Specific types of probability samples include area probability sample, simple random sample, and systematic sample.

proposal: Written plan identifying the major elements of a research study, such as the problem, purpose, and framework, and outlining the methods to conduct the study. A formal way to communicate ideas about a proposed study to receive approval to conduct the study and to seek funding.

purposive sample: A type of nonprobability sample in which the units to be observed are selected on the basis of one's own judgment about which will be the most useful or representative. Same as *judgment sample*.

qualitative analysis: The nonnumerical examination and interpretation of observations for the purpose of describing and explaining the phenomena that those observations reflect.

quantitative research: The use of applied mathematics to assist in the research process.

quasi-experimental designs: Research designs that have the characteristics of experimental design but lack randomization.

r^2: Coefficient of determination. Indicates the percent variance of y accounted for by x_1 and x_2 in combination.

random sample: A collection of phenomena selected such that each phenomenon in the population has an equal chance of being selected.

range: The highest score in a distribution minus the lowest score.

ratio scale: The assignment of numbers to identify ordered relations of some characteristic, the order having been arbitrarily assigned and at equal intervals, but with an absolute zero point. The ratio scale specifies values and differences that are applicable to arithmetic operations and to statements about phenomena. Age is a ratio measure (scale).

references: The specific items or units used as information resources for a study or written report. References can be texts, journal articles, individuals, and so on. They are generally noted in the body of a report and listed in the bibliography.

referential adequacy: A technique used by qualitative researchers in which they collect a separate set of data for comparison with the initial data.

rejection region (significance level): A level of probability set by the researcher as grounds for the rejection of the null hypothesis. If a calculated value of probability falls within the rejection region, the researcher will interpret the difference or relationship as statistically significant.

relative risk (RR): A ratio that represents the probability of developing an outcome within a specific period when a risk factor is present, divided by the probability of developing the outcome in the same period if the risk factor is not present.

reliability: The external and internal consistency of a measurement. In the abstract, whether a particular technique, applied repeatedly to the same object, would yield the same result each time.

representativeness: That quality of a sample having the same distribution of characteristics as the population from which it was selected. By implication, descriptions and explanations derived from an analysis of the sample may be assumed to *represent* similar ones in the population. Representativeness is enhanced by probability sampling and provides for generalizability and the use of inferential statistics.

research design: The plan, protocol, format, and parameters of a research project.

research hypothesis: A statement expressing differences or relationships among phenomena, the acceptance or nonacceptance of which implies the existence of a null hypothesis that is susceptible to a probability estimate.

research methods: The methods used in systematic inquiry into a subject in order to discover or revise facts, theories, and the like.

research proposal: Written proposal that provides a preview of why a study will be undertaken and how it will be conducted. It is a useful device for planning and is required in most circumstances when research is being conducted.

response formats: Types of replies allowed by questions (e.g., open-ended versus closed).

response rate: The number of persons participating in a survey divided by the number selected in the sample, in the form of a percentage; the percentage of questionnaires sent out that is returned.

robust: In terms of a statistic, remaining useful even when its assumptions are violated.

sample: A collection of phenomena selected to represent some well-defined population.

sample distribution: The frequency with which observations in a sample are assigned to each category or point on a measurement scale.

sampling bias: Inherent bias in a sample. Sources include nonrandom, systematic sampling; incomplete or inaccurate sampling frame; and nonresponse. Sampling bias causes systematic error not compensated for by increasing the size of the sample.

sampling distribution: The frequencies with which particular values of a statistic would be expected when sampling randomly from a given population.

sampling error: An estimate of how statistics may be expected to deviate from parameters when sampling randomly from a given population.

sampling frame: The source from which a sample is taken or a list of a population from which a sample can be taken.

sampling ratio: The proportion of elements in the population that are selected to be in a sample.

sampling size: The number of subjects, usually designated as n, in each category, group, or the like used in a research study.

sampling statistics: Calculated values that represent how sample characteristics are likely to vary from population characteristics.

scale: A specific scheme for assigning numbers or symbols to designate characteristics of a variable. Nominal, ordinal, interval, and ratio are examples of scales. Scales can be single-item or multiple-item measures.

scatterplot: A two-dimensional dot plot that places data in an x and y grid.

secondary analysis: A form of research in which the data collected and processed by one researcher are analyzed (often for a different purpose) by another. This is especially appropriate in the case of survey data.

significance: The level of calculated probability that is sufficiently low to serve as grounds for rejection of the null hypothesis.

skewed: Unusual or odd distributions.
snowball sample: A nonprobability sampling method often employed in epidemiology research. Each person interviewed may be asked to suggest additional people for interviewing. One use is to track down the source of a communicable disease.
specification: Explanatory and clarifying comments about the handling of difficult or confusing situations that may occur with regard to specific questions in a questionnaire.
standard deviation (SD): The square root of the mean of the squared deviation scores about the mean of a distribution; more simply, the square root of the variance. SD gives a basis for estimating the probability of how frequently certain scores can be expected to occur in a sample.
standard error of the mean: The standard deviation of a distribution of sample means; describes the likely deviations of sample means about the population mean.
standardized score: A value that results from methods of converting values from different distributions into scores that can be compared.
statistic: A characteristic of a sample. Statistics are mathematical models that provide a framework for reasoning so that generalized statements can be made about the data. Types include descriptive and sampling statistics.
statistical inference: The process of estimating parameters from statistics.
statistical power: The probability of rejecting a null hypothesis that is, in fact, false.
statistical significance level: The level of probability that an association between two (or more) variables could have been produced by chance. Expressed as a P value and referred to as the level of significance. Arbitrarily set by the investigators, but commonly set at the .05 or .01 level.
statistical test: A test that addresses the question, "Could the observed relationship between x and y have occurred by chance?" Statistical tests state the relationship between variables by some specified degree.
stratification: The sorting of the units composing a population into homogenous groups (strata) before sampling.
survey techniques: Research methods to collect data from populations. These include face-to-face interviews, survey questionnaires (by mail or in person), telephone interviewing, and group interviewing.

systematic sample: A type of probability sample in which every kth unit in a list is selected for inclusion in the sample: for example, every 25th patient visiting a clinic.
***t* table:** A statistical table of percentage points of the t distribution. Used with statistical analyses that produce a t value.
***t*-test (student's *t*-test):** Test of the difference between two population means, based on the observed difference between two sample means and their distribution.
thick description: A technique used by qualitative researchers that reveals the lived experience of participants in a way that evokes a human response and meaningful interpretation.
two-tailed test: A nondirectional hypothesis test that incorporates rejection regions in both tails of the probability curve used for a given statistic. Also known as nondirectionality tests.
type I error: Rejecting a null hypothesis when it should have been retained.
type II error: Retaining a null hypothesis when it should have been rejected.
unitization: The breaking down of qualitative data into separate pieces of meaning that can stand alone.
units of analysis: The *what* or *whom* being studied, such as individual people.
univariate analysis: The examination of the distribution of cases on only one variable at a time. Usually reported in the form of frequency distributions, central tendencies (averages), and dispersions (ranges and standard deviations).
validity: The degree to which a scale is in fact consistently measuring the variable that it was designed to measure.
variable: An observable characteristic of an object or event that can be described according to some well-defined classification or measurement scheme.
variable, dichotomous: A variable with only two values. Also known as *binary* and *dummy*.
variance: The mean of the squared deviation scores about the mean of a distribution.
weighted mean: A procedure for combining the means of groups of different sizes.
Wilcoxon test: A nonparametric test for use with related samples.
Wilks lambda: A commonly used test for group mean equality in multivariate tests.
***x*-axis:** The horizontal axis on a graph, also called the abscissa.

***x* variable:** Variable plotted on the horizontal axis, usually the independent variable

***y*-axis:** The vertical axis on a graph, also called the ordinate.

***y* variable:** Variable plotted on the vertical axis, usually the dependent variable.

***z*-score (lowercase *z*):** A commonly used standard score that gives a measure of relative location in the distribution.

***Z*-score (uppercase *Z*):** A standard score, based on manipulation of the *z* score, where the mean of the distribution is 50 and the standard deviation is 10.

Index

Note: Page numbers followed by *b*, *f*, and *t* indicate materials in boxes, figures and tables respectively.

A

abstracts, 202
action-oriented community diagnosis (AOCD), 115–117, 115*b*
adverse events (AEs), 19–20, 137–138
Agency for Healthcare Research and Quality (AHRQ), 46, 49*t*
AMA writing style, 186, 194–195, 198
American Psychological Association (APA), 37, 41
 writing style, 186–187
analysis of covariance (ANCOVA), 153
analysis of variance (ANOVA), 150, 153, 156
analytic studies, 68–69
analyze, systematic review
 assess limitations, 55
 recommendations for action, 55
 strength of the evidence, 55
ANCOVA. *See* analysis of covariance
annotated bibliography, 188
ANOVA. *See* analysis of variance
AOCD. *See* action-oriented community diagnosis
APA. *See* American Psychological Association
applied research, 6*t*
appraisal process, review
 evaluating screening, 52
 evaluation, 52
 methods of articles, 52
 screening, 51–52, 52*t*
approaches to publication, 199
association, measures of, 149, 149*f*
attrition effect on internal validity, 65–66
audit trail, 108
author–date styles, 187–188
authors and authorship
 assignment and determination of, 209–210
 reputation and affiliations of, 218–219

B

bar graph, 172, 173, 175*t*
baseline visit procedures, 136
Bayesian meta-analysis, 55
Belmont Report, 12, 12*t*
benefit *vs.* risk, 16
bias control, 63
bibliographic databases, 34–35
 searches
  de-duplicate and translate for other databases, 50–51
  develop, 49
  evaluating, 49–50
  in MEDLINE, 50*t*
  MeSH tree for body weight, 51*f*
  number of articles with obesity as concept in various fields, 51*f*
  save and document, 50
 bibliographies, 188
Biomed Central, 36
blinded reviews, 208
body of manuscript, clinical reviews, 42–43
Bonferroni correction, 161
book reviews, 201
Box's test, 166
brainstorming, 7

C

case-control study design, 69
case report forms (CRF), 135
case reports, 200–201
causality, defined, 79–80
CBPR. *See* Community-based participatory research
CCIA. *See* Chatham Communities in Action
Centers for Disease Control and Prevention (CDC), 125
central tendency measurement, 146
Centre for Reviews and Dissemination (CRD), 46
CFR. *See* Code of Federal Regulations
chart reviews, 15
charts used in results section of report, 171–172, 174–176
Chatham Communities in Action (CCIA), 124
Chicago writing style, 186–187
CI. *See* confidence interval

citations. *See also* references documentation
  for Internet sources, 198–199
  searching, 52–53
  style of, 197
  tools for, 40–41
clinical investigations, 14
  adverse events, 137–138
  baseline visits, 136
  follow-up, 137
  meeting inclusion and/or exclusion criteria, 136–138
  overview, 133
  phases of clinical research, 138–139
  randomization, 136–137
  research process, 134–138
  termination of study, 138
clinical research, 6*t*
clinical research associates (CRAs), 135, 136
clinical reviews, 41
  articles for, 200
  body of manuscript, 42–43
  systematic review of literature, 200
"clinically significant," 170
closed questions and responses, 120
coauthors, 209–210
Cochrane Handbook, 46, 48, 49, 53, 55
Cochran's Q test, 153
Code of Federal Regulations (CFR), 135–138
coding database, 104, 106*f*
coding, systematic review, 53
coefficient of determination, 178
Cohen's *d*, 158
cohort study design, 69
comadres, 126
common cardiac murmurs, 171, 174*t*
Common Rule regulation, 12–14, 16
communications
  IRB reports, 19–20
  with publication personnel, 207
community-based participatory research (CBPR), 111–131
  advantages, 113*t*
  AOCD. *See* action-oriented community diagnosis
  case study, 124–126
  design types, 114–121
  focus groups, 100, 117–118
  in-depth interviews, 119–121
  initiating process. *See* initiating process
  overview, 111–112, 112*b*, 113*t*
  photovoice, 118–119, 119*b*
  principles and values, 113–114
  qualitative study designs, 114–121
  quantitative study designs, 121
  research paradigms, 112–113
community forum, 117, 123
community guide, 53

complex multisite clinical trials, 149
conclusions subsection of research report, 180–181, 180*t*–181*t*
concurrent validity, 65
conference proceedings, 35
confidence interval (CI), 54, 95, 95*b*, 222–223, 223*f*
confidence levels, 95, 95*b*, 222–223, 223*f*
confirmability, 108
consensus construction of reality, 113
construct validity, 65
constructivist paradigm, 98
constructivist research paradigm, 113
continuous data, 144*t*, 149, 149*f*, 151
control groups, 107
  posttest-only designs, 74–75
  pretest-posttest designs, 74–75
controlled vocabulary, 36
convenience samples, 95
Copyright Act, 188
copyrighted material, 188–189, 209
covariates, 162
cover letters for surveys, 82, 83*t*
CRAs. *See* Clinical research associates
CRD. *See* Centre for Reviews and Dissemination
credibility
  persistent observation, 107
  prolonged engagement, 106–107
  triangulation, 107
CRF. *See* case report forms
criteria
  for discussion section, 180*t*
  for IRB approval, 17, 17*f*
criterion validity, 65
cross-sectional studies, 69
Cumulative Index to Nursing and Allied Health Literature (CINAHL) database, 36–37
curiosity, 5–6

D

data abstraction. *See* coding
data analysis, 143–154
  continuous data, 144*t*, 149, 149*f*, 151
  descriptive statistics, 145–147, 153
  hypothesis testing, 147–149
  inferential statistics, 147
  interval and ratio data, 70, 144*t*, 146*f*, 150
  meta-analysis, 150–151
  overview, 143–144
  for qualitative studies, 104–106, 121
  for quantitative studies, 121
  results presentation, 169–176, 174*f*–175*f*
  statistical test selection, 151–152
  statistical test types, 220

  statistical tests, 152–153
  statistics for, 95
data collection, 103–104
data management, 104–106
data types, 70–71, 100
database
  searches, 35–36, 38, 39*f*
  types of, 47
deficits-based approach to research, 115
demographic data, 88–89, 88*b*, 89*b*
demographic profile for PA class of 2012, 171, 171*t*
dental x-rays, 16
dependability, 108
dependent variable, 153
descriptive research, 6*t*
descriptive statistics, 145–147, 152
descriptive studies, 68
design factors, 63–65
design strategies, 34, 220
design types, 69–77, 114–121
design validity, 65
direct plagiarism, 199
discussion section of research report, 177–181
  conclusions subsection, 180–181, 180*t*–181*t*
  discussion subsection, 179
  implications subsection, 177–178
  limitations subsection, 178–179
  overview, 177
  recommendations subsection, 180
discussion subsection research report, 179
dissertations, 36
  databases, 48
documentation for informed consent, 17. *See also* references documentation
double-blind studies, 74–75
Duncan range test, 153

E

early termination/withdrawal from studies, 138
editorials, 201
editors, working with, 205
educational research practices, 15
electronic journals, 199
electronic sources of documentation, 190–191, 199
email surveys, 80, 80*t*
"emergent design," 103
emic (insider) data, 116–117
endnotes, 187
environmental threats to external validity, 67–68
epidemiological studies, 71, 148–149
equity in risk-benefit, 16
errors in measurement, 63–64
ethics in research, plagiarism, 199

Index | 243

etic (outsider) data, 116–117
evaluating reference sources, 189
evidence-based medicine (EBM), 221–224, 222t–224t, 223f–224f
evidence-based practice, role in research and, 46
evidence-level ratings, 223, 224t
exclusion criteria in clinical investigations, 136–138
exempt and expedited status studies, 14–16
experiment-related threats, 65, 67–68
experimental designs, 71, 74–76, 112–113
experimental research, 6t
experimental validity, 65
external validity, 65, 67–68

F
F ratio, 159
face validity, 65
factorial ANOVA, 162–163, 164f
fair use of copyrighted materials, 188
FDA. *See* Food and Drug Administration
FDA-regulated research, 14
field notes, 104, 105, 116
figures used in reports, 171–176, 171t–173t, 174f–175f, 175, 176t, 203
findings of research, 169–176, 174f–175f
first-in-human research studies, 139
fixed effects analysis, 54
focus group moderator's guide, 117, 124
follow-up
 to clinical investigations visits, 137
 to surveys, 83–84
Food and Drug Administration (FDA), 12–14, 16, 18, 20, 137–139
 Code of Federal Regulations (CFR), 135–136
footnotes, 187
forced response in surveys, 93
framework synthesis, 54

G
GCP. *See* Guideline for Good Clinical Practice
general approach to literature interpretation, 224–225
generalizable knowledge concept, 13
"going native," 107
Google Scholar database, 37–38
graduate projects and papers, 205
graphs, 171–172, 174f–175f, 175–176
graphs, guidelines for developing, 171, 176t
gray literature, 53, 53t
grounded theory approach, 117
group authorship, 210

groups, comparing, 156
Guideline for Good Clinical Practice (GCP), 134, 137–138

H
handbook, defined, 55
handsearching, 53
harm, defined, 15
hawthorne effect, 68
health care
 exploring statistics comparing differences in, 155–168
  comparing groups, 156
  factorial ANOVA, 162–163, 164f
  Hotelling's T2, 165–166
  MANOVA, 166–168
  one-way ANOVA, 159–162, 160f
  overview, 155–156
  paired t-test (matched t-test), 158–159
  repeated measures ANOVA, 163–165, 165t
  t-test (student t-test), 156–158, 157f
 qualitative research in
  design and implementation, 103–106
  flow of, 102f
 quantitative studies *vs.* qualitative research. *See* qualitative research, *vs.* quantitative studies in healthcare
Health Insurance Portability and Accountability Act (HIPAA) of 1996, 135–136
healthcare professionals, 24, 29–31
healthcare professions, research and students of, 4, 5
HHS. *See* U.S. Department of Health and Human Services
HIPAA of 1996. *See* Health Insurance Portability and Accountability Act of 1996
histograms, 171–173, 175f
HIV. *See* human immunodeficiency virus
HoMBReS case study. *See* Hombres Manteniendo Bienestar y Relaciones Saludables
Hombres Manteniendo Bienestar y Relaciones Saludables (HoMBReS case study), 124–126
Hotelling's T2, 165–166
human immunodeficiency virus (HIV), 125–126
human subjects
 accessibility to study, 67
 regulatory protection of, 11–22, 12t, 13f, 17f, 18t
 training for research on, 21
 treatment interactions, 67
hypothesis development, 26–29, 27f, 31
hypothesis testing, 147–149

I
ideas for research problem, sources of, 30
 need for study, 31
 stating the research question, 31
illustrations used in reports, 203
implications subsection of research report, 177–178
in-depth interviews, 119–121
inactivation of IRB studies, 20
inclusion criteria in clinical investigations, 136–138
inferential statistics, 147
influential community advocates, 117, 119
informed consent, 16–17, 18t, 135–136
initiating process
 build trust, 122–123
 maintain relationships, 123
 negotiate partnerships, 123–124
 network, 121–122
institutional review board (IRB), 12–19, 13f, 17f, 18t, 123, 209
instrument reliability, 64
insufficient acknowledgment as plagiarism, 199
integrative review, 46
integrative synthesis, 54–55
inter-rater reliability, 64
intercorrelations among educational outcomes for PA students, 171, 172t
internal validity, 65–67
Internet
 as documentation source, 190–191, 199
 surveys via, 85–86
interval data, 70, 144t, 146f
interviews
 in-depth, 119–121
 personal interview surveys, 86–87, 87t
 as research technique, 104
 structure of, 119–120
intrarater reliability, 64
inverse of the covariance matrix, 166
investigator's responsibilities, 19–21
 inactivation, 20
 reporting noncompliance, 20
 responsibilities, 20–21
 tracking adverse events and reporting UPIRSOs, 19–20
IRB. *See* institutional review board

J
JBI. *See* Joanna Briggs Institute
Joanna Briggs Institute (JBI), 46
job profiles for PA classes of 2011 and 2012, 171, 172t

journals
  electronic, 199
  medical, 211, 218
  selection process for, 202

K
Kendall's rank correlation test, 153
keywords. *See* controlled vocabulary
Kruskal-Wallis test, 153

L
laboratory research, 6t
Latino community case study, 124–126
letters to the editor, 201–202
Levene's test, 166
Likert Scale, 91–92, 92b, 92t
limitations subsection of research report, 178–179
line graph, 172, 174f
line of no effect, 54
literature interpretation, 215–225
  evidence-based medicine, 221–224, 222t–224t, 223f–224f
  general approach to, 224–225
  overview, 215–216
  questions to ask and answer, 217–221, 218t
  scientific method of, 217
literature review, 33–43
  CINAHL database, 33–43
  citation tools, 40–41
  clinical reviews, 41–43
  database search hints, 38, 39f
  designing research strategy, 34
  elements of successful, 34
  Google Scholar database, 37–38
  MEDLINE database, 35–36
  overview, 33–34
  PsycINFO database, 37
  resources selection, 34–35
  search results, 30–40, 40f, 220–221
  systematic review of, 200
  Web of Science database, 38, 39t
  writing review, 41
longitudinal studies, 69

M
magnetic resonance imaging (MRI), 15
Mahalanobis distance (D^2), 166
main effect, 162
Mann-Whitney Test, 153
MANOVA. *See* Multiple analysis of variance
manuscripts
  flaws to prevent publication, 211–212, 212t
  revisions to, 197
  submission of, 208–209
matched data results, 152

matched t-test, 158–159
maturation effect on internal validity, 65–66
Mauchley's test, 163
mean, defined, 146
mean squares (MS), 159
mean vectors, 165
measurement effects on internal validity, 65–66
measurement factors in design, 63–65
measurement, levels of, 144–145, 144t, 146f
measurement validity, 64–68
median, defined, 146
medical journals, 211
Medical Subject Headings (MeSH) controlled vocabulary, 36
MEDLINE database, 35–36
member checking technique, 107
Men Maintaining Wellness and Healthy Relationships (HoMBReS case study), 124–126
meta-analysis, 45, 48, 54, 54f, 55–56, 56f, 150–151
methodology, 61–77
  design factors, 63–65
  experimental designs, 71, 74–76, 112–113
  external validity threats, 67–68
  internal validity threats, 65–67
  methods section of project, 62–63, 62t
  overview, 61–62
  pre-experimental designs, 71–74
  quasi-experimental designs, 71, 76–77
  study types, 68–71
minimal risk, defined, 15
mixed-methodological study, 97
mode, defined, 146
modifications to IRB approved studies, 19
modified group authorship, 210
monitoring data collection, 17–18
mosaic plagiarism, 199
MRI. *See* magnetic resonance imaging
MS. *See* mean squares
Mujeres Juntas Estableciendo Relaciones Saludables (MuJEReS), 126
multiple analysis of variance (MANOVA), 166–168
multiple regression analysis, 153
multivariate regression techniques, 149

N
narrative synthesis, 54
National Institutes of Health (NIH), 18, 21, 36
navegantes, 125–126
needs assessment, 115, 115b
negative case analysis, 107

network, 121–122
Newman-Keuls test, 153
NIH. *See* National Institutes of Health
95 percent confidence interval calculation, 222–223, 223f
nominal data, 70, 144–145, 144t, 147–149
noncompliance reporting, 20
nonequivalent control group design, 62t, 76
nonnumerical data studies, 68, 70
nonparametric analyses, 152
nonparametric data, 70–71
note takers in focus groups, 118, 124
null hypothesis, 156–157
  development, 26–29, 31
number needed to treat (NNT) calculation, 222, 223t
numerical data studies, 68, 70–71

O
observations, 98, 106, 107
Office for Human Research Protections (OHRP), 14, 20
omega-squared (ω^2), 161
one group pretest–posttest designs, 62t, 72–73
one-shot case study design, 62t, 72
one-way ANOVA, 159–162, 160f
Online Writing Lab (OWL), 41
open-ended questions, 89, 89b, 120
OR and AND operators, 38, 39f
oral presentations, 204
ordinal data, 144–145, 144t, 151
original articles, 200
original data, 70
original research abstracts, 202
OWL. *See* Online Writing Lab

P
paired data results, 152
paired t-test, 158–159
parametric analyses, 152
parametric data, 70–71
paraphrase plagiarism, 199
participant selection, sampling strategies for, 103, 103t
partnership negotiations, 123–124
Patient Oriented Evidence that Matters (POEM) format, 223
Paulo Freirian-based questioning, 119
Pearson's product moment test, 153
Pearson's x^2 test, 153
peer debriefing, 107
peer reviews, 189, 207–208, 218–219
Peer Reviews Electronic Search Strategies (PRESS), 50
persistent observation, 107
personal interview surveys, 86–87, 87t

phases of clinical research, 138–139
photovoice, 118–119, 119b
pilot testing surveys, 94
PIs. *See* principal investigators
plagiarism, 188–189, 199
population-related threats to external validity, 67
population samples, 95, 220
position papers, 201
positivist and postpositivist paradigms, 112–113
poster presentations, 202, 203f
posttest-only control group design, 62t, 74–75
pre-experimental designs, 71–74
pre-screen informed consent form, 136
preclinical studies, 139
predictive validity, 65
Preferred Reporting Items for Systematic Reviews and Meta-Analyses (PRISMA), 48, 55–56, 56f
PRESS. *See* Peer Reviews Electronic Search Strategies
pretest–posttest
　control group designs, 62t, 74–75
　one group designs, 72–73
　separate sample design, 76–77
primary sources of documentation, 188
principal investigators (PIs), 19–21, 134, 135
PRISMA. *See* Preferred Reporting Items for Systematic Reviews and Meta-Analyses
privacy protection, 18
privacy rule regulation, 12
project development, 6–9
　defining process, 7
　scientific process approach, 8f
prolonged engagement, 106–107
Proquest's Dissertations & Theses database, 35
prose revision, 197
prospective *vs.* retrospective designs, 69–70
protocol and practice (two P rule), 64
PsycINFO database, 37
public domain documents, 188
PubMed Central (PMC) database, 36
PubMed website, 36
pulmonologist, 26
pure research, 6t

Q

qualitative data analysis, 104–106
qualitative data management, 104–106
qualitative design and implementation, 103–106
qualitative investigations, 98, 100
qualitative investigators, 100, 108

qualitative research, 97–109
　data analysis, 121
　in health care, 101–106
　　design and implementation, 103–106
　　flow of, 102f
　mixed-methodological, 97
　overview, 97–98
　philosophy of, 98
　quality assessment, 106–108
　vs. quantitative studies in healthcare, 98–101
　data types, 100
　key characteristics of, 99t
　methodology, 100
　reporting, 101
　researcher's role, 99
　rigor and validity in, 99t
　sampling, 100
　settings, 100
　research techniques, 106–108
　sampling strategies for, 103, 103t
　steps for, 101–103
　study designs, 114–121
　trustworthiness criteria of credibility. *See* credibility
　dependability and confirmability, 108
　member checking, 107
　negative case analysis, 107
　peer debriefing, 107
　referential adequacy, 107
　reflexive journal, 107–108
　transferability, 108
　validity of, 99f, 106, 108
qualitative review, 46
qualitative synthesis, 53–54
quantitative data analysis, 121
quantitative studies, 98, 100
　vs. qualitative research in healthcare, 98–101
quantitative synthesis, 54, 54f
quasi-experimental designs, 71, 76–77
quasi-experimental research designs and methods, 113
question development for surveys, 87–88, 87t
questioning techniques, 119, 119b

R

random effects analysis, 54
random errors, 63
randomization phase of clinical studies, 74–75, 136–137
range (variability measure), 146
rankings of survey responses, 91, 91b
ratio data, 70, 144t, 145, 146t, 150
Rausch analysis, 150
"real-world concerns," 31

realist synthesis, 54–55
recommendations subsection of research report, 180
refereeing, defined, 34
reference lists, 197–198
reference searching, 52–53
references documentation, 185–191
　acknowledgment of all materials used, 188–189
　documentation sources, 187–188
　electronic and Internet-based sources, 190–191, 198–199
　evaluating sources, 189
　overview, 187
　writing styles, 185–187
referential adequacy, 107
reflexive journal, 107–108
regression analysis, 153
regulatory protection of human subjects, 11–22
　institutional review board approval, 12–19, 18t
　investigator's responsibilities, 19–21
　overview, 11
　regulatory definitions, 12–19, 13f, 17f, 18t
　research approved, 12, 12t
relationship maintenance, 123
relevant reviews, 47–48, 47t
reliability of measurements, 64
repeated measures ANOVA, 163–165, 165t
replication, study, 24, 31
reprint requests, 207
requests for proposals (RFPs), 31
research, 3–9
　applications, 5
　curiosity and, 4–5
　and evidence-based practice, role in, 46
　fear of unknown, 5
　forms of, 5–6, 6t
　importance of, 4–5
　overview, 3–4
　project development, 6–9, 8f
　students of healthcare professions and, 4, 5
　types, 6t
research design, 63–65
research papers, 196–199, 203
research paradigms, 112–113
research problem development and refinement, 23–32
　getting started, 25, 25b
　identification of, 25–29, 27f
　overview, 23–24
　process, 24
　question focus of, 29–30, 29t, 219
　sources of ideas, 30–32
　topics for, 24–25, 25t, 28b

research questions
　focus of, 29–30, 29t
　prioritizing, 25b
　stating, 31
research reports
　bibliographies, 188
　charts used in results section of report, 171–172, 174–176
　conclusions subsection, 180–181, 180t–181t
　discussion section, 177–181
　　conclusions subsection, 180–181, 180t–181t
　　discussion subsection, 179
　　implications subsection, 177–178
　　limitations subsection, 178–179
　　overview, 177
　　recommendations subsection, 180
　implications subsection, 177–178
　limitations subsection, 178–179
　recommendations subsection, 180
　results section, 169–176, 174f–175f
　subsections, 177–181, 180t–181t
　tables used in, 171–172, 171t–173t, 174f, 176, 176t, 203
　titles used in in, 203–204
research techniques, 106–108
research topics
　origins, 24–25, 25t
　revising from general to more specific, 28b
resources
　for literature review, 34–35
　for writers, 207
respiratory therapist (RT), 26–27
response rates, 81–82
results of literature review, 30–40, 220–221
　evidence pyramid, 40f
results section of research report, 169–176, 174f–175f
　overview, 169–170
　tables and figures, 171–176, 171t–173t, 174f–175f, 176t
　text, 170–171
retrospective *vs.* prospective designs, 69–70
review databases, 47, 47t
review of reviews, 46
RFPs. *See* requests for proposals
risk assessment, 16
root-cause questioning technique (SHOWED), 119, 119b
rosenthal effect, 68
RT. *See* respiratory therapist

S
SAEs. *See* serious adverse events
sample size, 95, 220
sampling, 100
　effect on internal validity, 66
scientific method of literature interpretation, 217
scoping review, 46
screening, 51
　evaluating, 52
　questions, 52, 52t
SD. *See* standard deviation
search techniques, systematic review
　gray literature, 53
　handsearching, 53
　reference/citation, 52–53
　request studies, 53
secondary sources of documentation, 188
SEM. *See* standard error of the mean
semi-structured interviews, 119–120
serious adverse events (SAEs), 135, 137–138
sexually transmitted disease (STD), 125
signal-to-noise ratio, 157
significant, defined, 170
simple main effects, 162
Solomon four-group design, 62t, 75–76
Spearman's rho, 153
SR. *See* systematic review
SSB. *See* sums of squares between
SSBT. *See* sums of squares between treatments
SSE. *See* sums of squares error
SST. *See* total sums of squares
SSW. *See* sums of squares within
stackholders in communities, 122
standard deviation (SD), 146
standard error of the mean (SEM), 147
static group comparison design, 62t, 73–74
statistical analysis, 220
statistical regression effects on internal validity, 67
"statistically significant," 170
statistics, 70
status reports to IRB, 19
STD. *See* sexually transmitted disease
steps of systematic review
　analyze and write, 55–56
　appraisal, 51–52
　bibliographic database searches, 49–51, 50t, 51f
　code and synthesize, 53–55, 54f
　define and plan, 46–49

free review databases, 47t
question and criteria, 47t
software for various processes, 49t
expanded search techniques, 52–53, 53t
strengths-based approach to research, 115
structured interviews, 120
student t-test, 156–158, 157f
study coordinators, 134–135
study monitors, 135
study types, 68–71
style manuals, 185–187, 194–195, 194t
styles of writing
　for citations, 197
　for references, 185–187
subinvestigators (sub-I), 134–135, 137, 138
subject-specific databases, 47
subsections of research report, 177–181, 180t–181t
sums of squares between (SSB), 159
sums of squares between treatments (SSBT), 165
sums of squares error (SSE), 165
sums of squares within (SSW), 159
surveys, 79–96
　cover letters for, 82, 83t
　demographic data, 88–89, 88b, 89b
　error in, 63–64
　exempted example of, 14–15
　follow-up for, 83–84
　format of, 89–91, 89b, 90b, 90t
　instrument for, 89–93
　internet surveys, 85–86
　overview, 79–80, 80t
　personal interview, 86–87, 87t
　pilot testing of, 94
　planning for, 80–81
　population sample for, 95
　pre-experimental designs, 71–74
　putting together, 94
　rankings, 91, 91b
　statistics for, 95
　survey item construction, 87–88, 87t
　telephone surveys, 86, 86t
　types of, 80, 81t
　verbal frequency scales, 91–93, 92b, 92t, 93b
　web-based, 84–86, 85t
synthesize, systematic review, 53–55, 54f
systematic errors, 63
systematic investigation, 13–14

systematic review (SR), 45–57, 200
    development, organizations leading, 46
    overview, 45–46
    role in research and evidence-based practice, 46
    steps, 46–56
    types, 46

T
t-test, 152–153, 156–158, 157f
tables used in reports, 171–176, 171t–173t, 174f, 174f–175f, 175, 176, 176t, 203
telephone surveys, 86, 86t
temporal effects on internal validity, 65–66
termination of studies, 138
test order effect on external validity, 68
test validity, 65
testing effect on internal validity, 66
thematic saturation, 100
thematic synthesis, 54
themes in qualitative data, 121
theses and dissertations, 35
time-based effects on internal validity, 65–67
time limits for IRB approvals, 19
time series design, 62t, 77
titles used in reports, 203–204
total sums of squares (SST), 159

training on human subjects, 21
transferability, 108
triangulation, 107
true experiment, defined, 69
trust building, 122–123
Tukey test, 153
two P rule (protocol and practice), 64

U
unanticipated adverse events (UAEs), 135
Unanticipated Problem Involving Risks to Subjects or Others (UPIRSO), 19–20
unstructured interviews, 119
UPIRSO. *See* Unanticipated Problem Involving Risks to Subjects or Others
U.S. Department of Health and Human Services (HHS), 12

V
validity of measurements, 64–68
validity of qualitative research, 108
Vancouver writing style, 186–187, 197
variability, measures of, 146
variables, 153
    description, 67
verbal frequency scales, 91–93, 92b, 92t, 93b
vulnerable populations, 18–19

W
waiver of consent, 16–17
web-based surveys, 84–86, 85t
Web of Science database, 38, 39t
Wilcoxon rank sum test, 153
windshield tour of community, 115–116
withdrawal from studies, 138
write, systematic review, 53–56, 56f
writing and publishing, 193–214
    challenges in, 210–211
    graduate projects and papers, 205
    importance of writing, 195–196, 196t
    manuscript flaws, 211–212, 212t
    options for new writers, 200–203, 203f
    oral presentations, 204
    overview, 193–194
    publication approaches, 199–200
    publication steps, 205–210
    research papers, 196–199
    rules for aspiring authors, 213
    steps in process of, 213
    style manuals, 194–195, 194t
written consent, 135–136
written informed consent, 16–17, 18t

X
X-rays, dental, 16